EXCELLENT CARE
FOR CANCER SURVIVORS

**Recent Titles in
the Praeger Series on Contemporary Health and Living**

EXCELLENT CARE FOR CANCER SURVIVORS

A Guide to Fully Meet Their Needs in Medical Offices and in the Community

KENNETH MILLER, MD, EDITOR

The Praeger Series on Contemporary Health and Living
Julie K. Silver, MD, Series Editor

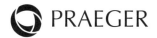 PRAEGER

AN IMPRINT OF ABC-CLIO, LLC
Santa Barbara, California • Denver, Colorado • Oxford, England

Library of Congress Cataloging-in-Publication Data

Excellent care for cancer survivors : a guide to fully meet their needs in medical offices and in the community / Kenneth Miller, editor.
    p. ; cm. — (Praeger series on contemporary health and living)
  Includes bibliographical references and index.
  ISBN 978-0-313-39786-8 (alk. paper) — ISBN 978-0-313-39787-5 (eISBN)
1. Cancer—Patients—Services for. 2. Cancer—Psychological aspects. I. Miller, Kenneth D., 1956- II. Series: Praeger series on contemporary health and living. 1932–8079
    [DNLM: 1. Neoplasms. 2. Survivors—psychology. 3. Community Health Services. QZ 200]
  RC262.E96 2012
  362.196'994—dc23   2011027586

ISBN: 978-0-313-39786-8
EISBN: 978-0-313-39787-5

16 15 14 13 12   1 2 3 4 5

This book is also available on the World Wide Web as an eBook.
Visit www.abc-clio.com for details.

Praeger
An Imprint of ABC-CLIO, LLC

ABC-CLIO, LLC
130 Cremona Drive, P.O. Box 1911
Santa Barbara, California 93116-1911

This book is printed on acid-free paper ∞

Manufactured in the United States of America

CONTENTS

Contents

Series Foreword

Contemporary Health and Living

Over the past 100 years, there have been incredible medical breakthroughs that have prevented or cured illness in billions of people and helped many more improve their health while living with chronic conditions. A few of the most important 20th century discoveries include antibiotics, organ transplants, and vaccines. The 21st century has already heralded important new treatments including a vaccine to prevent human papillomavirus from infecting and potentially leading to cervical cancer in women. Polio is on the verge of being eradicated worldwide, making it only the second infectious disease behind smallpox to ever be erased as a human health threat.

In this series, experts from many disciplines share with readers important and updated medical knowledge. All aspects of health are considered, including subjects that are disease specific and preventive medical care. Disseminating this information will help individuals to improve their health, researchers to determine where there are gaps in our current knowledge, and policy makers to assess the most pressing needs in healthcare.

Series Editor Julie K. Silver, MD
Assistant Professor
Harvard Medical School
Department of Physical Medicine and Rehabilitation

FOREWORD

This year, an estimated 1.5 million people in the United States will hear the words, "you have cancer." Due to advances in screening, early detection and treatment, there are more than 12 million cancer survivors in the United States today. While we should be encouraged that so many people are now surviving cancer—a relatively new phenomenon—the harsh truth is that for many individuals, being cured marks the beginning of life-long emotional, day-to-day and physical challenges related to cancer and its treatment.

At LIVE**STRONG** we recognize that while cancer may leave your body, it never leaves your life. Many cancer survivors find themselves unable to work, have children, or perform the daily activities they did before cancer. Some face debilitating medical and emotional problems they cannot conquer on their own. Cancer survivors need support throughout their lives to ensure they have appropriate medical care, including screening for secondary cancers and recurrences, access to services that address emotional concerns, and opportunities to engage as active participants in their health.

The 2006 Institute of Medicine (IOM) report, "From Cancer Patient to Cancer Survivor: Lost in Transition" provided a critical look at the issues experienced by survivors and recommended next steps to improve outcomes for them. The report recommends establishing post-treatment survivorship as a distinct phase of the cancer continuum for all survivors and their families. In recent years, a movement to embrace this challenge and provide effective care to the growing survivor population has taken shape. Yet, as the field of survivorship is relatively new, there is still much work to do in understanding how to develop a survivorship program, what cancer survivors are experiencing when treatment ends, and how different cancer types impact survivorship.

This book takes a comprehensive approach in addressing all three of these areas, providing not just information about what to expect but also practical advice on how to meet the needs of survivors and their families.

In developing a survivorship program, getting started can be one of the biggest obstacles. The authors thoughtfully address many of the hurdles, such as how to identify funding and finding the right team. Readers who are starting or currently evaluating survivorship programs will find particular relevance in the chapters addressing different models of care and different settings for care including an academic cancer center, a major urban hospital, and community health centers. The authors make recommendations about engaging many levels and members of the health care team and note the importance of understanding the specific needs of the survivor and their loved ones. Their insights on developing successful survivorship programs are a road map toward achieving the noble goal of providing survivors all over the country excellent care.

Historically, little attention has been paid and scant resources offered to post-treatment survivors. Thus, perhaps most relevant is the picture painted in these pages of what life is like after cancer. The disease impacts all aspects of an individual's life, often leaving a survivor—when help is available—in a complicated maze of providers and professionals to address their medical, emotional, and day-to-day needs. This book addresses many of these issues such as cancer fatigue, infertility, sexuality and intimacy, psychosocial issues, and fear of recurrence. Importantly, this book also addresses ways to empower survivors to participate in their care. By utilizing tools, such as survivorship care plans, as well as interventions and information, such as how to eat well and exercise after treatment ends, survivors can become active participants in improving their long-term outcomes.

As there are more than 100 different types of cancer, understanding the unique needs of survivors and the opportunities to improve treatment and long-term care by disease type is extremely relevant, especially as science moves forward to more targeted therapies. These chapters include critical information about the successes achieved in improving outcomes for nine cancer types as well as recommendations for how best to overcome challenges facing them.

As two individuals who have heard the words, "you have cancer," we were impressed by the breadth of focus on the complex issues that occur after treatment ends. Both through personal experiences, and through LIVE**STRONG**'s comprehensive research with cancer survivors, we have uncovered the same challenges detailed hereafter. The emphasis placed on the role of the survivor and their loved ones as partners in care is vitally important. As the number of individuals surviving cancer over the long-term is on the rise, now is the time to provide effective patient-centered care for all cancer survivors.

Doug Ulman
President & CEO
Ruth Rechis, PhD
Director, Research & Evaluation
LIVE**STRONG**

1

An Overview of
Cancer Survivorship

Kenneth Miller, MD, Brittany Algiere, BS, and Binja Basimike, BS

In 1985, Dr. Fitzhugh Mullen wrote an article in the *New England Journal of Medicine* titled "Seasons of Survival: Reflections of a Physician with Cancer" describing his physical emotional challenges during cancer treatment.[1] Dr. Mullen also wrote about his experience after treatment ended and defined "three seasons of survival": (1) acute survival including the time of diagnosis and initial treatment, (2) extended survival defined as a period of surveillance, and (3) permanent survivorship when the risk of recurrence and the fear of recurrence are low.

Many aspects of cancer care have changed since 1985, including:

1. The increased use of cancer screening and the diagnosis of cancer at an earlier stage.
2. The use of pre-operative (neoadjuvant) and post-operative (adjuvant) chemotherapy and radiation therapy.
3. Improved management of the acute toxicities of chemotherapy and radiation therapy.
4. The introduction and growing use of biological and targeted therapies such as Imatinib and Rituximab.
5. Increasing use of high dose chemotherapy with autologous stem cell transplantation or allogeneic transplantation including for older patients who were previously considered ineligible.
6. More patients living with cancer as a chronic disease.
7. More patients living long enough to develop second malignancies or secondary malignancies related to their previous chemotherapy or radiation therapy.

As a result of this progress the number of cancer survivors in the United States is growing and may reach close to 20 million by the year 2020 (see Figure 1.1).[2] Many of these cancer survivors are now 10 or more years

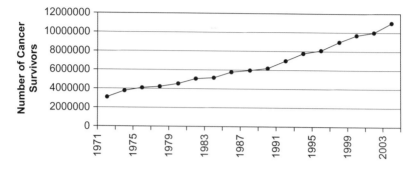

Figure 1.1. Estimated Number of Cancer Survivors in the United States from 1971 to 2007. (Adapted from SEER, 2004.)

beyond their diagnosis, and this number is increasing as well. An analysis of SEER data in 2002 demonstrated that 17% of breast cancer survivors were 10–15 years post-diagnosis, 10% 15–20 years, 6% 20–25 years, and 8% more than 25 years post-diagnosis.[3]

THE SEASONS OF SURVIVORSHIP

The seasons of survivorship described in 1985 include acute survivorship, extended survivorship, and permanent survivorship. Updating this model recognizes the concept of transitional survivorship at the end of treatment during which some of the acute toxicities of treatment are resolving. Chronic survivorship describes a growing group of patients who are "living with cancer." Finally, this model recognizes the heterogeneity in permanent survivorship.

The seasons of survivorship in this updated model include[4]

Acute Survivorship:
This is the period that includes the diagnosis of cancer and its treatment. Some of the acute toxicities of treatment have been reduced but nonetheless this is typically a physically and emotionally difficult time.

Transition at the End of Acute Survivorship:
This season begins at the completion of acute treatment although some of the effects of treatment may persist. The challenges that cancer survivors face include transitioning back to previous responsibilities including work and family.

Extended Cancer Survivorship:
There are a large number of cancer survivors who are in remission after surgery, radiation therapy, or chemotherapy. Extended survivorship is a time of careful observation and surveillance.

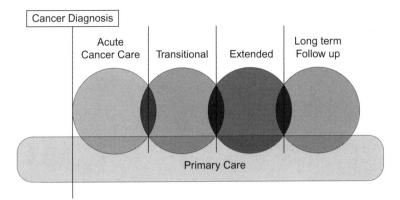

Figure 1.2. Opportunities for Survivorship Care. (Adapted from Richard Boyajian, RN, MA, APRN.)

Chronic Survivorship:

This encompasses the growing number of cancer survivors who are "living with cancer" as a chronic disease. Women who have metastatic estrogen receptor positive breast cancer are one example. Similarly, some cancer survivors are in a maintained remission while taking Imatinib or a hormonal therapy.

Permanent Survivorship:

Anecdotally, the majority of long-term cancer survivors can be described as "cancer-free and free of cancer" and cancer may represent a relatively small note as part of their past medical history. In contrast, unfortunately, other cancer survivors are cancer-free but suffer from some late or long-term effect of treatment. This might be the development of a cardiomyopathy following treatment with an anthracycline, pulmonary fibrosis, a painful neuropathy, or post-traumatic stress. Some survivors go on to develop second or secondary malignancies, and they essentially re-enter acute survivorship. Finally, end of life, as a part of living, is also a part of the cancer survivorship experience. Similarly, Welch-McCaffrey and colleagues describe multiple groups of cancer survivors including survivors who:

Live cancer free for many years and then die from natural causes.
Live cancer free for many years but then die after a late recurrence.
Live cancer free but then develop a second cancer.
Live with intermittent periods of remission and active disease.
Live with persistent disease.
Live after expecting to die of cancer.

THE TASKS OF CANCER SURVIVORSHIP

Typical oncology follow-up visits focus attention on surveillance for disease recurrence. More broadly, though, the tasks of cancer survivorship care include:

- Promotion of a smoother transition from acute survivorship to a "new normal."
- Coordination of care.
- Addressing the psychosocial needs of cancer survivors and secondary survivors.
- Surveillance for cancer recurrence.
- Surveillance for the development of late and long-term effects as well as risk identification, management, and mitigation.
- Surveillance for second and secondary cancers and important routine health care maintenance.
- Health and wellness promotion for cancer survivors.
- In addition, efforts directed at secondary prevention through cancer risk reduction.

PROMOTING A SMOOTHER TRANSITION

As cancer treatment ends, many cancer survivors face a difficult period including the withdrawal of the treatment team and the need to adjust to temporary or permanent physical and emotional changes. The Institute of Medicine report on cancer survivorship in 2005 titled "From Cancer Patient to Cancer Survivor: Lost in Transition" details many of these challenges for cancer survivors and their care providers.[5] Some challenges that cancer survivors face during transitional survivorship are in multiple domains: physical, psychological, social, and spiritual.

Cancer survivorship programs can focus on medical and psychosocial symptom identification and management after treatment has ended. They can also help cancer survivors navigate the complexities of the care community and coordinate this care.

COORDINATION OF CARE

For cancer survivors, coordination of their care is often not optimal. In a study of more than 47,000 breast cancer survivors and controls, Snyder et al. found that survivors were less likely to receive preventive care than the controls. However, survivors who visited both a PCP and oncology specialist were most likely to receive recommended care. Similarly, in another large study, Earle et al. reported that 5,965 elderly breast cancer survivors who continued to see oncology specialists were more likely to receive appropriate follow-up mammography for their cancer, but those who were monitored by primary care physicians were more likely to receive all other non-cancer-related preventive services. Those who saw both types of practitioners received more of both types of services.[7] Among survivors of colorectal cancer the same observations have been made. Snyder reported that survivors who visited both a PCP and oncology specialist were most likely to receive each preventive care service.[8] This study has concluded that involvement by both PCPs and oncology specialists can facilitate appropriate care for survivors.[9]

There are undoubtedly many factors contributing to the under-use of necessary services by cancer survivors. One of these factors is the lack of clarity about what services are needed and differing expectations of who is responsible for providing this care. In a study of approximately 1,000 cancer survivors and 600 physicians that compared patients with their oncologists, expectations were highly discrepant for screening for cancers other than the index one (agreement rate, 29%), with patients anticipating significantly more oncologist involvement. Between patients and their PCPs, expectations were incongruent for primary cancer follow-up (agreement rate, 35%), with PCPs indicating they should contribute a much greater part to this aspect of care than patients had expected. In the case of primary cancer follow-up, both PCPs and oncologists indicated that both should carry substantial responsibility for this task.[10]

Some of the anxiety that patients experience when completing treatment may be related to this lack of clarity regarding follow-up care. Care coordination is an integral component in the treatment of cancer survivors and survivorship programs help to delineate and optimize the cancer specialists and the primary care providers' roles and responsibilities.

ADDRESSING THE PSYCHOSOCIAL NEEDS OF CANCER SURVIVORS

During the period of transition between "cancer patient" and "cancer survivor," cancer survivors report varying degrees of depression, anxiety, and feelings of loss of control. The fear of recurrence varies in both duration and intensity and perceived risk may be directly or indirectly proportional to the actual risk. Helping cancer survivors move through and beyond the fear of recurrence may help them with reintegration into their home, work, and social environment.

SURVEILLANCE

The majority of cancer survivors experience a decrease in the risk of recurrence over time. For example, the risk of recurrence in the first three years after treatment of colon cancer is generally greater than the subsequent years. However, while the risk of recurrence decreases, the risk of late and long-term effects, including second and secondary cancers, simultaneously increases (see figure 1.3).

Cancer survivors may not have adequate knowledge about the risk of recurrence or the signs of recurrence. The IOM report cites that only 22% of colon cancer survivors could identify symptoms or signs that might indicate a recurrence.[5] In addition, after the initial therapy has been completed, compliance with follow-up visit or testing schedules may diminish over time.

Cancer surveillance guidelines for follow-up care have been developed. For example, the American Society of Clinical Oncology (ASCO) created a Breast Cancer Survivorship Care Plan.[12] ASCO guidelines take the form of a simple chart that can be filled out by the clinician, which details the plan and schedule for sequential history and physical examinations, post-treatment

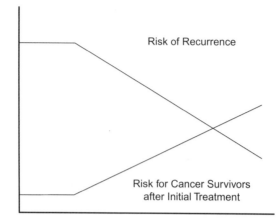

Figure 1.3[11]. Risks for Cancer Survivors after Initial Treatment. (Credit: Kenneth Miller.)

mammography, breast self-examination, and pelvic exams. ASCO guidelines also incorporate a coordination of care discussion and referrals for genetic counseling, as needed. These specific guidelines help to ensure the quality of care as well as assist in the process of care coordination.

SURVEILLANCE FOR LATE AND LONG-TERM EFFECTS

Cancer survivors may be unaware of some of the late and long-term effects they may face. The IOM Report cites that female adult survivors of Hodgkin's disease who received mantle field radiation have an increased risk of developing breast cancer but that only 47% report having a mammogram within the past two years.[5] Similarly, many breast cancer survivors had little knowledge about lymphedema risk and prevention.

The risk of developing late and long-term effects depends on many factors, including the type of cancer therapy that the patient received as well as the cancer survivors' age, gender, genetics, lifestyle, medical care, environmental exposures, and pre-morbid conditions. Cancer survivors have different levels of risk for late and long-term effects. Women treated for non-invasive breast cancer or men treated for early stage prostate cancer are at relatively low risk. Survivors treated for lymphoma who received combined modality radiation and chemotherapy are at greater risk. Finally, those who undergo allogeneic bone marrow transplant may be at the highest risk. There is a wide range of late and long-term effects that have been reported" (see Table 1.1). Broadly viewed these effects are physical, psychological, social, and spiritual (See figure 1.4).[13]

It is not possible to reverse the impact of treatment once it has been given, but being aware of these risks does provide the opportunity to identify these effects early. This allows for opportunity to minimize other contributing factors and to intervene in an attempt to change the natural history of these problems.

TABLE 1.1 COMMON LONG-TERM AND LATE EFFECTS

Surgery	Radiation	Chemotherapy
Loss of function	Xerostomia	Secondary leukemia
Pain	Cataracts	Amenorrhea
Erectile Dysfunction	Cognitive changes	Neuropathy
	Pulmonary fibrosis	Cognitive changes
	Infertility	Cardiomyopathy
	Osteoradionecrosis	

Adapted from Children's Oncology Group, 2008.

HEALTH PROMOTION

"Cancer is a teachable moment" is a commonly used expression in cancer survivorship. In fact, physical wellness is one of the fastest growing areas related to all cancer patients and survivors. The main focus of survivorship wellness is the encouragement of regular physical activity. Considering how difficult maintaining an exercise routine is in general, the challenge is magnified for those who are actively undergoing or who have recently gone through treatment. According to a 2004 Agency for Healthcare Research and Quality (AHRQ) evidence report, increased physical activity showed positive outcomes on vigor and vitality, cardiorespiratory fitness, quality of life, depression, anxiety, and fatigue/tiredness.[5] The Institute of Medicine's report, "From Cancer Patient to Cancer Survivor: Lost in Transition," advises that moderate to intense aerobic activity should be performed "3 or more days a week, for 10 to 60 minutes per session."[14] It is unclear if physical activity directly affects cancer recurrence or survival, but this is suggested by several studies.

Multiple cancer organizations report that there is not enough information available to recommend specific exercise regimens. However, the consensus is that physical activity appropriate for each patient is healthy and helpful. This activity can be taught in survivorship care programs using the expertise of health educators, physical therapists, or personal trainers such as Certified Cancer Exercise Trainers (CET). These trainers specialize in helping those who have just been diagnosed and are not yet receiving treatment, those who are in the process of receiving treatment, those who have finished treatment, and those who are experiencing late and long-term effects due to their finished treatment. Certification from the American College of Sport Medicine allows a trainer to "perform appropriate fitness assessments and make exercise recommendations while demonstrating a basic understanding of cancer diagnoses, surgeries, treatment, symptoms and side effects"[15] (go to www.acsm.org for more information).

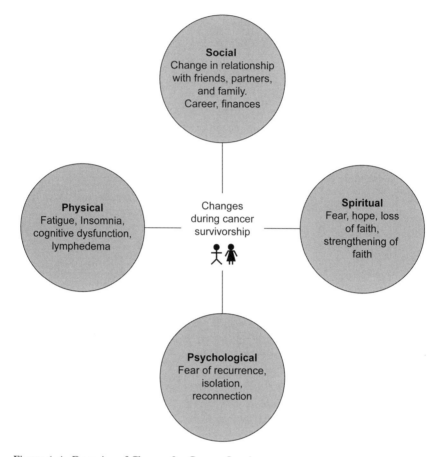

Figure 1.4. Domains of Change for Cancer Survivors.

The concept of wellness after cancer also emphasizes the great importance of nutrition. Nutritional education and guidelines have been encouraged for the generally healthy public, but are crucial for cancer survivors as well. A key aspect of nutritional education is the management of a healthy weight. Excess weight has been shown to increase the risk of cancer recurrence and decrease overall quality of life. The IOM reported "there is convincing evidence that obesity is associated with an increased risk of several cancers, including cancers of the colon, breast, and endometrium."[5] Generally, nutritional counseling has been neglected in the development of many cancer survivorship programs. For example, in a recent study, the 2010 Oncology Roundtable Member Survey[16] targeted programs that were expanding services for active patients to survivors, and questioned if certain survivorship services were provided. The results concluded that 80% of the 69 programs surveyed did not make nutritional counseling available. Registered dietitians are a crucial part of the survivorship program and are able to counsel patients on what foods are "cancer friendly."

CONCLUSION

The total number of cancer survivors is growing as is the number of long-term cancer survivors. Cancer diagnosis and treatment is still the most crucial phase of cancer care, but after treatment there is hope for years and decades of cancer survivorship. Most cancer survivors are doing well and are "cancer-free and free of cancer" while others have late and long-term effects of treatment or develop second or secondary cancers.

There are gaps in the continuum of care for cancer survivors. Cancer survivorship programs can be designed to directly provide some of these services and to coordinate this care by other members of the health care team.

REFERENCES

1. Mullen F. Seasons of survival: reflections of a physician with cancer. *New England Journal of Medicine.* 1985; 313(4) 270–3.

2. U.S. Bureau of Census. Estimated number of cancer survivors in the United States from 1971 to 2007. Altekruse SF, Kosary CL, Krapcho M, Neyman N, Aminou R, Waldron W, Ruhl J, Howlader N, Tatalovich Z, Cho H, Mariotto A, Eisner MP, Lewis DR, Cronin K, Chen HS, Feuer EJ, Stinchcomb DG, Edwards BK, editors. SEER Cancer Statistics Review, 1975–2007, National Cancer Institute. Bethesda, MD, http://seer.cancer.gov/csr/1975_2007/, based on November 2009 SEER data submission, posted to the SEER website, 2010.

3. Boyajian R. Presented to Oncology Nursing Society—unpublished.

4. Hewitt M, Greenfield S, and Stovall E, editors. From cancer patient to cancer survivor: lost in transition. *Institute of Medicine Report.* 2006; 01–506.

5. Rechis, R. How cancer has affected post-treatment survivors: a Live**STRONG** report. June 2010. Published Survey.

6. Earle CC, Burstein HJ, Winer EP, Weeks JC. Quality of non-breast cancer health maintenance among elderly breast cancer survivors. *J Clin Oncol.* 2003 Apr 15; 21 (8):1447–51.

7. Snyder CF, Earle CC, Herbert RJ, Neville BA, Blackford AL, Frick KD. Preventive care for colorectal cancer survivors: a 5-year longitudinal study. *J Gen Intern Med.* 2008 Mar 23(3):254–59.

8. Snyder CF, Frick KD, Kantsiper ME, Peairs KS, et al. Prevention, screening, and surveillance care for breast cancer survivors compared with controls: changes from 1998 to 2002. *J Clin Oncol.* 2009 Mar 1; 27(7):1054–61. Epub 2009 Jan 21.

9. Cheung WY, Neville BA, Cameron DB, Cook EF, Earle CC. Comparisons of patient and physician expectations for cancer survivorship care. *J Clin Oncol.* 2009 May 20; 27(15):2489–95.

10. Figure 1.3. Kenneth D. Miller. Unpublished communication.

11. ASCO cancer treatment summaries. Cancer.net. http://www.cancer.net/patient/Survivorship/ASCO+Cancer+Treatment+Summaries. Accessed February 15, 2011.

12. Long-term follow-up guidelines for survivors of childhood, adolescent, and young adult cancers. Children's Oncology Group website. http://www.survivorshipguidelines.org. Children's Oncology Group; 2008 Oct. 4 p.

13. Hewitt M, Greenfield S, and Stovall E, editors. From cancer patient to cancer survivor: lost in transition. Washington, DC: National Academies Press; 2005.

14. ACSM/ACS certified cancer exercise trainer (CET), 2007. American College of Sports Medicine website. http://www.acsm.org/AM/Template.cfm?Section=ACSM_ACS_Certified_Cancer_Exercise_Trainer.

15. Oncology Roundtable, 2010. Delivering on the promise of patient centered care. The Advisory Board Company. http://www.advisory.com/Research/Oncology-Roundtable/Studies/2011/Delivering-on-the-Promise-of-Patient-Centered-Ca.

2

Survivors' Experience with Living after Cancer: Results from the LIVESTRONG Survey for Post-Treatment Cancer Survivors

Ruth Rechis, PhD, Stephanie Nutt, MA, MPA
and Binja Basimike, BS

In the United States during the past 30 years, the number of cancer survivors has more than tripled to nearly 12 million people (Ries et al., 2008). As the number of cancer survivors has increased, the late effects caused by cancer and its treatment have come to the forefront (U.S. Department of Health and Human Services [HHS], 2004). These late effects can take many forms. Post-treatment, some cancer survivors will experience very few late effects, while others will face life-altering symptoms (National Cancer Institute, 2007). These effects can occur months or even years after treatment ends. Cancer survivors may face medical as well as non-medical late effects (Hoffman, McCarthy, Reckiltis, & Ng, 2009). The medical late effects cancer survivors experience vary but may include psychological distress, sexual dysfunction, infertility, impaired organ function, cosmetic changes and limitations in communication, mobility, and cognition (Hewitt, Greenfield, & Stoval, 2006). Non-medical late effects can include issues such as employment discrimination, debt, and loss of insurance (Wolff et al., 2005).

A poll conducted in 2004 on behalf of the Lance Armstrong Foundation (LIVE**STRONG**) revealed that about half (49%) of the cancer survivors who responded felt that their non-medical needs were not being met. Further, of this group, 70% indicated that their oncologists did not offer support in dealing with their non-medical needs. The remaining 30% responded that their physicians were willing to talk about their needs but did not have the resources to address them (Wolff et al., 2005). Although post-treatment cancer survivors may have many needs, research on these needs and how they are met is limited (Hewitt et al., 2006; Rowland & Bellizzi, 2008). As the number of cancer survivors continues to increase, it is imperative that a system of care be developed to understand what the needs of cancer survivors are and how those needs are (and are not) being met (Rowland, Hewitt, & Ganz, 2006).

The Institute of Medicine (IOM; Hewitt et al., 2006) released a report titled "From Cancer Patient to Cancer Survivor: Lost in Transition," which focused on survivors of adult cancer during the phase of care that follows primary treatment. In this report, the IOM made recommendations for follow-up care for cancer survivors and addressed those issues that need to be studied further to ensure better care for post-treatment survivors. The IOM report (2006) noted that "too many survivors are lost in transition once they finish treatment. They move from an orderly system of care to a 'non-system' in which there are few guidelines to assist them through the next stage of their life or help them overcome the medical and psychosocial problems that may arise." Often cancer survivors are unaware of the late effects that may be caused by their treatment, and even for those who are aware, their needs are often unmet. Further, the IOM report recommended that private voluntary organizations, such as nonprofit organizations, need to increase their support of survivorship research and expand mechanisms for its conduct. Future research initiatives should include populations that represent the diversity of cancer survivors in terms of types of cancer and treatments as well as their sociodemographic and health care characteristics (Hewitt et al., 2006).

LIVESTRONG Survey for Post-Treatment Cancer Survivors

In late 2006, in response to the IOM recommendations, LIVE**STRONG** launched a survey designed to capture data to provide insight into the needs of post-treatment cancer survivors. The mission of LIVE**STRONG**, a nonprofit organization, is to inspire and empower people affected by cancer. To this end, LIVE**STRONG** provides people with resources and support they need to fight cancer head-on and finds innovative ways to raise awareness, fund research, and end the stigma that many cancer survivors face. In addition, LIVE**STRONG** empowers people and communities to drive social change and calls for state, national, and world leaders to help fight this disease. The LIVE**STRONG** Survey for Post-Treatment Cancer Survivors (LIVE**STRONG** Survey) was designed to comprehensively assess the physical, emotional, and practical needs of survivorship post-treatment. Further, the survey gathered information about why some post-treatment survivors did not receive care and, if they did receive care, who provided it.

Survey Design and Characteristics

The survey instrument was designed through a process that engaged both cancer survivors and experts in the field of survey methodology and oncology through peer review, three focus groups, and a pilot test. The concerns used in the survey were initially selected and included for the following reasons: (1) they had been used in other surveys, (2) they were concerns that had been identified by experts as known late effects of cancer, and/or (3) they were areas of concern addressed by LIVE**STRONG** educational resources. Concerns and related answer choices were included in the final instrument only if they were recognized as effects known or options used by the participants in the cancer survivor focus group and pilot test. This was done intentionally to ensure that the survivor voice was the driving force behind all aspects of this survey. The survey instrument was divided into five sections that covered (1) physical concerns, (2) emotional concerns, (3) practical concerns, (4) positive experiences with cancer, and (5) resources and information provided by LIVE**STRONG**.

The positive experiences section and the resources and information provided by LIVE**STRONG** section included dichotomous statements to which respondents indicated whether or not they agreed. (For example, "I have appreciated life more because of having had cancer.")

The other three sections of the survey (physical, emotional, and practical concerns) were further organized into groups of related items, which will be referred to as "collections" throughout the rest of this chapter. For example, one collection contained four items related to energy and fatigue and another collection contained four items related to sadness and depression. There were a total of 27 collections addressing a broad range of concerns such as heart problems, insurance issues, and spirituality.

For each collection participants were asked to respond to the following statement: "Since completing treatment, have any of the following statements been true for you as a result of your experience with cancer?" For almost all collections, the statements that followed included both a simple description of the concern and a selection related to a doctor having told the survivor that he or she had a particular condition. Participants were then provided with a list of one or more options that were relevant to a particular collection. If individuals did not select "yes" for any concerns within a collection, they were directed to the next collection. If individuals selected "yes" for any of the concerns within the collection, they were then asked to answer if the concern had occurred before their experience with cancer, since their cancer diagnosis and within the last six months or since their cancer diagnosis but not within the last six months. If respondents had experienced the concern before cancer, they were directed to the next collection. This was done to try to ensure that responses were related to the post-treatment cancer experience. If respondents chose either of the latter answer choices, they were then asked to complete a statement about whether they had received care or help for these concerns. Depending on whether an individual received care, the respondent was sent down one of two paths: care received and care not received.

The concerns included in the physical collections included topics such as heart problems, fatigue, and lymphedema. The concerns included in the emotional collections included topics such as fearing a recurrence, feeling sad or blue, and worrying about social relationships. The concerns included in the practical collections included topics such as issues related to debt, health insurance, and employment. A full list of the collections is included in Appendix A.

METHODOLOGY

The survey was opened on March 30, 2006, following analysis of three focus groups and a pilot test. The survey remained open through February 2007 and was available both online and in paper form. The survey was intended for individuals who had been diagnosed with cancer who were currently finished with treatment or managing cancer as a chronic condition. This included those still taking medication, such as tamoxifen, to prevent a recurrence as well as those still seeing a doctor to check for new or returning cancers. The study was reviewed and approved by the University of Texas Institutional Review Board.

The survey instrument was available on LIVE**STRONG**.org to anyone who was interested in taking the survey. LIVE**STRONG** constituents were notified about the survey through the LIVE**STRONG** newsletter and emails. Additionally, LIVE**STRONG** reached out to all of its community and national partner organizations and all state cancer coalitions to provide information about the survey. Of note, just less than half of respondents (42%) reported having used an educational resource or being engaged with a LIVE**STRONG** program.

DATA ANALYSIS

To assess the prevalence of physical, emotional, and practical needs of post-treatment survivors, the mean percentages of those survey respondents who answered a particular question or answered all reported questions in a particular collection were used. This number varied from question to question, and collection to collection. Additionally, respondents were often able to select more than one item; that is, they could have sought multiple sources for help, or experienced concerns both before treatment and since.

Most collections used a dichotomous selection to choose either a positive, "yes, I have experienced this concern," or a negative, "no, I have not experienced this concern." Once a selection was made whether a respondent experienced a particular physical, practical, or emotional aspect of the cancer experience, follow-up questions were given. Because not all respondents answered every question in a collection, averages for each section were estimated using the available data. Likewise, not all respondents answered all questions in each area of physical, emotional, or practical needs and estimations were made using the available data. Additionally, all percentages were rounded to the nearest whole percent.

RESULTS

Sample Size, Demographics, and Medical Characteristics

A total of 2,568 individuals accessed the survey. Of these, 261 participants were ineligible to continue because they were still on some form of treatment for cancer or were under the age of 18. A total of 2,307 individuals were included in the survey analysis. Demographics for the sample are reported below. In several cases below, the demographics of the participants in this survey were compared to estimates of the demographics for all U.S. cancer survivors provided by the Surveillance Epidemiology and End Results (SEER) Program. SEER is a program of the National Cancer Institute that collects population-based data on cancer incidence and survival from state cancer registries in the United States. There are many notable differences between those who took this survey and the overall survivor population as captured by SEER.

Gender

The majority of survey respondents were females (67%). See Figure 2.1.

Race/Ethnicity

The majority of survey respondents (92%) identified themselves as white.

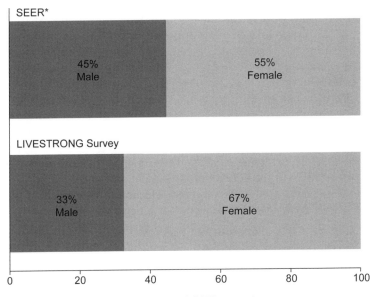

*Based on U.S. Prevalence Counts for 2006; Horner et al. (2009)

Figure 2.1. Gender of LIVESTRONG Survey Compared with SEER. (Based on U.S. Prevalence Counts for 2006; Horner et al., 2009.)

TABLE 2.1 FIVE MOST COMMON CANCERS AMONG **LIVESTRONG** SURVEY
RESPONDENTS

Type of Cancer	LIVESTRONG Survey Respondents' Percentages
Breast	32%
Testicular	7%
Lymphoma, non-Hodgkin	6%
Colorectal	6%
Lymphoma, Hodgkin	5%
Total	56%

Age at Diagnosis

The majority of survey respondents were younger at the time of diagnosis when compared to the SEER incidence cases—with the majority diagnosed between ages 20 and 54. Most notably, the median age of the LIVE**STRONG** Survey at time of diagnosis is 43 while the median age of the SEER incidence cases is 67.

Cancer Type

Based on SEER data, in the United States the five most prevalent types of cancer, based on the total number of people living with cancer at any point in time, are breast, prostate, colorectal, gynecologic, and hematologic. The five most commonly selected types of cancer from the LIVE**STRONG** Survey were as follows: Breast (32%), Testicular (7%), Lymphoma, Non-Hodgkin (6%), Colorectal (6%), and Lymphoma, Hodgkin (5%). See Table 2.1.

CANCER EXPERIENCE

The following section includes information about the treatment experiences of the LIVE**STRONG** Survey respondents.

Time since Last Treatment

While some respondents had not been treated for cancer for more than 5 or 10 years, the majority of respondents (73.4%) had received treatment within 5 years of taking the survey (see Figure 2.2).

Type of Treatment

The majority of respondents used traditional methods for treatment. Additionally, 830 respondents (36%) reported receiving a second or third opinion for cancer, cancer treatment or late effects of cancer. Of this group, 21% of

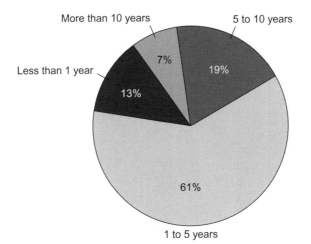

Figure 2.2. Time since Last Treatment.

respondents followed the second or third opinion, but 79% did not. Also, the majority of respondents (62%) also used at least one type of alternative or complementary therapy for cancer or late effects of cancer.

While the results of this survey cannot be generalized to the experiences of all post-treatment cancer survivors, the findings provide important information and help to build the body of literature on the needs of post-treatment cancer survivors. The results of this survey also provide insight about a less-studied population of cancer survivors—those diagnosed under the age of 55.

PHYSICAL, EMOTIONAL, AND PRACTICAL CONCERNS EXPERIENCED

Cancer survivors who responded to this survey experienced effects in their lives that were multidimensional. While respondents had varied experiences in terms of type of cancer, type of treatment, time since treatment, and a number of other characteristics, for these survivors life after a cancer diagnosis continued to bring changes and challenges. As one respondent noted, "Going into and during treatment, I had tremendous medical support, but I feel that my issues as a survivor have not been well-addressed by the medical community. I knew what to expect in treatment, but I have muddled through as a survivor."

Almost all respondents (99%) experienced at least one concern after cancer treatment ended. Overall, the emotional collections were selected the most, while the practical collections were selected the least. This may be due in part to the fact that most respondents in this particular survey were employed and insured during their experience with cancer.

Overall, there were stark differences related to receiving help. While the majority of survey respondents who had experienced at least one physical concern did receive care, just over half of those who experienced emotional concerns received help. Almost half, 45% (996), of those with post-treatment emotional concerns reported that they had not received help for any of their

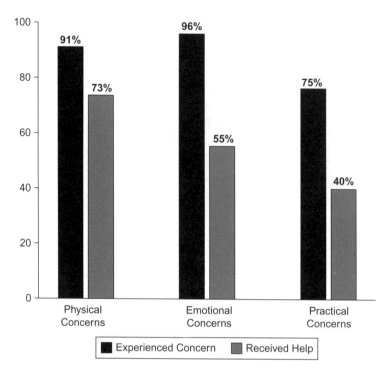

Figure 2.3. Percentage of Individuals Who Experienced Concerns and the Percentage Who Received Care for Those Concerns.

post-treatment emotional concerns. Likewise, the majority of those with practical concerns did not receive help. Of the respondents with practical concerns since treatment ended, only 40% (784) indicated they had received help with one or more practical concerns (see Figure 2.3). As one respondent noted in the following quote, survivors are not always aware that what they are experiencing is due to cancer, "Many of the symptoms I experienced were not addressed because no one told me that they were side effects of treatment."

Those cancer survivors who did receive help indicated they received it from professionals, loved ones, other survivors, and themselves. The most frequently selected providers across all collections were (1) medical specialists such as dentists or fertility specialists, (2) oncologists, and (3) primary care physicians (see Figures 2.4–6). Interestingly, the providers of care or help received varied greatly by collections. While medical professionals were most selected for the physical concerns, they were not for the emotional and practical concerns.

Encouragingly, across all of the collections, the majority of those who did receive help indicated that many of their needs were met. Across all of the collections, the reasons cited for not receiving help varied but were primarily related to the survivor's willingness to address the concern on their own. The top three reasons across collections for not getting help were (1) I have learned to live with this concern, (2) I have addressed this on my own, and

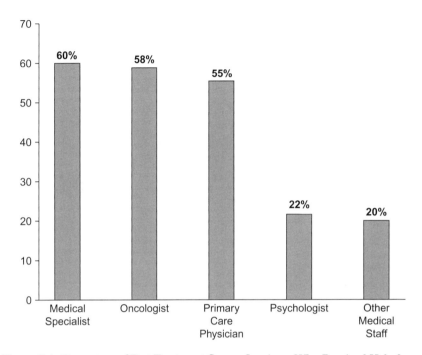

Figure 2.4. Percentage of Past-Treatment Cancer Survivors Who Received Help from the Medical Field.

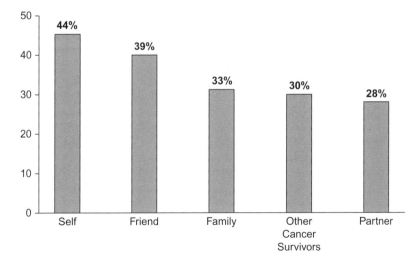

Figure 2.5. Percentage of Past-Treatment Cancer Survivors Who Received Help from Personal Sources.

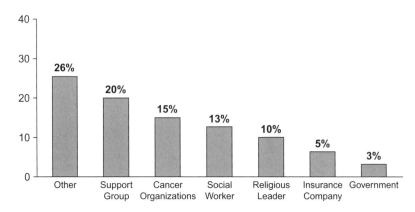

Figure 2.6. Percentage of Past-Treatment Cancer Survivors Who Received Help from Other Sources.

(3) I was told this was a side effect that would go away with time. A full report of the survey results is available at http://www.livestrong.org/What-We-Do/Our-Approach/Reports-Findings/LIVESTRONG-Survey-Report.

Discussion

Understanding the impact of cancer on long-term survivorship has never been a more relevant topic to address. The LIVE**STRONG** Survey was created to better understand the experiences of cancer survivors after treatment is completed—specifically, the constituency of survivors who engage with LIVE**STRONG.**

The findings of this survey indicate that cancer has impacted many facets of these 2,307 post-treatment cancer survivors' lives. While the results of this survey may not represent the experiences of all post-treatment cancer survivors, the findings make an important contribution to the scientific understanding of the needs of post-treatment cancer survivors.

Based on the LIVE**STRONG** Survey results, LIVE**STRONG** encourages the cancer community, including all of those who work with people with cancer, to consider the following:

1. **Cancer survivors' post-treatment concerns should be addressed and understood more fully.**

   For the survivors in this survey, in particular for emotional and practical concerns, many did not receive help for their post-treatment concerns. The survivors in this survey indicated most often that they chose not to receive help because they had learned to live with their concerns. Even for those who received help, across the collections 78% indicated that not all of their needs were met. Interestingly, in this survey, other cancer survivors were frequently selected (30%) as a support mechanism—often times over medical professionals and family members. Additionally, many of these survivors reported that they either have helped or have the desire to help other cancer survivors. Identifying ways to meet all of survivors' post-treatment needs through effective existing or new evidence-based programs and resources, especially for emotional and practical concerns, is a critical step in ensuring positive outcomes for survivors. Further, understanding the role that all providers and support systems play in cancer survivors' lives can provide insight in all aspects of survivorship care.

To address some of these issues, in 2010 LIVE**STRONG** launched the LIVE**STRONG** Survey for People Affected by Cancer. This new survey was similar to the last version, but also included a section open to anyone who has been impacted by cancer to better understand the role of advocacy, engagement, health communication, and stigma on the cancer experience. Additionally, the survey was made available in Spanish.

2. **Health care providers should engage with their patients to understand the multifaceted nature of survivorship.**

Cancer impacted almost all aspects of these survivors' lives. Most survivors experienced at least one concern and many experienced physical, practical, and emotional concerns. Across these concerns, survivors received help from as many as 17 different types of providers. For some, receiving help from multiple providers was challenging. As one respondent noted, "Addressing difficulties following treatment is something none of us anticipated. Each physician I met was wonderful but they addressed the problem in their field. Period." Finding ways to understand and address the full scope of the survivors' experiences with cancer, including both the negative and positive outcomes, could help to better meet the needs of cancer survivors. Survivors should be engaged as active partners in their care strategies and be provided with sufficient information to make challenging decisions and to facilitate meaningful discussion with health care providers. Survivorship care plans can help health care providers and survivors to coordinate care and address the complexities of surviving cancer (Hewitt et al., 2006).

3. **Research should be conducted to better understand the survivorship experience, especially of underserved populations including adolescent and young adult (AYA) cancer survivors.**

Further research is needed to more fully understand the post-treatment cancer experience, especially studies across the cancer continuum that engage cancer survivors in study design, implementation, and dissemination of research results. Research should include minority and medically underserved populations as well as individuals who represent the diversity of cancer survivors in terms of type of cancer and treatment. The results of this survey differ from other research in post-treatment survivorship in part because more than 30% of the LIVE**STRONG** Survey respondents were AYA cancer survivors, individuals diagnosed between 15 and 39 years of age. AYA cancer survivors represent an underserved and under-studied population (Adolescent and Young Adult Oncology Progress Review Group, 2006). By conducting further research, appropriate interventions and programs can be created to support these vulnerable populations. Survivors and their loved ones as well as health care providers need quality, evidence-based information to ensure the best quality of life and long-term outcomes for cancer survivors.

References

Adolescent and Young Adult Oncology Progress Review Group. (2006). *Closing the Gap: Research and Care Imperatives for Adolescents and Young Adults with Cancer.* Bethesda, MD: National Cancer Institute.

American Cancer Society. (2009). *Cancer Facts & Figures 2009.* Atlanta, GA: American Cancer Society.

Hewitt, M., Greenfield, S., & Stoval, E. (2006). *From Cancer Patient to Cancer Survivor: Lost in Transition. National Cancer Policy Board, Committee on Cancer Survivorship: Improving Care and Quality of Life.* Washington, DC: National Academy Press.

Hoffman, K. E., McCarthy, E. P., Reckiltis, C. J., & Ng, A. K. (2009). Psychological distress in long-term survivors of adult-onset cancer: Results from a national survey. *Archives of Internal Medicine, 169*(14), 1274–1281.

Horner, M. J., Ries, L. A. G., Krapcho, M., Neyman, N., Aminou, R., Howlader, N., Altekruse, S. F., Feuer, E. J., Huang, L., Mariotto, A., Miller, B. A., Lewis, D. R., Eisner, M. P., Stinchcomb, D. G., & Edwards B. K. (eds.) (2009). SEER Cancer Statistics Review, 1975–2006, National Cancer Institute. Bethesda, MD, http://seer.cancer.gov/csr/1975_2006/, based on November 2008 SEER data submission, posted to the SEER website.

National Cancer Institute. (2007). *Facing Forward: Life after Cancer Treatment.* U.S. Department of Health and Human Services.

Rechis, R. (2008, March). *Post-Treatment Cancer Survivors' Concerns and Help Seeking Choices.* Poster presented at the American Psychosocial Oncology Society Annual Conference, Irvine, CA.

Rechis, R., & Shaw, K. (2009, August). *Health Information Needs: Results from the LIVESTRONG Survey for Post-Treatment Cancer Survivors.* Poster presented at the Third Annual National Conference on Health Communication, Marketing and Media, Atlanta, GA.

Ries, L. A. G., Melbert, D., Krapcho, M., Mariotto, A., Miller, B. A., Feuer, E. J., Clegg, L., Horner, M. J., Howlader, N., Eisner, M. P., Reichman, M., Edwards, B. K. (eds.) (2007). SEER Cancer Statistics Review, 1975–2004, National Cancer Institute. Bethesda, MD, http://seer.cancer.gov/csr/1975_2004/, based on November 2006 SEER data submission, posted to the SEER website.

Ries, L. A. G., Melbert, D., Krapcho, M., Stincomb, D. G., Howlander, N., Horner, M. J., Mariotto, A., Miller, B. A., Feuer, E. J., Altekruse, S. F., Lewis, D. R., Clegg, L., Eisner, M. P., Reichman, M., Edwards, B. K. (eds.) (2008). SEER Cancer Statistics Review, 1975–2005, National Cancer Institute. Bethesda, MD, http://seer.cancer.gov/csr/1975_2005/, based on November 2007 SEER data submission, posted to the SEER website.

Rowland, J. H., & Bellizzi, K. M. (2008). Cancer survivors and survivorship research: A reflection on today's successes and tomorrow's challenges. *Hematology Oncology Clinics of North America, 22,* 181–200.

Rowland, J. H., Hewitt, M., & Ganz, P. A. (2006). Cancer survivorship: A new challenge in delivering quality cancer care. *Journal of Clinical Oncology, 24,* 5101–5104.

U.S. Department of Health and Human Services. (2004). *A National Plan for Cancer Survivorship: Advancing Public Health Strategies.* Centers for Disease Control and LIVESTRONG.

Wolff, S. N., Nichols, C., Ulman, D., Miller, A., Kho, S., Lofye, D., Milford, M., Tracy, D., Bellavia, B., & Armstrong, L. (2005). *Survivorship: An Unmet Need of the Patient with Cancer—Implications of a Survey of the Lance Armstrong Foundation.* Poster presented at the American Society of Clinical Oncology Annual Meeting, Chicago, IL.

APPENDIX A: SURVEY ITEMS

Physical Concerns

- I have had trouble with my heart.
- I have been told by a doctor that I have heart problems.

- I have had trouble breathing.
- I have been told by a doctor that I have damage to my lungs.
- I have had trouble seeing.
- I have been told by a doctor that I have problems with my vision or sight.
- I have had trouble hearing.
- I have been told by a doctor that I problems with my hearing.
- I have had problems with my mouth.
- I have had problems with my teeth.
- I have been told by a doctor I have problems with my mouth.
- I have been told by a doctor I have problems with my teeth.
- I have been told by a doctor that I have graft-versus-host disease.
- I have had swelling in my legs, arms, or other areas of my body.
- I have been told by a doctor that I have lymphedema.
- I have lost feeling or had strange sensations in my hands or feet.
- I have experienced dizziness, such as when getting up from a chair.
- I have been told by a doctor that I have neuropathy.
- I have been told by a doctor that I have a thyroid condition.
- I have not been able to control when I urinate.
- I urinate more frequently than I used to.
- I have been told by a doctor that I have urinary incontinence.
- I have been pregnant or fathered a pregnancy since cancer treatment ended . . .
  - No, because my partner is infertile or has fertility problems.
  - No, a doctor has told me that I am infertile because of my cancer diagnosis or cancer treatment.
  - No, I have been unable to get pregnant, maintain a pregnancy, or father a pregnancy for more than a year.
  - No, because _____
- I have been bothered by difficulty or inability to function sexually.
- I have been dissatisfied with my sex life.
- I have avoided sexual activity or lacked interest in sex.
- I have had difficulties with impotence.
- I have had aches or pains for long periods of time.
- I have had pain that kept me from doing the things I wanted to do.
- I have had difficulty doing activities that require concentration.
- I have been bothered by having a short attention span.
- I have had trouble remembering things.
- I have been bothered by forgetting what I started to do.
- I have had "chemo brain."
- I have not had the energy to do the things I wanted to do.
- I have felt tired a lot.
- I have had trouble getting the rest that I need.
- I have had trouble sleeping for several nights in a row.

Emotional Concerns

- I have felt that I have lost a sense of security in my future.
- I have felt that I have lost a sense of my identity.
- I have felt grief about the death of other cancer patients.
- I have felt guilt over the death of other cancer patients.
- I have felt that I have lost a sense of my faith or spirituality.

- I have felt that my faith or spirituality has been negatively affected.
- I have been preoccupied with concerns about cancer.
- I have worried about dying from cancer.
- I have worried about cancer coming back.
- I have been reluctant to start new relationships.
- I have not wanted to participate in social gatherings.
- I have not wanted to be around people because I worried about germs.
- I have not wanted to be around my friends.
- I have been reluctant to meet new people.
- I do not go to events that I used to enjoy.
- I have received the support that I need from my partner.
- I have received the support that I need from my friends.
- I have received the support that I need from my children.
- I have received the support that I need from my family.
- I broke up with, separated from or divorced my partner.
- I have not wanted to tell others that I have had cancer.
- I have worried about whether my family members should have genetic tests for cancer.
- I have worried that my family members were at risk of getting cancer.
- I have worried about whether my family members might have cancer-causing genes.
- I have felt unattractive.
- I have felt people have treated me differently because of changes to my appearance.
- I was bothered by hair loss from cancer treatment long after treatment ended.
- I was bothered by the amount of weight I lost.
- I was bothered by the amount of weight I gained.

Practical Concerns

- I have been affected at my job because of my cancer diagnosis in the following negative ways: (Please check all that apply.)
  - I lost my job.
  - I left my job.
  - I am unable to work at all now.
  - I am unable to work full time now.
  - I am unable to work in the same way I did before my cancer diagnosis.
  - I have been treated poorly on the job.
  - I have received a decrease in pay.
  - I have experienced employment discrimination.
  - I have felt that my employer would not make reasonable changes or accommodations in my job to help me.
  - I was passed over for a promotion.
  - I have returned to work at a lower level than I was at before my diagnosis.
  - I have stayed in my job because I did not want to lose my health insurance.
  - I have stayed in my job because I did not want to lose my life insurance.
  - I had difficulty with the return to work.
  - I had to take on a second job because of debt due to cancer.

- I have felt that I did not get a job because of my cancer diagnosis.
- Other_____
- I have been affected at my school because of my cancer diagnosis in the following ways: (Please check all that apply.)
  - I left school.
  - I missed a large amount of school.
  - I have had difficulty keeping up with my school work.
  - I have had trouble with my classmates since receiving a cancer diagnosis.
  - I did not have any special accommodations while I was in school.
  - I had to drop out of school because of debt.
  - I was unable to attend college.
  - Other_____
- My loved ones or I have had financial problems because of cancer, treatment or late effects of cancer.
- Since my cancer diagnosis, I have: (Please check all that apply.)
  - Led a healthier lifestyle.
  - Participated in regular physical activity (for example, you participate in some type of physical activity at least two–three times a week).
    Increased the amount of physical activity I participate in.
  - Quit smoking.
  - Attended regular medical appointments.
  - Received screenings for secondary cancers.
  - Tried to take care of my health.
  - Other_____
  - Led a less healthy lifestyle.
  - Not changed the amount of physical activity I participate in.
  - Decreased the amount of physical activity I participate in because of pain.
  - Decreased the amount of physical activity I participate in because of I'm afraid of being injured.
  - Decreased the amount of physical activity I participate in because I have no time.
  - Decreased the amount of physical activity I participate in because I'm not sure what level of exercise is appropriate.
  - Decreased the amount of physical activity I participate in because of fatigue.
  - Continued to smoke cigarettes.
  - Started to smoke cigarettes.
  - Needed help with everyday tasks that I did not need help with before cancer.

Positive Experiences

- I have appreciated life more because of having had cancer.
- I have felt that cancer helped me to recognize what is important in life.
- I have a renewed sense of spirituality because of having had cancer.
- I am willing to share my story if it can help other cancer survivors.
- I have helped other cancer survivors through their cancer experience.
- I think that cancer will always be a part of my life.
- I speak up more now about screening for cancer.
- I would like to do more to help other cancer survivors.

3

THE CANCER SURVIVORSHIP TEAM

CHRISTIAN MCEVOY, MPH, AND KENNETH MILLER, MD

Cancer surveillance and follow-up are typically provided by surgical, radiation, and medical oncologists. Cancer survivorship care can also be provided by individual care providers including oncology nurses, advanced practice nurses, physician's assistants, PCPs, and oncologists. In some settings, a survivorship clinic is available to provide this type of care and could include a team of clinicians whose efforts hopefully complement each other's, including:

1. Survivorship clinic medical director: primary care physician or oncologist
2. Program administrator or coordinator
3. Advanced practice nurse or RN
4. Mental health provider
5. Nutritionist
6. Exercise trainer/rehabilitation specialist

A survivorship clinic is built on the premise that an informed patient is a healthier patient. Some cancer survivors visit the clinic once, others on an 'as needed basis', and finally still others return annually. During a visit, the survivor/patient will see as many of the complementing clinicians as possible. The clinicians will individually review each survivor's case before the visit, and the clinicians will meet after the visit to develop consensus recommendations for continuing care. These recommendations might include, but are not limited to, cognitive therapy, advanced screenings, nutritional adjustments, increased or modified exercise regimens, physical therapy, financial counseling, and/or basic life and habit modifications. The goal of the clinic visit is to provide a road map for the survivor for the foreseeable future.

As a good example, the Connecticut Challenge Survivorship Clinic at the Yale Cancer Center was created in 2007 to provide this type of multidisciplinary care. At its core, the Connecticut Challenge Cancer Survivorship Clinic is a health promotion program for people with a recent diagnosis of cancer. The program promotes basic health and wellness for survivors in light of the diagnosis and treatment already received. The intervention was designed to serve survivors soon after they finished treatment. Indeed, the intention was to bridge the gap between acute treatment and long-term care defined and described in the 2005 Institute of Medicine report, "From Cancer Patient to Cancer Survivor: Lost in Transition." "Despite the increase in survivors, primary care physicians and other health care providers often are not extremely familiar with the consequences of cancer, and seldom receive explicit guidance from oncologists." The Yale Cancer Center Survivorship Clinic connects the two opposing cliffs of the cancer survivorship gap—medical oncology and primary care/health and wellness promotion.

THE CLINIC STAFF

The coordinator: The coordinator for the clinic "is the voice of the clinic, as people call in." She explains how the clinic works, sends out the intake forms, and makes appointments. On clinic day, she creates a schedule for each patient and clinician, prints the pertinent records, and prepares a folder of information for the patient. These tasks are more difficult than one might originally assume. The difficulty associated with this position is a symptom of a systemic challenge in cancer survivorship—the need for individual treatment summaries. A treatment summary is simply a summary of all cancer treatments received by a patient including therapy names, dosages, dates, and quantitative as well as qualitative response data. In an ideal world, each survivor visiting the clinic would simply forward his or her treatment summary to the coordinator before the visit. Unfortunately, in current practice, most survivors do not receive a treatment summary, so the coordinator spends a great deal of energy tracking down the sometimes disparate components of a survivor's treatment. This can be especially difficult, yet probably even more important if the survivor has been treated for multiple cancers or in more than one location by more than one treatment team.

In the ideal setting, the coordinator would simply facilitate the transfer of the treatment summary from the oncologist's records to the clinic's records, and the survivor's initial visit would coincide closely with the end of treatment, and eventually this will be the case. But as survivorship clinics are developing and opening, a prevalent population of cancer survivors who have been out of treatment for many years would clearly benefit from the education and empowerment the clinic can offer. These are the challenges facing the coordinator, and the reason Scott Capozza, the Yale Cancer Center Survivorship Clinic's physical therapist and an 11-year cancer survivor, says, "from a personnel standpoint, the success of the clinic truly rests on the coordinator. It is the toughest and most important job in the clinic."

Nurse practitioner/medical director: The nurse practitioner or the medical director meets with each patient for approximately 30 minutes to talk about any of the actual short-term or current side effects that they are experiencing as well as potential late and long-term effects. This person also discusses risk identification and mitigation, health promotion, and the importance of cancer screening. This is often a broad-stroke planning meeting between the supervising clinician and the survivor. The survivor will delve into deeper planning and education with each subsequent and specialized clinician, and the topics to be covered in the specialized meetings, in large part, emanate from this meeting.

While epidemiologic data may suggest risks for recurrent or subsequent cancers and side effects of treatments, each survivor should understand his or her individual risk profile. In order for a clinician to communicate this individual risk profile accurately and effectively, a comprehensive study of the survivor's complete medical, family, and behavioral history is required. This data forms a unique risk profile for each survivor. The NP or MD prepares for the visit by reviewing these histories, provided to him or her by the coordinator; however, the NP/MD also conducts a short interview to fill in gaps in the information. These gaps may not be apparent from a careful perusal of the survivor's charts before the visit. For example, on the surface it might be assumed that a young testicular cancer survivor might benefit from fertility counseling with his partner; however, an interview might inform the clinician that the survivor is in a same-sex partnership and has plans for adoption, so a fertility counseling recommendation would be unnecessary. The investigative nature and broadstroke planning goals require more than a "quick visit"; thus, the meeting between the NP/MD and the survivor is scheduled for at least 30 minutes.

The mental health provider: A social worker meets with each patient to "hear his or her story." It is important to distinguish this meeting from psychotherapy. In an ongoing counseling or therapy session, the patient and clinician operate in continuity from one session to the next, and the clinician "treats" the patient. In contrast, the goal of the survivorship clinic meeting between the mental health care provider and the survivor is diagnostic and therapeutic. The clinician listens to the survivor's story and may make suitable evidence-based recommendations for further treatment including ongoing counseling therapy, consideration of pharmacologic therapy, and/or self-care practices such as meditation and relaxation. Many survivors who visit the Yale Cancer Center Survivorship Clinic identify this component as one of their favorite parts of the visit.

Cancer survivors have an opportunity to share any trauma they experienced, their insights, and their growth. This speaks to the need many survivors have for ongoing therapeutic counseling and to the genuine benefit survivors feel from airing their experiences with an unbiased professional.

The nutritionist: A registered dietician meets with each patient to assess their dietary habits and their lifestyle. Again, this is an educational opportunity. The nutrition expert uses the time to learn about the survivor and to teach the survivor about "fighting cancer with a fork". A nutritionist serving this role will likely come up against a few obstacles, the greatest of which is incomplete information available to the pubic. Advertisements, so-called experts, and rumors proffering the latest cancer-fighting diets, nutritional supplements, and special diets are ubiquitous. The associations between the foods and supplements touted and the reduction of cancer risk and/or side-effect risk are rarely based in good science. In the best case scenario, following such a plan can be just expensive; however, unfortunately sometimes these dietary plans are actually harmful to a survivor's health. In the clinic, the nutritionist is an educator, and in that capacity a myth de-bunker. To that end, the Yale Cancer Center Survivorship Clinic's nutritionist's counsel is based on the new dinner plate model. The well-known dinner plate pyramid, officially adopted by the United States Department of Agriculture in 1992, usually depicts the components of a recommended healthy diet based in lean fruits, vegetables, whole grains, and lean protein. These are the building blocks of solid nutrition, and from this base, the nutritionist can help a survivor identify key areas. For example, head and neck cancer survivors often experience limitations with difficult-to-chew foods. The nutritionist can suggest ideas for soft and liquid nutrition that satisfy the nutritional needs of the survivor as well as provide variety and enjoyment. The nutritionist must work closely with the other clinicians because the meetings between the survivor and the other clinicians greatly inform the nutritional needs of the survivor (e.g., calorie intake, weight loss/gain goals).

The cancer exercise trainer or physical therapist: This person assesses each cancer survivor's level of activity, figures out their limitations, and designs an exercise prescription for them. Many cancer survivors have some ongoing problem such as a reduced range of motion or pain and referrals are commonly made for ongoing rehabilitation services. The American College of Sports Medicine and the American Cancer Society recently collaborated to develop the Cancer Exercise Trainer (CET) Certification. A CET is a fitness professional who trains cancer survivors at any stage of survivorship. The CET performs appropriate fitness assessments and makes exercise recommendations while demonstrating a basic understanding of cancer diagnoses, surgeries, treatments, symptoms, and side effects (American College of Sports Medicine, 2007).

A traditional physical therapist is a rehabilitation specialist who aims through therapy to restore an individual to functional physical abilities. The definition of functional is uniquely defined on an individual level by parameters such as previous capabilities and occupational requirements. The physical therapist is trained to assess the survivor's limitations and suggest therapy while a CET is trained to design exercise regimens for cancer survivors given the limitations identified by the physical therapist.

The Yale Cancer Center Survivorship Clinic is fortunate to have a certified CET and a licensed Physical Therapist in the same person. This combination is beneficial because the clinician can diagnose and suggest physical therapy regimens for the physical direct and side effects of cancer and treatment, and can also suggest an exercise regiment that works within the physical limitations of the survivor. The importance and power of this combination cannot be overstated. Cancer survivorship research is in its infancy, but evidence suggests that exercise is an important component of healthy living as a cancer survivor. The exercise can be as moderate as walking to the mailbox or as goal-oriented as completing an Ironman triathlon depending on a number of factors, including the most obvious one—the presence of any physical limitations. This meeting is especially important if these limitations are due to cancer or therapy to combat cancer. This means that the survivor might have to re-learn how to exercise. For example, a breast cancer survivor who swam for exercise before diagnosis, surgery, and treatment may experience lymphedema after surgery and be unable to swim as well. This type of problem solving is generally required in a cancer survivorship clinic and specifically by the physical therapist and CET on staff.

The CT Challenge Yale Cancer Center Team Has Noted Several Lessons Learned

Lesson One:

Some patients may not completely understand why they are coming, or the nature of their visit, and some are too close to diagnosis and treatment to benefit from the visit. Under-informed patients may not realize that a clinic visit is an educational opportunity rather than another treatment. They might expect to have their problems fixed. The disappointment associated with the reality of the situation may lead a survivor to tune out the very valuable information he or she receives during the visit.

Lesson Two:

It is important to gather medical records and to have patients complete an intake form prior to the visit. Again, the role of the coordinator cannot be overestimated. Health and wellness as a cancer survivor is a product of the confluence of preexisting comorbidities, the specific cancer a person was treated for, the treatment to combat the cancer, and health behaviors during and after treatment. In other words, many disparate data points must be considered when developing a survivorship care plan. Some of this data can and/or must be provided by the survivor (e.g., behavioral history), but other data is most reliable when obtained directly from the oncology care provider (e.g., dosage and timing of chemotherapeutic agents).

Lesson Three:

Internal marketing is important both before a survivorship program starts and on an ongoing basis. The long-term goal of an embryonic survivorship program should focus on developing a flow of patients originating from local treatment centers. The survivorship clinic should be the next step patients take as they finish treatment. This ideal will not be the likely situation at the outset. For one, unless there is an institutional mechanism in place to ensure this ideal flow (e.g., a patient navigator assigned to discharge each patient from treatment who sets up the clinic visit at discharge), this plan hinges on referrals made by the surveillance/treatment team. In other words, unless the oncologist says, "You are finished with treatment. I really recommend that you visit the Survivorship Clinic as soon as possible. Here is the number. Call the coordinator, [coordinator name]; she is expecting to hear from you," a survivor is not likely to visit the clinic soon after treatment. The Survivorship Clinic team must market the program to the very busy treatment team. There is no roadmap for this; it requires institutional knowledge and, frankly, a bit of charisma.

Lesson Four:
Automating the production of an end of treatment summary and care plan for patients would be helpful and should pull together the recommendations of each member of the team. This lesson is really a solution to challenges presented in Lessons Two and Three. Comprehensive end of treatment summaries are integral to a great survivorship program, and in order to make them ubiquitous, the survivorship clinic team must urge the cancer treatment team to produce them. Discussions have been had on the national, regional, state, and intuitional levels regarding the automation and standardization of a treatment summary for all survivors. Until the standard summary is a reality, the clinic team must advocate for survivors within their own community. The key document for the clinic team to produce is a survivorship care plan. This document would be a roadmap for the survivor that should remind him or her of the key points covered in each of the components of the clinic visit.

Lesson Five:
Having a family member, partner, or spouse participate in the survivorship clinic visit is often beneficial. Meeting with a number of clinicians can be overwhelming. It would be easy to forget questions one might want to ask, and it would certainly be easy to lose key bits of information. Clinic staff (most likely the coordinator) should stress the importance of preparation to each patient before the visit. Reminding survivors to think about and write down questions in advance of their visits is key. It may also be helpful for survivors to bring a family member or close friend to the clinic visit. That person may be able to help the survivor digest information; moreover, the family member or friend may gain a deeper understanding of the cancer experience for the survivor.

Lesson Six:
Measuring outcomes and operating in iterations is crucial to improvement. The field of survivorship care is young, and so the clinic team learns as it grows. The clinic at Yale is associated with faculty members in the Department of Epidemiology at the Yale School of Public Health. Measuring outcomes is also important on the individual level. Ideally, survivors return to the clinic annually. Measuring the success of their wellness behavior can be a huge motivator. The clinic staff should also encourage each survivor to measure his or her own success on a regular basis (e.g., weight loss, happiness scale test, productivity scale test, or exercise goals such as a distance to run/walk).

A Team Approach to Survivorship Care

Cancer survivors present individual problems and challenges to the team, but there are common themes that have emerged for the clinic team including those noted in Figure 3.1. The benefit of a team approach is to provide cancer survivors with many different methods and strategies.

Below are two examples of a multidisciplinary approach to cancer survivorship care.

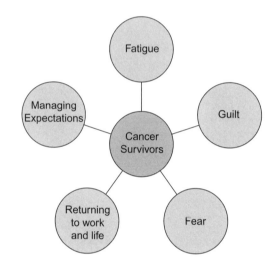

Concern or Question	Theme
I'm worried about the cancer coming back. Is there anything I can do?	Fear of recurrence
I'm so Tired!	Fatigue
I must have brought this on myself somehow	Guilt
I'm starting back to work soon. I'm looking forward to it but I'm nervous, too. What if my boss expects too much of me at first? I've developed some healthy habits after my treatment and I'm afraid I won't have time or will get too busy to continue them.	Concerns about returning to work
Other people have these expectations of how I should be and act and feel now that I'm "over" the cancer. They really don't get it.	Managing (unrealistic) expectations of others

Figure 3.1. Five Common Patient-Centered Themes. (Reprinted from Capozza, S., Chase, L., Harrigan, N., Quinn, T., & Miller K. [2009]. "What We Hear: A Conversation with Survivors." *Creating a cancer survivorship program* [p. 24]. Copyright © 2009 by Bike Across America Inc., dba the Connecticut Challenge. Reprinted with permission.)

Theme One: The Survivorship Team Members' Perspective on Fear of Recurrence

Physical Therapist (Scott Capozza, PT): "Exercising five times a week for 30 minutes may reduce one's risk of a recurrence or developing a second cancer by 40–70% depending on the diagnosis. Additional benefits of exercising after cancer treatment include weight reduction, improved musculoskeletal strength, and improved mood. Exercising not only reduces one's risk of a recurrence of cancer but it also decreases one's risk for other chronic diseases such as diabetes and high blood pressure and reduces your risk of stroke and heart attack"

Social Worker (Lina Chase, LCSW): "Fear of recurrence is very common. It is important to realize that fear of cancer returning is a projection into the future . . . we are imagining the future in a negative way. I suggest that if we are going to use our imagination, then it is helpful to use it in a positive way and imagine ourselves as healthy. (There are visualizations and affirmations that can be helpful in projecting into the future.) Best of all, there are techniques to assist in keeping us in the present."

Nutritionist (Maura Harrigan, RD): "There is no food that will trigger a recurrence. In fact, eating a healthy diet may help prevent recurrence. In addition, a nutritious diet will manage your weight, improve cardiovascular health, and help manage your blood pressure, cholesterol levels, blood glucose levels, and even your mood." Some specific recommendations include:

Eat a predominantly plant-based diet
Eat a rainbow of colors of fruits and vegetables
Limit consumption of processed and red meats
Emphasize omega-3 fatty acids
Limit consumption of alcohol
Observe food safety precautions

Medical Director (Kenneth Miller, MD): "If any of us told you that there was a zero percent risk of recurrence you probably wouldn't believe it because everyone who has had a diagnosis of cancer has some risk of recurrence. Fortunately, often the risk of recurrence is lower than you might have estimated and has been lowered even more by the treatment that you have received. In addition, as each month passes some of your risk of recurrence may be lessened as well. Hope is an important partner. Some cancer survivors like to have quantitative information on risk and some don't. Ask your primary oncologist if you want more specific information."

Theme Two: The Survivorship Team Members' Perspective on Fatigue

Physical Therapist (Scott Capozza, PT): "During and following surgery, radiation therapy, and chemotherapy, your body may feel fatigued as it is healing from these treatments, and thus you do not feel like exercising. A vicious cycle can be created: you feel tired, so you don't exercise, and then you become more fatigued because you have not been able to increase your energy level by exercising, and so on. The journey of 1,000 miles begins with a single step (Capozza, 2010). Begin slowly and keep things in perspective. "If you were exercising before you began your treatments, it will take you time to regain your previous fitness level; if you did not exercise before your cancer diagnosis, you will see improvements at a faster rate."

Social Worker (Lina Chase, LCSW): "First of all, please know that your concern is felt by most cancer survivors. Frankly, as a non-medical professional, my answer will be one of an observer. It appears that most medical professionals want to reassure cancer survivors and tend to underestimate the amount of time it takes to return to a previous level of energy. My suggestion is to trust your body and attune to what you can do. In yoga, it is called 'the edge' meaning to go to the edge of what you can do, without pushing so hard that you go over (the edge)" (Chase, 2010).

Nutritionist (Maura Harrigan, RD): "Cancer survivors often say that they are too tired to shop for food, cook, even at times to eat." As explained above with exercise, the same vicious circle can be created; you feel tired so you skip meals then you become more fatigued because you are not giving your body enough fuel and nutrients. Eating five to six smaller meals throughout the day helps sustain your blood glucose levels, which make you feel more energized. It is important to have a source of protein at every meal (cheese, skim milk, nuts, peanut butter, eggs, fish, or lean meat). Also have two types of high-fiber foods at every meal (Harrigan, 2010).

Oncologist (Kenneth Miller, MD): "Fatigue after cancer treatment is very common. There are probably many things that contribute to this including for some cancer survivors problems with deconditioning, poor nutrition, lack of exercise, sleep problems, and anxiety. Generally, this improves over time, and typically energy levels return to normal or near normal, though for some the fatigue persists. It is important to go through your list of medications carefully and to think about other medical causes of fatigue. Ultimately, it is really important to gradually increase your activity level and to exercise. This is a proactive plan to try to maximize your recovery."

CONCLUSION

An individual's experience of cancer differs greatly and is related to many factors including diagnosis and treatment but also age, education, and cultural and religious background. Cancer survivors have needs after treatment that are physical, emotional, and practical to varying degrees. In addition, many tasks of survivorship are important including surveillance for recurrence and also (for second cancers) late and long-term effects and health and wellness education and promotion. A team approach to survivorship care is ideal, when possible, to meet the needs of the diversity of survivors. The medical needs of cancer survivors are a priority but optimum recovery to a new normal can be facilitated by the efforts of social workers and other mental health professionals, nutritionists, physical therapists, and exercise physiologists and trainers.

REFERENCES

American College of Sports Medicine. (2007). *ACSM/ACS certified cancer exercise trainer (CET).* Retrieved from http://www.acsm.org/AM/Template.cfm?Section=ACSM_ACS_Certified_Cancer_Exercise_Trainer. Accessed on January 26, 2011.

Capozza, S. (2010, September). Survivorship themes: fatigue. *Yale Cares Newsletter, 4*(8). Retrieved from http://archive.constantcontact.com/fs079/1102000702257/archive/1103684316644.html. Accessed on January 26, 2010.

Harrigan, M. (2010, September). Survivorship themes: fatigue. *Yale Cares Newsletter, 4*(8). Retrieved from http://archive.constantcontact.com/fs079/1102000702257/archive/1103684316644.html. Accessed on January 26, 2010.

Hewitt M, Greenfield S, and Stovall E, editors. From cancer patient to cancer survivor: lost in transition. Washington, DC: National Academies Press; 2005.

Lina, C. (2010, September). Survivorship themes: fatigue. *Yale Cares Newsletter, 4*(8). Retrieved from http://archive.constantcontact.com/fs079/1102000702257/archive/1103684316644.html. Accessed on January 26, 2010.

4

THE DOLLARS AND SENSE OF CANCER SURVIVORSHIP CARE

CHRISTIAN MCEVOY, MPH, KENNETH MILLER, MD, AND BINJA BASIMIKE, BS

Survivorship care is a relatively new field, and quality interventions are still being developed, implemented, tested, and redesigned. Health care administration models suggest broad relationships between costs, revenues, and subjective value; however, because so few survivorship programs exist, in vivo data from different communities and survivorship clinic settings are not yet available.

The costs of and the revenues from survivorship care are not particularly easy to determine or to predict. Widely variable health status before cancer treatment, varying responses to treatment, and conditions unique to each survivor all complicate any econometric prediction models. In addition, the subjective or indirect value of quality survivorship care is very difficult to quantify.

THE COST OF SURVIVORSHIP CARE

Practically, the cost of any clinical program is determined by the largest single cost: the cost of staff. If post-treatment care is comprehensive, the costs can be extraordinary because many clinicians will be required to meet the need. Survivorship programs may hire an administrator, a physician, a nurse, navigator, or health educator. Some survivorship programs offer mental health services and groups; some employ or collaborate with medical subspecialists or a nutritionist or exercise trainer. A research program on survivorship brings its own staffing needs as well.

Estimated Costs for Full-Time Employees Include:

Oncologist: $134,717–$257,040[1]
Primary Care Physician: $134,959–$222,949[2]
Advanced Practice Nurse: $77,431–$94,035[3]

Registered Nurse: $54,535–$97,303[4]
Administrator: $39,208–$59,194[5]
Nutritionist: $31,460–$73,410[6]
Exercise Trainer: $24,420–$50,304[7]
Social Worker: $28,727–$41,043[8]

Modified and Adapted from Oncology Roundtable interviews and analysis.
© 2010 The Advisory Board Company

SHARING RESOURCES

It is important to keep in mind that cancer programs may have existing resources in mental health, nutrition, and physical therapy and coordinating the efforts of existing personnel may be less expensive then hiring new staff. Similarly, some survivorship tasks can be accomplished by expanding the role of existing staff, which may reduce the need for hiring new staff. For example, if the mission of the program is to provide only an end of treatment summary, this might be incorporated into the educational function of the oncology nurses or other staff members.

REVENUE

Reimbursable Services

Visits to survivorship programs can be billed to major insurers using a History of Cancer code, if the provider of the service and the type of service is covered. In many settings a physician's or mid-level provider's care may be covered, but not that of a registered nurse. Similarly, nutrition counseling may be covered by some insurers for specific conditions, such as diabetes, but not covered when it is for health and wellness education.

If a survivorship program is focusing on transferring cancer survivorship care to a follow-up survivorship team, then a very busy clinician may be able to cover a significant portion of the cost. A recent pro forma analysis by the Advisory Board revealed that a nurse practitioner seeing five patients each week would generate approximately 21% of their salary calculated at $100,000/year. In many cities nurse practitioners' salaries are higher, and the benefits are calculated at more than 30%, so unfortunately it is not likely that reimbursement for clinical services will support a survivorship program in full (see Table 4.1).[9]

Another Perspective on Revenue: Increased Access
for New Patients Just Diagnosed with Cancer

For an oncologist just starting in practice, most or all of their patients are new patients and many have been just diagnosed with cancer. Over the course of years, referrals of new patients typically increase, and so do the number of patients who are long-term cancer survivors. A significant portion of oncologists' time can be spent on follow-up care. The percentage of clinical hours

TABLE 4.1 SAMPLE PRO-FORMA FOR A NURSE PRACTITIONER

Total Revenues	
Comprehensive New Patient Visit-Level 5 Charge for a Nurse Practitioner	$220
Number of New Patient visits/year	250
Charges ($220 x 250)	$55,000
Collections (50% of charges)	$27,000
Total Costs	
Nurse Practitioner Salary and Benifits	$100,000
% FTE for Survivorship (250 visits @ 1.7 hours/visit)	21%
Portion of salary	$21,000

Adapted from the Oncology Roundtable interviews and analysis. © 2010 The Advisory Board Company—21344C.

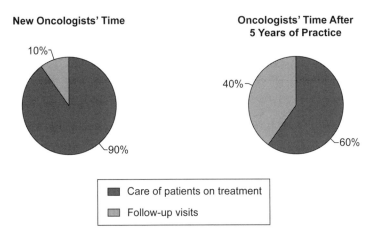

Figure 4.1. Change in Oncologist Practice Over Time- A Theoretical Perspective.

spent seeing follow-up patients usually will increase over time (see Figure 4.1). In the meantime, the demand for oncology care is exceeding the supply of oncology hours and appointments (see Figure 4.2). In some centers, patients newly diagnosed with cancer are seen promptly, while others may have a delay related to the availability of appointments. Anecdotally, some programs report that there is a fall in the waiting time due to availability of survivorship care services. In this setting, one option is for cancer survivorship programs to assume some or all of a cancer survivor's follow-up care, allowing for new patients to be seen more promptly.

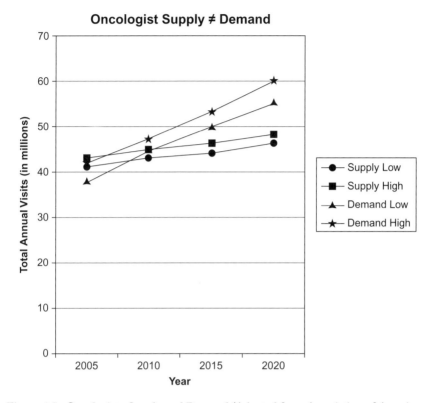

Figure 4.2. Oncologists: Supply and Demand (Adapted from Association of American Medical Colleges, 2007.)

Downstream Revenues

One goal of any survivorship program should be to gain institutional support by demonstrating direct revenue or considerable downstream revenues.

A survivorship program is partially, at its core, a patient education program. Survivors meet with clinicians and learn about future screenings and ongoing clinical care (e.g., cognitive therapy, physical therapy, occupational therapy) that might mitigate risks and long-term and late effects. These educational services may be partially reimbursed as a component of clinical care. Medical screenings and ongoing clinical visits are all potential sources of revenue for the institution, especially if a strong and efficient inside referral program is implemented. For example, most cancer centers and hospitals offer the additional services that cancer survivors need, including physical and occupational therapy, complementary and alternative medicine, nutrition counseling, genetic testing, and fertility services. Hence, a survivorship clinic may not be self-supporting but the additional revenue from providing important care to patients may help to justify the need for survivorship care. At Vanderbilt University it is estimated that 167 survivorship clinic visits resulted in $177,450 of additional charges.[10]

Vanderbilt Survivorship Clinics

FY 2010

Survivorship Clinic	Visits	Downstream Changes
Clinic for survivors of pediatric cancers	196	$378,493
Clinic for survivors of adult cancers	167	$177,450

Case in Brief: Vanderbilt University Medical Center

- 858 bed academic medical center located in Nashville, Tennessee

- Clinic for survivors of pediatric cancers opened in 2007; Clinic for survivors of adult cancers opened in 2009

- Billing manager reviews records for each patient seen on survivorship clinic to track downstream changes; notes technical charges associated with each encounter on same date as clinic visit

Figure 4.3. "Downstream Charges" Associated with Cancer Survivorship Care (Adapted from Vanderbilt University Medical Center, Nashville, TN; Oncology Roundtable interviews and analysis. © 2010 The Advisory Board Company.)

INCREASED COMPLIANCE WITH FOLLOW-UP CARE WITHIN THE HOSPITALS CARE NETWORK

Ongoing treatment for cancer compliance is reinforced by physicians, nurses, social workers, and others on the oncology team. After the completion of treatment, the oncology team typically emphasizes the importance of post-treatment follow-up care. Nonetheless adherence to follow-up care may diminish for a variety of reasons. (See table 4.2).

Similarly, compliance with screening for other cancers may also be suboptimal. A large study of female colorectal cancer survivors found that during the first year after treatment only 55% had screening mammograms and 19% had cervical cancer screening, and that these numbers then decreased over the next four years.

The 2005 Institute of Medicine report "Lost in Transition" describes the experience of transition from patient to survivor at the end of active treatment as "being dropped off a cliff." Studies of cancer survivorship programs have still not been done to determine if compliance with follow-up care or cancer screening is improved but this is hypothesized to be the case. A survivorship program can be a mechanism to keep patients engaged and compliant with follow-up in the institutional care system.

TABLE 4.2 POST-TREATMENT PATIENTS COMPLETING FOLLOW-UP BY YEAR POST-TREATMENT

		Year 1	Year 2	Year 3
14 percent of patients completed only one follow-up visit with their oncologist during their first post- treatment year	0 visits	9%	12%	29%
	1 visit	14%	27%	25%
	2 visits	14%	20%	21%
	3 visits	20%	15%	15%
	4 visits	13%	9%	10%
	>4 visits	30%	17%	9%

Adapted from Thomas Johns Cancer Hospital, Richmond, VA; Oncology Roundtable interviews and analysis. © 2010 The Advisory Board Company.

PHILANTHROPY

Philanthropy can supplement institutional support and potentially serve as part most of the support for a survivorship program. Typically, any fundraising effort includes individual giving, individual major gift giving, planned estate giving, corporate support, and foundation support. Relying on philanthropy can be difficult, however, because the priorities of donors and their commitment to survivorship as a cause may change over time.

THE INTANGIBLE BENEFITS

Patients who undergo surgery or are treated with radiation or chemotherapy at a hospital can be referred directly to the survivorship program. In the survivorship program services can be provided to meet their individual post-treatment needs. The goal is to facilitate the combination of optimal oncology and primary care.

A cancer survivorship program can provide many benefits to cancer survivors. It provides primary care providers with comprehensive information about their patients' cancer care and the support services to facilitate their care. More broadly, survivorship programs also benefit a cancer center or program. Survivorship is a value-added service that contributes to a program's reputation. It adds to the meaningful perception by the community that the program, which treated cancer patients, remains committed to them as cancer survivors.

REFERENCES

Cbsalary. (2007, December 18). *Registered nurse salary.* Retrieved from http://www .cbsalary.com/industries/nursing/. Accessed January 2011.

Nutritionist-World. (2011). *Nutritionist annual salary percentiles.* Retrieved from http:// www.nutritionist-world.com/nutritionist_salaries.html. Accessed January 26, 2011.

PayScale. (2011, January 11). *Salary snapshot for physician/doctor, oncologist jobs.* Retrieved from http://www.payscale.com/research/US/Job=Physician_%2F_Doc tor,_Oncologist/Salary. Accessed January 2011.

PayScale. (2011, January 15). *Salary snapshot for social worker jobs.* Retrieved from http://www.payscale.com/research/US/Job=Social_Worker/Salary. Accessed Janu ary 26, 2011.

PayScale, Initials. (2011, January 16). *Salary snapshot for network administrator, IT jobs.* Retrieved from http://www.payscale.com/research/US/Job=Network_Admin istrator,_IT/Salary. Accessed January 26, 2011.

PayScale. (2011, January 20). *Employees with an advanced practice registered nurse-board certified (aprn-bc) certification.* Retrieved from http://www.payscale.com/research/ US/Certification=Advanced_Practice_Registered_Nurse-Board_Certified_(APRN-BC)/Salary. Accessed January 26, 2011.

PayScale. (2011, January 22). *Hourly rate snapshot for fitness trainer or aerobics instruc-tor jobs.* Retrieved from http://www.payscale.com/research/US/Job=Fitness_Train er_or_Aerobics_Instructor/Hourly_Rate.

"Potential for NP-Clinic to break even," by Oncology Roundtable interviews and analy-sis, 2008, Patient centered care, p. 225. © 2010 The Advisory Board Company—21344C.

Salary.com. (2010). *Physician-family practice.* Retrieved from http://www1.salary.com/ Physician-Family-Practice-salary.html. Accessed January 26, 2010.

5

STARTING TO PROVIDE SURVIVORSHIP CARE

KENNETH MILLER, MD, AND BRITTANY ALGIERE, BS

Cancer survivorship is a distinct phase of cancer but many (or perhaps most) cancer survivors and care providers are unclear if and how survivorship services differ from typical follow-up care. Presently, there are no standardized metrics defining the elements of cancer survivorship care. Some survivorship programs assume the care of survivors and primarily provide follow-up and surveillance once the diagnosis and treatment phases have been completed. Others programs focus on providing "value added" services including psychosocial support, nutrition, and exercise education.

Prior to developing a program to provide cancer survivorship care there are several questions to ask:

1. Are there gaps in the existing cancer care system?
2. Who is in need of survivorship care in your community?
3. What services will you provide and when?
4. Who will "buy-in" (Encourage and promote) and who will "push-back" (discourage or delay), and what are the practical issues that a survivorship program will face?

ARE THERE GAPS IN EXISTING CANCER CARE SYSTEM?

Most cancer programs pride themselves on having an excellent medical staff, state-of-the art technology, and cutting-edge care. Surveillance for cancer recurrence is typically very good but not distinctive. In other words, cancer programs usually do not advertise that patients should receive care with a particular team because the follow-up care is special.

Oncologists typically provide ongoing follow-up focused on surveillance for cancer recurrence. In broader terms, however, the "tasks" of post-treatment care also include identification, mitigation, surveillance for late and long-term risks, screening for and treatment of late and long-term effects, psychosocial support, and wellness education. If a cancer care system believes that such gaps exist in their post-treatment care, then a survivorship program may serve to fill these gaps by providing these services. Survivorship programs may also nurture collaborative efforts within the cancer program and health care system to provide these services for their patients.

WHO IS IN NEED OF SURVIVORSHIP CARE AND WHEN?

The definition of cancer survivorship, embraced by the National Cancer Institute (NCI), "covers the physical, psychosocial, and economic issues of cancer, from diagnosis until the end of life" (cancer.gov). Some survivorship programs serve anyone with a cancer diagnosis at any time during their cancer journey. Other programs begin to provide services after the completion of initial therapy, and finally still others provide care for survivors who have completed treatment and have no evidence of disease.

There is no one single correct decision regarding who should receive survivorship care services. If the non-medical, psychosocial, spiritual, and other needs of patients with cancer are not consistently met during their diagnosis and treatment, then cancer survivorship may become a broader part of a supportive oncology program to provide care throughout the cancer continuum. If, on the other hand, patients' needs are well-met during acute treatment, then a survivorship program might better focus on post-treatment care. Similarly, a survivorship program could provide services for patients who are living with cancer, for those in remission, or for both groups.

Cancer survivors' needs change throughout the seasons of survivorship. A few cancer survivorship programs assume the long-term care for cancer survivors after the initial treatment, as well as a pre-determined oncology follow-up period. In this setting, survivorship programs continue surveillance for disease recurrence, but also focus on surveillance for late and long-term effects and other ongoing needs. In many cancer programs, patients continue to receive care from their primary oncology team and the survivorship program provides "value added" services including subspecialty care such as cardiology, neurology, pulmonary, survivorship counseling, and sexual health counseling, for example.

WHAT TYPE OF SERVICES WILL YOU PROVIDE AND WHEN IN SURVIVORSHIP?

One of the key elements of cancer survivorship care is providing cancer survivors with an end of treatment summary (TS) and survivorship care plan (SCP). The Institute of Medicine's (IOM) report in 2005 described the key elements of a cancer survivorship end of TS and SCP:

The TS is a personalized document, which can be produced by several different members of the cancer care team including the oncologists (surgical, medical, and radiation), a midlevel provider, or an oncology nurse. Similarly, the SCP is also customized and can be provided to cancer survivors in a special transition visit at the end of treatment. It can also be provided in support groups, educational programs, or resource centers.

Survivorship programs can provide the core service of developing a TS and SCP for each cancer survivor including a list of local resources to address these needs. Programs may directly provide some of these services including psychosocial counseling and supportive care, long-term surveillance for late and long-term effects along with risk identification and early intervention. Some also provide subspecialty care such as oncocardiology or onconephrology, or oncofertility.

LEVELS OF CANCER SURVIVORSHIP CARE

It is helpful to conceptualize four levels of cancer survivorship care.

Level One:
Providing a TS and SCP.

Level Two:
Providing a TS and SCP, as well as associated education and support services at transition from acute to extended survivorship.

Level Three:
Providing a TS and SCP, associated education and support services, counseling at transition, as well as late and long-term risk identification, stratification, risk management and mitigation.

Level Four:
All of the above, but also provision of subspecialty care including cardiology, pulmonary, and so on.

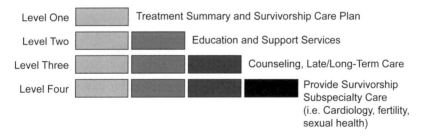

Figure 5.1. Levels of Survivorship Care.

LAUNCHING A PROGRAM: BUY-IN

It is helpful to identify early adopters who are particularly supportive of survivorship care. Some may be physicians, nurses, and others who are cancer survivors or friends or relatives of survivors. Others perhaps embrace some aspect of survivorship care such as the psychosocial or integrative care, or the wellness emphasis. A small number of providers may feel comfortable with the concept of transferring a patient's care to a long-term survivorship program staff.

Push-Back from Providers

Many new programs are met with uncertainty, apathy, or antipathy. Clinicians' uncertainty can lead to questions such as, What is survivorship? and How is it different than usual care? Apathy may result in statements such as, "I'm glad that they offer it, but I probably will not refer anyone." And antipathy has the potential to evoke statements such as, "It is unnecessary, a duplication of services, and will be confusing to the patients," "I do survivorship care already," "I want to be seeing my own patients when they come in for follow-up care," and "Survivorship is competition and will take away my patients."

Push-Back from Cancer Survivors

Some patients are resistant to say that they are cured of cancer, but rather that they are in remission. Cancer survivors may be hesitant to be seen in a survivorship program as well. Similarly, many people do not embrace the title cancer survivor and are unclear about the meaning of survivorship care. They may feel that their oncologist is providing all the care that they need, and may even feel that seeking care in a survivorship program is somehow disloyal to their physician.

The Practical Issues: Lack of Guidelines about Different Issues

One of the benefits of cancer survivorship is coordination of care, but in the process survivorship programs may seem to add another layer of complexity. Stated more simply, cancer survivorship may further confuse providers and patients unless its role is well-defined. Unfortunately, although there are NCCN and ASCO guidelines for follow-up care after cancer treatment, there is a lack of clear guidelines in screening for late and long-term effects. The difficulty in providing guidelines also contributes to the push-back, though at the same time there is push-back to developing guidelines when they might be construed as limiting individual providers' choices and recommendations.

The Children's Oncology Group has developed a detailed consensus-based document, which adult oncology groups are lacking. Despite the lack of a definitive document for adult survivorship, surveillance for late and long-term effects is important and survivorship programs can serve to raise awareness, so these problems are identified early. This also will be of help to cancer survivors who may otherwise feel, "Lost in Transition" as so titled by the IOM. Clearly stating the specific tasks in the patient's care, and deciding who is doing what among oncologists and primary care physicians, is helpful once these have been decided on a local level.

OTHER CHALLENGES: LACK OF FUNDING AND LACK OF SPACE

Some cancer survivorship services are reimbursable, and there are down-stream revenues from survivorship programs: goodwill, patient loyalty, and perhaps some prestige for a program. On the other hand, depending on the level of services provided, survivorship care is often a cost center and not a profit center. Philanthropic support can be helpful in sustaining survivorship programs, though cancer programs and hospitals have many competing needs and survivorship is only one of them. Similarly, hospitals and cancer centers may have limited space to house new or unique programs.

THE FUTURE OF SURVIVORSHIP CARE

It is anticipated that the number of cancer survivors will reach 20 million by 2020, but already in 2010 the number of new patients diagnosed with cancer may be starting to exceed the capacity of the workforce. These work-force issues may enhance the role of survivorship care particularly for patients who are living beyond the principal risk period for recurrence. At the same time, increased attention to psycho-oncology and a growing understanding of late and long-term effects of treatment, including the risk of secondary cancers, may promote the development of cancer survivorship programs. The adoption of palliative care as a separate and important field has taken close to two decades. Cancer survivorship is likely to take many years, as well, to reach greater acceptance.

6

SURVIVORSHIP CARE: GETTING STARTED

USHA THAKRAR, MPH

The NCI projects that by the end of the decade, there will be 20 million cancer survivors in the United States. Many of these survivors complete their cancer treatment and face lifelong complications and health risks related to the therapy they received. As the population of cancer survivors continues to grow, the need for comprehensive survivorship care has become more apparent. Cancer care institutions of all sizes face the challenge of setting up appropriate programs and maximizing resources to provide appropriate services to this population. These challenges beg the question—what are the important components in setting up a survivorship program? Below is a toolbox of critical questions that must be answered as part of any program development.

CRITICAL FACTORS OF SUCCESS

Before addressing any of the nuts and bolts of developing a program and delivering survivorship care, it is important to understand several key factors of success.

- There are as many definitions of cancer survivor as there are shades of blue. The survivorship needs of patients just completing therapy are very different than those of long-term survivors. Defining the target population is a critical first step. This decision will drive almost everything about the structure of the program. There is no right answer. The size of the institution, the demographics of the patient population and the availability of resources all drive this definition.

> **Q: Who are the patients this program is intended to serve?**

- There are many models for providing survivorship care. As these are explored elsewhere in this book, the important point here is the model that is chosen. This is a key point. Again there is no correct answer. The choices of service delivery model depend on a range of factors including staffing, space, geographic location and, of course, funding.

Q: What is the clinical service model?

- No survivorship program is going to thrive unless it has both institutional and disease center support. Historically, survivors have been cared for within their disease group. There are many models for caring for these patients going forward, but all of them involve a commitment from the treating oncologist.

Q: Who are the key stakeholders whose support is needed? (consider leadership, clinical staff, patients, primary care physicians)

- Supportive care is as important are clinical care. While not all cancer survivors suffer late-effects. most want information about their survivorship and the opportunity to meet other survivors. Educational and support programs can be as successful and as necessary as clinical care.

Q: What are the key services this program will provide? (consider medical, psychosocial, educational, wellness)

STAFFING

The staffing needs of a survivorship program fall into two major categories—clinical and administrative. Regardless of the clinical model of the program, certain administrative staffing is necessary. Caring for cancer survivors requires complex, multidisciplinary care and strong communication among patients, survivorship providers, oncologists, and primary care. It is critical that any program include a staff member who can both schedule patient appointment and ancillary visits as well as ensure that survivorship documentation (treatment summaries and care plans) are distributed appropriately. In addition, depending on volume, this person can be utilized to create treatment summary documentation.

Q: Who is the primary point of contact for patients?
How do appointments get scheduled?
What survivorship documentation will you provide (e.g. treatment summaries; care plans) and when? (e.g. at the visit or after)
Who will generate documentation?
Who will schedule follow up appointments?

Unless one has the luxury of having a free-standing survivorship program, a critical piece of success is integration with existing institutional clinical systems. This includes utilizing scheduling systems, electronic medical records, laboratory ordering, and billing, among other items. Coordinating those operations is a key role in any program. Depending on the size of the program, the operations role can be combined with other critical administrative roles including fiscal management, personnel management, and program development.

Q: What institutional systems exist?
Do they include the information needed for survivorship care (e.g., part medical history)?
Who is going to manage the day-to-day operations of the program?
Are there existing personnel who can be leveraged for some of these roles?

Clinical staffing depends entirely on the clinical model of care. Regardless of which model is used, developing a survivorship program requires strong clinical leadership. While a number of models exist, they are essentially variations on either a centralized or decentralized approach.

The **centralized approach** consolidates multidisciplinary clinical services in one physical location. Clinical staff can include nurse practitioners, psychosocial providers, and subspecialty providers such as endocrinologists, cardiologists, and nutritionists. Depending on the volume, most clinical staff is likely to be part-time (either shared with other programs or as contract employees). In addition to providing clinical services, all staff are likely involved in developing educational materials and programming for patients and families.

The **decentralized approach** develops mini survivorship clinics within disease centers or with partner primary care locations. Survivorship services are not provided by a survivorship clinic staff but instead the survivorship staff provides care for patients in different locations. This model generally uses pieces of nurse practitioners and psychosocial staff time within disease centers rather than having individual dedicated staff. This approach generally refers patients to subspecialists outside the program as appropriate. Depending on the level of disease center commitment, this model can be more fiscally sustainable as it leverages existing resources.

Q: Who is going to see patients?
How will the program ensure clear clinical communication about patient care, deliver consistent information to the patient, and manage communication with the PCP?
If the model is decentralized, how does the program maintain cohesion?

FISCAL ISSUES

As with any clinical program, the single largest cost is the staff. Regardless of which model is chosen, there will be fixed costs of clinical and administrative staff, not all of which can be billed to insurance. Annual visits to a survivorship clinic are reimbursed by most major insurers, as are most screening tests. In general most visits can be billed between Levels 3 and 5 using a V-code (History of Cancer).

One significant difference between survivorship care and oncology treatment is the potential revenue sources. All oncology care has high staffing costs, however, on-treatment care can off-set those costs with revenues from infusion services and other treatment-related services. Revenue for clinical survivorship care is limited to reimbursement for patient visits. Depending on the structure of the institution, there may be additional revenue realized from billing for ancillary services (e.g. scans, mammograms, subspecialty visits). In general, comprehensive, multi-disciplinary survivorship programs are not self-sustaining and must rely on other sources of funding. Historically, philanthropy has been the single largest source of support for developing survivorship programs. As the need for this type of care becomes more apparent, some cancer centers are devoting institutional resources to these efforts. However, anyone involved in the early stages of building a program must include plans for fundraising.

> **Q: What are the key expenses? Sources of revenue?**
> **Are their existing resources that can be leveraged?**
> **How will the program be funded?**

> **Other Questions to Consider**
>
> **Q: Marketing—Who is the audience? (e.g., patients, oncologists, primary care providers)**
> **Type of care—Consultative service versus long-term follow-up care**
> **Resources—Many survivors need financial and support resources in their local community. How will the program support that need?**

FINAL THOUGHTS

Developing a comprehensive survivorship program that includes medical psychosocial and supportive care components is challenging and resource-intensive. As the field moves forward with the development of standards of care for this population, survivorship programs will need to tailor services accordingly. Those programs that are created with a solid operational and fiscal foundation and are well integrated into their institution will be best positioned to care for these patients long-term.

7

MODELS OF SURVIVORSHIP CARE

MARY MCCABE, RN

OVERVIEW

Cancer care is at a crossroads and entering a period of tremendous change. This change is driven by novel and increasingly successful approaches to cancer diagnosis and treatment, as well as the identification of unique long-term follow-up needs of the almost 12 million cancer survivors in the United States today. Cancer survivorship is being identified as a set of chronic diseases with an array of complex health care delivery issues that require unique medical and psychosocial services.

Increasingly, national organizations, professional societies, and federal agencies are acknowledging the need to pay attention to survivorship. In particular, a focus is being put on the period that includes the "phase of care that follows primary treatment."[1] The most influential discourse on the topic to date is the 2006 Institute of Medicine (IOM) report titled "From Cancer Patient to Cancer Survivor: Lost in Transition." In this publication, the recommendations all focus on the need to make post-treatment survivorship a distinct phase of cancer care for all patients and their families. This important standard remains a goal to be reached and is currently a work in progress.

Since the national attention being paid to survivorship is fairly recent, the development of new models of care lags behind the identified need that is developing. Therefore, the oncology community needs to rethink how to care for this growing population and overcome the unique challenges involved in establishing quality care standards for the survivorship period. These obstacles include an absence of evidence-based standards for follow-up surveillance, limited continuity of care between the oncology team and the community primary care physicians, lack of knowledge about the issues facing cancer survivors, and lack of consensus about how to proceed with survivorship care among the various professional and patient organizations.[2]

Fortunately, the IOM report has given some direction and has acknowledged that specialized survivorship clinics and programs are a promising concept to pilot and evaluate. Innovative models of care are being developed at an increasing rate in cancer centers, community hospitals, and private oncology practices around the country. Each model must adapt to various care facilities and survivor populations while also focusing on the unique needs of cancer survivors.

Ideally these clinics and programs provide attention to both psychosocial and medical consequences of the cancer and/or its treatment. However, survivorship care reaches beyond the clinic visit. There is a need for referrals to appropriate specialists, communication between the specialist oncology team and the community primary care physician, education about the importance of ongoing screening for new cancers, focus on diet and exercise, smoking cessation programs, and helping patients negotiate the health care system.[3] Regardless of the type of model the clinic or program adopts, the goal is to assure that cancer survivors achieve the highest quality of life post-treatment.

MODELS OF SURVIVORSHIP CARE

Survivorship care goals can be met in many different ways. Services can vary based on specific goals. However, clinical offerings may change based on the needs of the survivorship patients and their families. Because there is no one size fits all outcome for survivorship, it is best to make every effort to understand the expectations of patients, family members, health providers, and the community when creating a program. Although there are basic services that all survivors need, the most successful care models are ones that adapt to the culture, economics, and patient population of its community. Below are brief descriptions of some of the most common survivorship care models that are being implemented nationally.

MULTIDISCIPLINARY CLINICS

Based on a survivorship model developed decades ago by pediatric oncologists, this type of clinic incorporates a multidisciplinary model of care that allows the individual to be seen by multiple providers in one location. The grouping may include an oncologist, nurse practitioner (NP) and a mental health expert—often a clinical psychologist and/or social worker. Alternatively, the grouping could include an oncologist and nurse practitioner who have expertise in long-term and late effects of cancer treatment, and certain specialists like cardiologists, endocrinologists, or nutritionists. This amalgamation of specialized expertise benefits patients who have a variety of complications, and allows them to receive treatment that is otherwise resource intensive and non-reimbursable by insurance companies. Unfortunately, a limitation of this model is that it can only be used when caring for small populations such as pediatrics. Because of the intensity of the services and appointment time for each patient, it doesn't lend itself to high volume practices.

DISEASE-SPECIFIC CLINICS

Many groups have initiated survivorship services that focus on a particular population of survivors. A disease-specific model is most often used when there is a sufficient population of survivors that were diagnosed with one particular type of cancer. This is done because there is either an expressed interest on the part of the patient group, or there is an interest on the part of the clinicians and/or administrators.

This type of clinic is relatively easy to implement because its services are focused on only one type of survivor. This also allows the required expertise for the program to be strictly defined. Disease-specific clinics are often the first step taken by hospitals and private practices when creating a survivorship program. It allows a limited commitment of resources, time to figure out how best to deploy resources, the ability to let the institution's commitment to survivorship grow, and a focus on testing and evaluating the feasibility and quality of services before expanding the program to other disease groups.

However, the limitation of this approach is the inequality it creates within an institution that may be hard to change in a time of diminishing resources. Because the program will focus on only one or two disease-specific clinics, it will exclude some survivors with both the greatest need and the least amount of available resources.

CONSULTATIVE CLINICS

Another model that is being commonly used is the consultative clinic. This provides a survivorship consult for individuals who have completed treatment. These models are easy to establish, require limited resources, and do not change the relationship of the survivor with the primary oncology team. The survivorship clinic is staffed by an NP or PA and is commonly located in a facility separate from where the survivor is followed by their oncologist. The visit typically includes a general review of survivorship issues along with the development of a Treatment Summary and Care Plan.

The Treatment Summary and Care Plan documents are important communication tools that provide consistent information about the ongoing care needs of the survivor. Those documents are also provided to the survivor and shared with the patient's oncologist and primary care physician. For specific issues identified during the consult visit, referrals are made to specialists as necessary.

INTEGRATED CLINICS

This model of care allows a survivor to transition from their treating oncologist to a survivorship provider (like an NP or PA) while staying within the same clinic. The advantage of this model comes with the ability to imbed the survivorship provider within the treatment team. The patient is able to move seamlessly from the treatment period to the follow-up period without leaving the primary oncologist. A standard of care can also be easily developed. Because all the providers are working as one group, it eliminates the possibility that an oncologist will not refer their patient to survivorship at the risk of transferring their patient out of the practice.

The Integrated Clinic model also creates the opportunity to address the comprehensive needs of the survivor by focusing on more than the usual surveillance for cancer recurrence. These potential survivorship topics include addressing the long-term and late effects of treatment, screening for second cancers, the benefits healthy of living, and the development of a Treatment Summary and Care Plan. However, the major challenge of using this model is the need for additional space for the survivorship provider, and the creation of a business plan for how these visits can and should be reimbursed.

SURVIVORSHIP PROVIDERS

Just as there is no one size fits all model for survivorship clinic models, the same can be said for the professionals who staff them. Each of the clinical models discussed are being implemented and evaluated nationally and carried out with various health professionals as the lead providers. For example, in a multidisciplinary clinic caring for adult survivors of pediatric cancer, the lead physician could be a medical oncologist or a primary care physician. That decision is based on the focus of the clinical care, the needs of the survivor population, and the philosophy of the group supporting the clinic. Initially survivorship clinics were all staffed with oncology experts, but there is a move to include internists and family medicine practitioners because those clinicians also fit the needs of survivors.

The focus on using non-physician providers in survivorship programs is prevalent for a variety of reasons. These reasons include economic issues related to follow-up care, the growing number of patients seeking long term follow-up care, the need for oncologists to accommodate a higher volume of patients in their practices, the natural fit for NPs and PAs to focus on wellness and healthy living, and the need to focus on psychosocial issues of survivors.

COMMUNITY SERVICES

Although the first survivorship clinics were developed in academic medical centers, survivorship care and the services related to it now extend throughout community hospitals/clinics and private practices. This is a very important and challenging transition for survivorship. Most patients diagnosed with adult-onset cancers are treated in community health centers. While these health centers may not be able to sustain full-service survivorship clinics due to a lack of resources, they can formalize and provide access to much-needed services and redirect existing programs to have a survivorship focus.

An example of this is transforming a physical rehabilitation program to work with survivors facing mobility problems resulting from surgery or radiation. Another example would be reforming a diet and exercise program that was initially focused on elderly patients with cardiovascular disease and providing those services with a concentration on survivorship. The concept of reusing and recycling services can also include taking programs for patients in active treatment (like support groups and counseling) and modifying them to incorporate the needs of survivors. Services can be meshed together in a seamless and economical way that will result in an efficient program, and improve the quality of life of cancer survivors.

CHALLENGES

Over the last decade, major advances have been made in increasing the focus on survivorship as a formal period of care. Although there continue to be challenges, the outcome will assure that one day survivorship will become a standard of oncology care.

In figuring out where to start when creating a survivorship program, it's critical to do an assessment to determine the level of support from leadership (both clinical and administrative) for developing and formalizing a set of survivorship services. That information will be very important to determine whether the leadership of the institution will agree with the implementation of a survivorship program. Although it is evident that survivorship is a unique period of care requiring specific services, an already busy staff may not have the extra time or energy to attend to those needs. This change will also not come quickly or easily. Due to a general lack of knowledge about what a Survivorship Program entails, reluctance should be expected by clinical staff and administrators. Roadblocks will include:

1. Questioning the program's utility
2. Finding financial support
3. Reimbursement for services
4. Changes in the reimbursement system for oncology in general
5. Moving beyond the assumption that a survivorship visit is just an assessment and testing for cancer recurrence
6. Getting busy clinicians to adapt to changes created by a survivorship program

For these reasons, a draft plan should be developed and presented so all the identified stakeholders give input and support the changes made. Starting small with only the support of key stakeholders is better than having a grand plan destined to fail from a lack of support at the beginning.

OPPORTUNITIES

Despite the challenges and obstacles facing the Survivorship community, there is a growing wave of change that is building interest in survivorship nationally and internationally. The problem of how to take care of patients living beyond their cancer is a good problem to have, and it's important to realize that building a future for Survivorship needs help. National service organizations like the American Cancer Society and professional organizations such as the American Society of Clinical Oncology, the Oncology Nursing Society, and the National Cancer Centers Network are all making Survivorship a priority. Even survivors themselves are demanding access to needed services and want information on their risks and late effects that they can share with their health care providers.

It behooves everyone in the medical oncology community to work together and make use of resources big and small, new and old. The combination of these resources at the local and national level will provide the tools that over time will bring about an evidence-based approach to survivorship care, and result in the highest quality of life possible for all cancer survivors.

NOTES

1. Hewitt M, Greenfield S, Stoval E, editors. From cancer patient to cancer survivor: lost in transition. Washington, DC: National Academies Press: 2006.

2. Nissen M, Beran M, Lee M, Menta SR, Pine DA, Swenson KK. Views of primary care providers on follow-up care of cancer patients. Fam Med. 2007; 39(7): 477–482.

3. Grunfeld E. Primary care physicians and oncologists are players on the same team. *J Clin Oncol.* 2008; 26(14): 2246–2247; Earle CC. Failing to plan is planning to fail: improving the quality of care with survivorship care plans. *J Clin Oncol.* 2006; 24(320): 5112–5116; Findley P, Sambamoorthi U. Preventive health services and lifestyle practices in cancer survivors: a population health investigation. *J Can Surviv.* 2009; 3(1): 43–58.

REFERENCES

Glanz, K., Rimer, B.K. (1997) *Theory at a Glance: A Guide for Health Promotion Practices,* National Institute of Health. Accessed at http://oc.nci.nih.gov/services/Theo ry_at_glance/HOME.html.

Hudelson, P.M. (1994). *Qualitative Research for Health Programs.* Geneva, Switzerland: Division of Mental Health, World Health Organization (WHO/MNH/PSF/94.3).

Implementing Cancer Survivorship Care Planning. Workshop Summary. A National Coalition for Cancer Survivorship and Institute of Medicine National Cancer Policy Forum Workshop (2007).

Institute of Medicine. (2001). Organizations, communities, and society: Models and interventions. In *Health and behavior: The interplay of biological, behavioral, and societal influences.* Washington, DC: National Academy Press. Accessed at http://books.nap .edu/html/health_behavior/.

Kettner, P.M., Moroney, R.M., L.L. (1990). *Designing and Managing Programs: An Effectiveness–Based Approach.* Newbury Park: Sage Publications.

Morbidity and Mortality Weekly Report (MMWR): *Framework for Program Evaluation in Public Health;* Vol. 48/No. RR-11, 9/17/1999.

Scheirer, M.A. (1994). Designing and using process evaluation. In Wolely, J.S., Hatry, H.P., Newcomer, K.E. (Eds.) *Handbook of Practical Program Evaluation* (pp. 40–68). San Francisco: Jossey-Bass.

8

AN ACADEMIC CANCER CENTER SURVIVORSHIP PROGRAM

ALMA PETROVIC, MD, AND JOSEPH LEHRBERG, BA

PROGRAM OVERVIEW

The Dana-Farber Cancer Institute (DFCI) specializes exclusively in cancer research and care. It is an academic cancer center with a commitment to supporting
patients with all kinds of cancer and to finding a cure for the disease. Fortunately,
because of the excellent treatment currently being provided by DFCI and other
cancer centers, more patients are surviving cancer. For this reason, DFCI began
offering programs help survivors address the medical, emotional, psychological,
and physical challenges stemming from their past disease or treatments.

The initial attempts at survivorship were introduced with the creation of
the Pediatric Oncology Clinic for Survivors of Brain Tumors and the Perini Pediatric Survivorship Clinic in 2003. The Lance Armstrong Foundation along
with the Dana-Farber staff recognized the need for Adult Survivorship Care,
and established the LAF Adult Survivorship Clinic in 2005. Today, the clinic
offers care for patients of any diagnosis and offers consultations with nurse
practitioners who have expertise in post-treatment and survivorship care. It
was not an easy task and took many years to develop and refine.

Program History

In the beginning the clinic consisted of one NP, a medical director (10%
of his time), and one administrative coordinator. Without previous experience
in similar programs, the NP needed to rely on related literature and previous
cancer research experience. This allowed the NP to create and develop a comprehensive screening system based on protocols with certain criteria, which
filtered into a database. A spreadsheet was then drafted showing the connection between short and long-term toxicities and various treatments that could
have caused them. Finally the NP made a list containing recommendations
and possible screenings the patients might need, followed by chart audits, and
a risk assessment (based on what the treatment was). The spreadsheet was

then reviewed by an oncologist and the medical director to get constructive feedback regarding proposed recommendations.

All the information initially collected had been reviewed by the survivorship program, which was a self- contained unit with little or no input from experts. It was a great step toward the program implementation, but there was little collaboration with other Dana-Farber staff on important topics:

1. How to set up the database
2. What benchmark to reach
3. Expectations of the leadership
4. Recognizing the needs and wants of the clinicians
5. Specific goals and objectives
6. Forms of measurement other than volume
7. Vision and mission statement
8. Specific plan of how the providers visit should be

This left providers with the only option of creating something similar to what they already had in place, which was a template similar to pediatric survivorship.

PROGRAM DESIGN

Referring patients to the Adult Survivorship Clinic began as very simple process. Providers who heard about the program would send one or several of their patients out of curiosity, or the NP would go to different providers and ask them to refer their patients to the clinic. At the time, the service

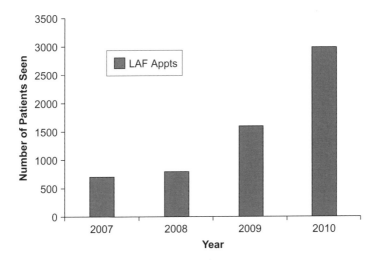

Figure 8.1. Dana-Farber Adult Survivorship Clinic Total Visits. (Illustration by Joseph Lehrberg.)

consisted of the NP's consultations with patients and recommendations for possible screenings. Space became an issue, and rooms had to be borrowed from clinics to hold consultation sessions.

Eventually the necessity for a new model of operations became painfully obvious. In order to move forward and grow, there needed to be an analysis of what had been done in the past, an identification of the challenges, and the creation of a list of recommendations for the future.

Today the LAF Adult Survivorship program has significantly expanded its medical services. The program also includes the launch of disease-based

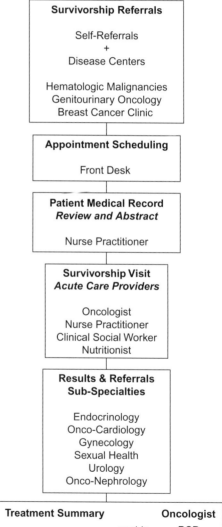

Figure 8.2. Academic Cancer Center Survivorship Program Flowchart. (Illustration by Joseph Lehrberg.)

integration and transition visits in addition to new subspecialties. Patient volume has considerably grown and in 2009 the clinic saw 623 patients and provided services in 1,053 patient visits. In 2010 the number of visits increased to over 3,000. (see Figure 8.2).

The DFCI clinic now has eight providers, an administrative coordinator, a medical assistant, a nutritionist, a clinical social worker, and a manager of operational procedures who is responsible for patient scheduling and compliance with Dana-Farber processes and procedures.

However, as the LAF clinic continues to develop and patient volume continues to grow, the clinic staff looks toward the future for areas of improvement and better ways to bring competent survivorship care to the DFCI community. The following is a list of projects and plans that are in development or have been included into LAF Survivorship standard of care.

1. **Implementation of the new model of care delivery**

   • **Transition visit and ongoing survivorship care**

The transition visit allows for patient care to move form the disease center's acute care provider to the survivorship providers seeing patients in the disease-based clinic. These visits occur when patients are completing active cancer treatment. During the visit the clinician and patient review the following:

- The treatment the patient received
- Any necessary follow-up care they will need (tests/scans)
- Contact information for their care team
- Educational information about healthy survivorship

2. **Implementation of disease center integration (*in progress*)**

In order for this to be successful it will require the presence of an NP in the disease centers who participates in the ongoing care of patients including cancer focused surveillance. The NP will also develop individualized care plans based on prior treatment exposure, and provide appropriate referrals for risk screening tests, specialty consults, and health and wellness education. These integrated services presently are provided in several disease centers including Hemtologic Malignancies, Genitourinary Oncology, and Bone Marrow Transplantation. More disease centers are expected to join the program.

3. **Development of End of Treatment Summary and Care Plans**

A two-phase process has been launched to ensure sustainability and success of the end of treatment summaries and care plans.

Phase One: The development of how an EOTSCP is redefined for survivors with different types of cancers. These will consist of a comprehensive and easy-to understand document that can be individualized for each patient based on his or her diagnoses and provider.

This document will include:

- A summary of treatment and exposures
- Standardized cover letter about transitioning off care, and the potential psycho-social impact that could result
- Wellness information including topics like nutrition and exercise
- Standardized follow-up documentation (using NCCN and ASCO guidelines) describing:
  - How often the patient should have follow up visits. For example:
    - This will be broken down by five-year intervals.
    - First year: every 3 months
    - Second year: every 4 months
    - Third year: every 6 months
    - Fourth year: every 6 months
    - Fifth year: every 12 months
  - How often the patient needs surveillance imaging
  - The labs or special testing that will be included with the follow-up visit
  - A list of symptoms of concern to help the patient recognize important symptoms
  - Contact information of the patient's care team members.

4. Addition of Subspecialty care services

During the past several years the clinic added a number of specialty care services to meet the unique needs of every patient. These included Endocrinology, Gynecology, Onco-Cardiology, Onco-Fertility, Onco-Neprhology, Sexual Health, and Urology.

5. Implementation of a Survivorship Counseling Program

The Survivorship Counseling Program aims to help survivors and their family members process the impact of their cancer experience. The intent is to create an action plan to help patients and their caregivers move forward and deal with emotional burden that their cancer experience placed on them.

6. Support Groups and Workshops

Support groups and workshops are a great resource for survivors encountering any kind of psychosocial distress after completing treatment. Transitioning out of a very attentive and detail oriented cancer care experience can also be lonely and frightening for some survivors. These groups and meetings can instill sense of community and togetherness during a turbulent time.

7. Educational Material Development

The LAF Clinic staff members have developed various educational materials that patients and their providers are able to use as a reference during their survivorship care. These documents include:

- Disease-specific survivorship education manual
- Protocol to survey patients and providers regarding their perceptions of the current state of survivorship care DFCI, and their expectations
- Survivorship Toolkit that addresses disparities in breast cancer prevention, detection, and treatment
- In addition, the clinic staff is also creating supplemental teaching sheets for survivors that cover a wide range of survivorship-related topics

CHALLENGES

1. Staffing
   - When setting up an initial survivorship program, a determination needs to be made regarding the appropriate amount of staff and the specific responsibilities each team member will have. This includes designating staff members for duties like screening patients for late effects, providing counseling for psychosocial issues, preparation of patient documentation, and appointment scheduling.
2. Finances
   - Before the survivorship team can see a patient in the clinic, the financing of the program needs to be established. Options include clinical revenue, philanthropy, research grants, and institutional support. Determining the critical stakeholders is also important.
   - Knowing patient demographics as well as understanding the typical "payor mix" for insurance reimbursement is important as well. Also determining what services provided by the survivorship program are reimbursable and at what level
3. To recognize survivorship as a distinct phase of cancer care
4. Changing the mindset of oncologists and encouraging them to buy into the survivorship program so they feel comfortable referring their patients
5. Clarifying what Dana-Farber, as an institution most needs from the Survivorship Program to consider it a success
6. Encouraging patients to use the services provided by the survivorship program including psychosocial counseling
7. Working without a national guidance for screening late effects. There is no consensus based guidance or research-based guidance
8. Increasing volume to warrant getting more space while dealing with the issue of not having enough space to increase volume

SUGGESTIONS FOR OTHER PROGRAMS

1. Focus on Incorporating and Integrating Survivorship Care Into Routine Patient Care Practices
2. Determining the difference between what objectives work well in theory, but not in practice
3. Developing a disease-based model and establishing collaboration with disease centers
4. Developing reasonable assessment process/tool so that all clinicians are comfortable with the standardization of clinical practices

5. Identifying what the "product is"!
6. Focusing each clinic on a particular aspect of care in the particular disease center
7. Clarifying measures and goals
8. Standardizing survivorship care and developing a system of documentation
9. Collaborating with other clinics to expand further
10. Setting up the infrastructure for the clinic
11. Identifying ways to reach more patients and providers through marketing and promotion
    - Newsletter (quarterly)
    - Presentations at the departmental meetings
12. Developing educational materials
13. Finding a way to get referrals from disease centers
14. Creating metrics in order to measure the success of the program
15. Asking patients what they want in terms of their care: They know!
16. Learning from other institutions that are blazing the trail of survivorship

NOTE

All information included in this chapter was compiled through various Dana-Farber Cancer Institute resources.

9

A Major Urban Hospital's Cancer Survivorship Program

ANDREW L. SALNER, MD, SHERRI STORMS, RN, MSN,
AND CARLY STROICH-EISLEY, RN, APRN

Hartford Hospital is a major tertiary care and community health care center that serves a statewide population. The Hospital's Centers of Excellence include regionally prominent clinical programs in Cancer Care, Cardiology, Emergency Services and Trauma, Mental Health, Stroke, Transplant, and Women's Health. Hartford Hospital is the largest surgical provider in Connecticut and one of the largest in New England. It is one of the major teaching hospitals for the University of Connecticut School of Medicine.

The *mission* of Hartford Hospital is "to offer comprehensive services in an environment where innovation and teaching are integral to care; where we are proud to serve patients and one another; where meeting the challenge of complex medical needs is viewed as a defining competency; and where quality and safety of care are a constant."

The *vision* of the Hospital is to be the regional destination provider of innovative and complex care.

Hartford Hospital's Helen & Harry Gray Cancer Center is a nationally recognized center that treats about 3,000 new cancer patients per year. The Helen & Harry Gray Cancer Center cares for 15–20% of all newly diagnosed cancer patients in Connecticut, offering cutting-edge technology where the well-being of patients and families comes first.

The Helen & Harry Gray Cancer Center was selected in 2007 by the National Cancer Institute (NCI) as one of the first 16 hospitals nationwide to participate in the pilot phase of a program that is helping to bring state-of-the-art cancer care to patients in community hospitals. Selection was based on several factors including the hospital's leadership role in excellent care delivery, clinical research programs, survivorship programs, cancer information systems, and outreach efforts. This collaboration researches new and enhanced ways to assist, educate, and treat the needs of underserved populations. Now a part of the NCI Community Cancer Centers Program (NCCCP), Hartford Hospital was the first hospital so designated in New England. The program, no longer a pilot, was expanded in 2010 to include 14 additional hospitals. The program focuses on seven pillar areas, including outreach, research, quality of care, survivorship, biospecimens, information technology, and advocacy. It has facilitated our development of a multitude of new survivorship offerings.

We pay special attention to assisting patients from underserved populations who have an especially difficult time finding appropriate resources. According to the 2000 U.S. Census, Hartford, Connecticut, is one of the state's largest cities with a population of 121,578 people. The population is diverse; racial data from the 2000 Census indicate that approximately 28% of the population is white and 38% is black; ethnicity data indicate that 41% of the population is Hispanic (of any race). The median income in the city is $24,800 with almost 30% of families living below the poverty line (per 2000 U.S. Census). We see over 3,000 newly diagnosed cancer patients each year, of which 15% are of an ethnic minority group, 28% are elderly (>75 years), and 6% are either without insurance, underinsured, or on Medicaid. Approximately 43% of the patients are in one or more of these underserved groups; this number rises to 62% when we include our Medicare population in our estimate. With a full implementation of a Survivorship Program our goal is to become a model program helping to bridge the gap between cancer patient and cancer survivor with a particular emphasis on assisting the underserved.

SUPPORT SERVICES FOR CANCER SURVIVORS

The construction of the new Gray Cancer Center was completed in 1990, recognizing the need for expansion of not only the treatment modalities and technology of medical oncology and radiation oncology, but also the inclusion of support staff and programs. Space was created for full-time dietary and social work presence in the center, as well as a reception function to help with cancer center navigation. A part time Cancer Center Director's role was created to help oversee programmatic development. Our first annual Celebrate Life event was held in June 1990, reaching approximately 200 patients and family members. Celebrate Life, one of the largest cancer survivor celebrations in the Northeast, is hosted annually by Hartford Hospital. Having grown over the years, the event attracts 1,200–1,300 attendees each year to share in a humor-focused day, with nationally recognized survivors serving as keynote speakers. The event also includes entertainment, music, food, and educational giveaways.

Several support groups were gradually created to help fill what was thought to be the need for both information and psychosocial support. Many of these groups were topic focused, such as groups on mind-body techniques including guided imagery, relaxation, and visualization, and "I Can Cope" or "Look Good . . . Feel Better." Others were site based, such as breast cancer, prostate cancer, brain tumors, and ovarian cancer. These site-specific groups were frequently created due to an articulated need by a cadre of patients and family members, and a specific interest on the part of nursing or social work staff to help implement the group. The first of its kind in the northeastern United States, the prostate cancer support group started in 1990 through a collaboration of the Department of Urology and the Cancer Center, and had more than 200 patients and family members at its first meeting! It continues to be a very active monthly group that includes an hour for a guest speaker on a topic of interest and a second hour of small breakout groups. In addition, a monthly group for advanced prostate cancer and a quarterly group for spouses was created. The entire program is guided by an advisory committee of patients, family members, physicians, and staff.

Hartford Hospital also offers New Beginnings, a unique six-week program designed to help adopt a healthy lifestyle following cancer treatment and cope with the stress and anxiety related to transition from active treatment back to normal life. In an intimate setting, women learn techniques such as yoga and tai chi, as well as healthy eating and exercise habits. All instructors are certified in their area of specialty and are assisted by an oncology social worker who assists women who may be dealing with fears of recurrence and changes that have developed as effects of cancer and/or treatment. We also offer Healthy Steps, moving you to better health with the Lebed Method, a gentle medically based exercise program with an emphasis on movement to music designed specially for cancer survivors.

The American Cancer Society (ACS) has developed a nationwide program of patient navigation, particularly focused on meeting the needs of patients who most need help on their cancer journey. Hartford Hospital was the first institution selected in New England for this exciting program. The Navigator works with hospital staff to ensure that newly diagnosed patients have access to information and resources available through both the ACS and Hartford Hospital. The ACS patient navigator particularly meets with patients who are underserved or who don't have support systems that help them through the complex journey of cancer diagnosis and care. She also meets with any patient needing rides, information on survivorship, information about their diagnosis, and help with finding resources. She triages patients to social service, pastoral care, nursing, patient accounts to help with financial issues, and others as needed.

Our Integrative Medicine Department offers relaxation and wellness through a variety of programs, including Reiki, Massage, Guided Imagery, Gentle Yoga, and Acupuncture/Acupressure. These services are offered to our patients free of charge, in part from a generous grant from Angie's Spa (a 501(c) (3) charitable organization) to support the spirit, the soul, and to enhance self-esteem. This therapy also may enhance the effectiveness of medical therapy and is truly embraced as a component of care.

Cancer Survivorship Services

Hartford Hospital's Helen & Harry Gray Cancer Center has a large patient volume and needs for provide comprehensive and exemplary survivorship services. Recognizing the need to enhance our survivorship care program, we focused on the importance of the treatment summary as a technique to empower patients and families with accurate and rich data about their cancer diagnosis, stage, grade, and treatment details. In addition, the summary should ideally include a monitoring plan for the treated neoplasm, a late effects monitoring plan, second neoplasm screening guidelines, and a wellness plan going forward. We were fortunate to work closely with the NCCCP survivorship committee and Dr. Julia Rowland on this treatment summary development. Our thinking reflected not only implementation but sustainability for such a program. We therefore applied for a community grant from the Lance Armstrong Foundation (LAF) to establish a Survivorship Patient Navigator Program (SPNP), initially focused on breast cancer, with the survivorship visit provided by an Advanced Practice Registered Nurse (APRN). This individual, in providing a comprehensive treatment summary and wellness plan, would complement the other members of the oncology team and provide some basis for coordination of this care and communication of all relevant data.

In 2008, we were selected by LAF as one of only eight organizations in the United States to be awarded a community grant for a three-year Breast Cancer Survivorship Navigator Program. Our initial work in year one was to recruit an APRN, develop the treatment summary product and determine how best to obtain all needed data from various electronic and paper health records from both hospital and physician office sources. We also presented the program to all of the treating physicians to gain their buy-in, considering that the introduction of another provider might threaten their control, independence, or involvement in the continued care of their patients. This was accomplished as the project was presented in a positive, inclusive, and collaborative fashion that suggested a win-win for all involved, most notably the patient and family. We have formed a Survivorship Advisory Committee, made up of survivors and staff, to help advise on this project and other components of our program.

Now in our second year, the Survivorship Patient Navigator (SPN) Program is growing and has had a positive impact on our patients. Currently, the SPN meets with the survivor within six weeks of active cancer treatment for an exit interview, the purpose of which is to:

- Provide the survivorship package, including the NCCCP Breast Cancer Treatment Summary, Treatment Plan, and Care Plan using the ASCO model including wellness and late effects;
- Review treatment summary and treatment plan with the patient (and family/ caregivers);
- Review Survivorship Care Plan with patient (and family/caregivers);
- Review signs and symptoms of recurrence, as well as potential late effects of treatment;
- Encourage adopting a healthy lifestyle through wellness programs;
- Identify immediate needs and refer to appropriate services;
- Assist with appointments with PCP and other health care professionals;
- Encourage participation in ongoing support programs; and
- Establish mutually agreeable goals for healthy living.

We are now expanding the program to provide this same comprehensive care to patients with other primary sites. We have a proven track record of quality survivorship care for our breast cancer patients.

In the current SPNP, cancer patients treated at Hartford Hospital participate in a visit with the SPN at the completion of their active treatment. The SPN is an APRN. It was decided to hire a nurse practitioner to fill the role of SPN. Utilizing a nurse practitioner in this role provides patients with high-level, specialized survivorship care. In addition, the ability to bill for the survivorship nurse practitioner's services creates a program model with the potential for self-sustainability and revenue generation.

Patients are currently provided with a Cancer Treatment Summary and Care Plan, outlining all of the cancer treatments they have received, diagnostic tests performed (including results), and informed about any potential side effects and late effects of their treatment. The tumor characteristics (e.g., site[s], stage and grade, hormonal status, and marker information) are part of this record. All dates of treatment initiation and completion, surgery, chemotherapy, radiotherapy, transplant, hormonal therapy, gene or other therapies provided (including agents used), treatment regimen, total dosage, identifying number and title of clinical trials (if any), indicators of treatment response, toxicities experienced during treatment, and complications of treatment are part of this record.

In addition, patients receive individualized education and counseling by the SPN regarding the contents of their Care Plan, as well as information about support services including coordination of care for medical and non-medical providers, appropriate screenings, wellness, and lifestyle modifications including ways to improve their overall health and well-being as they transition from cancer patient to cancer survivor. Specific recommendations for healthy behaviors include diet, exercise, maintaining a healthy weight, sunscreen use, virus protection, smoking cessation, and osteoporosis prevention. A description of recommended cancer screening and other periodic testing and examinations, and the schedule on which they should be performed, are in the electronic record. Information on possible signs of recurrence and second tumors are discussed as part of the survivorship visit, in addition to information on the possible effects of cancer on family and personal relationships, sexual functioning, work, parenting, and the potential future need for psychosocial support. The SPN is responsible for completing this Care Plan and reviewing it with the patient post-treatment.

Patients are screened for potential financial problems including employment concerns and referred to Hartford Hospital social workers, if needed, for assistance. Patients can also be referred to onsite Genetic Counselors if and when they are identified as high-risk. Patients are provided with information on all of the resources that are available to them through Hartford Hospital and in the community. In addition, Hartford Hospital has an onsite Patient Navigator from the ACS who is available to provide resources as well.

The SPN will serve as a point of contact for Cancer Survivors and will assist in coordinating the care they receive from their other health care providers, both at the Helen & Harry Gray Cancer Center and in the community setting. Providing specialized and individualized Survivorship Care will improve the quality of life of our Cancer Survivors, as well as their families and caregivers. The SPN will also provide greater continuity of care between oncologists, specialists, and primary care providers, ensuring that we meet our survivors' health needs by ensuring appropriate follow-up care.

Our Survivorship Program aspires to aid in the patient's navigation from the diagnosis and active treatment phase of their cancer experience to survivorship and wellness. The end of treatment is a very challenging time for many patients. With so many innovative opportunities available at the beginning of their journey, the Survivorship Program provides a transition and continuity of care for patients once they complete their active treatment. In addition, the Survivorship Nurse Practitioner will serve as an educator of the Cancer Center staff, to enlighten them about Cancer Survivorship issues and the unique aspects of survivorship care. This education will extend to include the nursing students, medical students and residents who rotate through Hartford Hospital, in order to incorporate survivorship education into providers' practice at all levels.

The administration at Hartford recognized the need for an electronic health record to support this effort and acquired a case management survivorship software package called EQUICARE CS developed by Cogent. Using this new survivorship software to deliver our treatment summary, treatment plan and care plan has taken survivorship to the next level. Using this survivorship software means that our patients, families, PCP, and oncology specialists are included in the survivorship plan. EQUICARE CS, an electronic web-based record, has clinical, operational, and technological advantages. EQUICARE CS follows guidelines developed using the American Society of Clinical Oncology (ASCO) treatment summary and care plan along with recommendations from NCI. See http://www.cogenths.com for further information on EQUICARE CS.

The web-based program allows an external portal for each member of the health care team to access patient information. This gives the physician immediate access to current information and allows patients access to their own personal record. For our patients, this system provides continuity of care and enhances accuracy of the patient record. As survivors, the electronic system enhances quality of life by accurately chronicling the care they have received as a cancer patient in the past and advising what to do in the future for health, as described in the survivorship care plan.

There are limited publications on the effectiveness of Survivorship Programs and patient outcomes. An added benefit to the electronic record is the ability to provide a methodology of collecting outcomes data from survivors, thus increasing the potential collection of data for future research in the survivorship arena. The Cogent software will allow us to track race and ethnicity thus improve reporting of our cancer population.

We have determined that the efficacy of this effort needs formal evaluation, so that we might learn from our experience and report it to others who might wish to establish or enhance their own Survivorship Program. This evaluation is comprised of several validated instruments measuring general quality of life and fear of recurrence, and a Patient Satisfaction Survey. The fear of cancer recurrence and quality of life is measured at project baseline and six months after the initial visit. Patient satisfaction concerning the SPN visit is measured immediately after the visit. Satisfaction is measured again at six months to ascertain longer lasting benefits of the visit and follow-up behavior. The specific tools used to measure fear of recurrence, quality of life and patient satisfaction are described below:

1. Fear of recurrence (Assessment of Survivor Concerns): The Cancer Worry Subscale of the Assessment of Survivor Concerns will be used to evaluate the degree to which SPN clients experience changes in fear of cancer at baseline and at six-month follow-up (Gotay et al. 2007). The Cancer Worry Subscale is a validated tool composed of three items asking respondents to rate the degree to which they worry about future testing, about other types of cancer, and about recurrence of the same cancer.
2. Quality of life (FACT-G): This is a multidimensional measure of quality of life in breast cancer patients that has been validated in breast cancer patients (Brady et al. 1997) that includes subscales addressing physical, social, emotional, and functional well-being.
3. Patient satisfaction: Both the visit and the six month satisfaction survey focus on whether information received concerning side effects, healthy behaviors, and screening was useful; whether physical and emotional needs are met, communication with health care providers, and whether patient's anxiety level was affected by the survivorship visit. The visit survey also includes questions on the SPN and scheduling and other aspects of the visit. The follow-up survey asks whether the patient followed up with the SPN, whether the program aided lifestyle goals, whether he or she would recommend the program and asks the patient to evaluate the timing of the visit. Additional open ended questions ask about the best thing about the program and for what the patient might try to change.

This information will be used to guide our program development as we expand our Survivorship Program to include more cancer diagnoses. We also hope to publish and disseminate the findings of our program evaluation, to expand the available resources on Cancer Survivorship, and to participate in the development of best practice models and guidelines for developing and providing Cancer Survivorship care in community institutions. Using new technology such as the Cogent survivorship software and seeking feedback from our survivors through the program evaluation will help us to continually improve and expand our program to best meet the needs of Hartford Hospital's Cancer Survivors.

Most recently, the Helen & Harry Gray Cancer Center was awarded additional NCI funding for survivorship to help augment this exciting treatment summary project and expand it to a broader patient population. We have participated actively in the development of an NCCCP whitepaper on survivorship. We are continually inspired by the spirit of our patients and families, and seek to meet their needs in new and creative ways which will facilitate their return to a new normalcy.

CHALLENGES AND SUGGESTIONS

- Perform an in depth analysis of existing survivorship services both at the institution and in the community.
- Determine where gaps might exist.
- Include patients in an advisory capacity in this assessment and in planning.
- Set up revenue process—work closely with hospital financial services and get appropriate CPT codes; explore philanthropic, governmental or foundation grants to help ensure sustainability.
- Education about and marketing the program to physicians and staff, and patients/families.
- Referral system for all aspects of program from providers, office staff, hospital staff, patients, and families.
- Space and resources—be creative and share existing space.
- Advice and buy in from physicians—show them the value as soon as possible and demonstrate win-win scenarios.
- Integrating into current care system.
- Staff education. Use every available meeting to provide continual updates and reminders. Add survivorship recommendations at multidisciplinary management conferences.
- Access to patient medical records—network with physicians and find advocates to help gather data.
- Network with colleagues. Find programs that are similar by attending conferences.

NOTE

This project has been funded in whole or in part with Federal Funds from the National Cancer Institute, National Institutes of Health, under Contract No. NO1-CO-12400. The content of this publication does not necessarily reflect the views or policies of the Department of Health and Human Services, nor does mention of trade names, commercial products, or organizations imply endorsement by the U.S. government.

Survivorship efforts described in this chapter are supported through a Lance Armstrong Foundation grant.

REFERENCES

American Society of Clinical Oncology. 2008. Focus on Quality, ASCO's Library of Treatment Plans and Summaries Expands. *Journal of Oncology Practice* 4(1): 31–36.
Brady MJ, Cella DF, Mo F, Bonomi AE, Tulsky DS, Lloyd SR, Deasy S, Cobleigh M and Shiomoto G. 1997. Reliability and Validity of the Functional Assessment of Cancer Therapy-Breast Quality of Life Instrument. *Journal of Clinical Oncology* 15(3): 974–86.
Gotay C and Pagano I. 2007. Assessment of Survivor Concerns (ASC): A Newly Proposed Brief Questionnaire. *Health and Quality of Life Outcomes* 5(15).

10

COMMUNITY ONCOLOGY PRACTICE SURVIVORSHIP PROGRAM: NEW HAMPSHIRE ONCOLOGY HEMATOLOGY

ALMA PETROVIC, MD, AND JOSEPH LEHRBERG, BA

PROGRAM OVERVIEW

New Hampshire Oncology Hematology (NHOH) is a community medical oncology practice that serves patients and their families in Manchester, Concord, Laconia, Exeter, and Derry. NHOH has more than 100 employees, including nine board-certified or board-eligible oncologists and hematologists. For more than 25 years NHOH has collaborated with the Dana-Farber Cancer Institute in Boston. They provide medical oncology and chemotherapy services as well as a wide range of services and programs developed for the unique needs of cancer patients and family members. These programs include pain and palliative care, complementary therapies, and psycho-social support.

Cancer Survivorship services are provided by NHOH to their patients through a collaborative effort with the LiveSTRONG Survivorship Center at Dana-Farber.

PROGRAM GOALS

The community-based survivorship program is designed to include clinical, educational, and research components to improve the standards of care for the region's cancer survivors. Services available to the community include conferences to improve physician education in survivorship issues, consultations and referrals, community education programs on survivorship, and survivor clinical trials.

The goal of this community based program at NHOH has been to identify and measure the components of the transition from oncology care to primary care by providing every patient and his or her primary care provider with a treatment summary and care plan. It also includes educational programs for both patients and primary care providers about a survivor's unique needs. The ultimate goal is to develop a self-sustaining program that can be replicated at five NHOH locations.

PROGRAM DESIGN

To establish the program, Dana-Farber is sending an Nurse Practitioner (NP) to NHOH in Londonderry, NH, once a month on an interim basis. In addition, Dana-Farber is providing administrative support until the program becomes self-sustaining. NHOH has a clinical social worker and a nurse who provide additional support to patients responding to their psychosocial and educational needs.

Patients are commonly self-referred to the clinic. They are also referred during their last treatment visit by their oncologists, mid-level provider, or RN. Their provider will review survivorship programs and encourage patients to

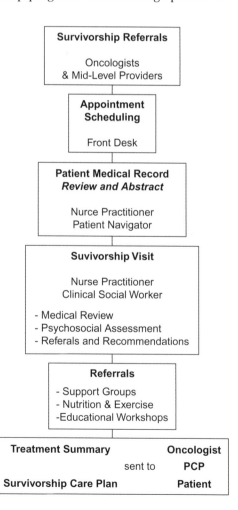

Figure 10.1. Community Practice Survivorship Program Flowchart. (Illustration by Joseph Lehrberg.)

make a survivorship appointment before leaving the clinic (preferably within the next three months).

A patient list is then generated by an RN Clinical Leader to identify patients who have not scheduled their survivorship appointment within three months of the end of the treatment date. The Executive Assistant will also follow-up by sending a letter to all patients who are newly off treatment and deemed by an Oncologist to be eligible for referral to the survivorship program. Finally the patients are called by the Executive Assistant 30 days after their letter has been mailed, and are invited to participate in the program. This list is updated and reviewed weekly. However, all patients may not be eligible due to provider preference and insurance.

Patients are also asked to bring a list of documents with them to their survivorship appointment. These materials include:

1. Surgical/operation reports
2. Path report from definitive/curative cancer surgeries
3. Infusion room flow sheets
4. Initial oncology consult note
5. Radiation treatment summary (if applicable)
6. Any note documenting intended duration of hormonal therapy
7. Any note documenting critical complications from chemotherapy:
   - Prolonged treatment delay (beyond one week) and duration
   - Hospitalization on treatment
   - Other intervening illness/diagnosis while undergoing treatment
   - Any grade three or four treatment toxicities.
8. Most recent clinic note

Patients then receive a Survivorship Tool Kit. This tool kit is a pamphlet that includes resources, frequently asked questions, and contact information relevant to survivorship care. It also contains details on the importance of treatment summaries and appropriate questions to ask the patient's oncologist upon first entering into survivorship. Along with the tool kit, patients are given the survivorship provider's business card.

These materials are handed out by an RN at the teaching visit or by an oncologist at one of the patient's early treatment visits. This way the patient is knowledgeable about the program in advance and is able to ask questions about a referral for a survivorship visit. The NP utilizes the OncoLinc web-based tool to create a LIVE**STRONG** Care Plan, which is transferred into an electronic medical record available to all clinicians with access to this system. Primary care physicians also receive a hard copy of the summaries and care plans.

After the patient's 60-minute appointment with the NP, they see a social worker for a half hour to address their potential psychosocial needs. A resource specialist/educator is also available to further answer questions they might have, and schedule follow-up appointments and additional screenings when needed.

In addition, the program offers periodic visits with educators from Dana-Farber, as well as educational workshops. Both of these programs provide in-depth education regarding the services available for cancer survivors. These include support groups, nutrition consults, and access to exercise specialists.

CHALLENGES

1. Standardizing clinical processes for survivorship
2. Changing the mindset of oncologists to make them feel comfortable referring their patients and not keeping them after treatment ends
3. Generating an adequate number of patient referrals

SUGGESTIONS

1. Creating focus groups with providers and patients as a way to increase their insight about the program
2. Developing a plan to educate the community about the program

NOTE

All information included in this chapter was compiled through various New Hampshire Oncology Hematology practice resources. This includes websites, interviews with clinicians and ancillary staff, written protocols, and documents endorsed by the survivorship program.

11

A COMMUNITY HEALTH CENTER CANCER SURVIVORSHIP PROGRAM: WHITTIER STREET HEALTH CENTER CANCER SURVIVOR NAVIGATOR PROGRAM

FREDERICA M. WILLIAMS, MBA, PRESIDENT AND CEO,
WHITTIER STREET HEALTH CENTER

CANCER SURVIVOR NAVIGATOR PROGRAM OVERVIEW

Whittier Street Health Center is a comprehensive community health center that provides primary care, wellness, education programs, and support services to more than 18,500 individuals from some of the most impoverished areas of Boston. Located in the Roxbury neighborhood of Boston, Whittier works closely with the community, its residents, and its leaders to provide holistic care to a community that faces significant disparities in health outcomes due to poverty, historical neglect, and negative social and environmental determinants of health. The communities that Whittier serves are at high risk for debilitating and costly chronic diseases and negative health outcomes. According to the Boston Public Health Commission's 2009 Health of Boston Report, among Boston's 16 neighborhoods, Roxbury has the highest rate of low birth weights, infant mortality, emergency room visits, hospitalizations for children under the age of five due to asthma, hospitalizations due to diabetes, and hospitalizations due to heart disease. Roxbury also has the second-highest rate of new HIV cases, obesity, and mortality due to substance abuse.

Significant racial and ethnic disparities exist within the communities served. Black residents of Boston are more than twice as likely to have diabetes as white residents. Black women have a mortality rate from breast cancer nearly twice that of white women. Black men in Boston have a mortality rate from prostate cancer nearly three times higher than white men. And 95% of the homicide victims in Boston are black or Latino.

Whittier works closely with the community not only to provide care to those facing these significant health issues but also to address the underlying causes of these disparities, including poverty, to make healthier communities for future generations.

Whittier Street Health Center's cancer survivor navigator program is designed to serve patients over 21 years old, who were treated for any type of cancer in the past to receive needed medical care, education, and emotional support. Whittier has found that patients accessing primary care at Whittier who are diagnosed with cancer are often disconnected from primary care, as they see their oncologist for cancer care. The overall goal of the survivorship program is to reengage cancer survivors with their primary care providers so that all aspects of health are once again monitored, not just cancer. For Whittier's population, which faces significant disparities in chronic diseases and often presents with comorbidities (e.g., diabetes, hypertension), this reestablishment of primary care is critical to manage overall health. Through a partnership with Dana-Farber Cancer Institute (Dana-Farber), Whittier successfully implemented the survivorship program in 2008.

CANCER DISPARITIES

For anyone, facing the trials of cancer requires strength and fortitude, and the battle must be approached with courage. From taking that first step of scheduling a screening, fearful of the potential results, to completing treatment and wondering what to expect next, every phase can be filled with anticipation and apprehension. While the fears associated with cancer are harrowing for anyone to confront, those in our community who have a limited access to care, a lack of social safety nets, cultural/linguistic barriers to health care, and are facing poverty, extra support is often needed for success and cancer survival. This support is especially needed when patients transition to different institutions for varying cancer-related clinical and social needs.

Serving Boston's most impoverished and racially and ethnically diverse neighborhoods, the data indicate that for those who make up Whittier's patient population, cancer survivor rates are particularly low. According to data from the Boston Public Health Commission's Health of Boston 2010 report, black non-Hispanic residents of Boston die from cancer at a rate 44% higher than white non-Hispanic residents. This disparity is most pronounced among men in Boston with prostate cancer. Black non-Hispanic men in Boston die from prostate cancer 3.3 times more often than white non-Hispanic men.

Disparities in cancer mortality rates in Boston are not typically due to higher incidence rates. In fact, for most types of cancer, white non-Hispanic residents are diagnosed more often, yet black non-Hispanic residents die from the disease more often. Perhaps most alarming is how these disparities plays out for breast cancer incidence and mortality in Boston. White non-Hispanic women in Boston are diagnosed with breast cancer 33% more often than black non-Hispanic women, yet black women die from the disease twice as often. This is partially due to an historical disparity in access to regular screenings, education, diagnosis, and follow-up. Because of this disparity, black women are often diagnosed and treated during a later stage. Therefore, while new cases of breast cancer are highest among white women, historical access to screening services allows for earlier diagnosis and a lower mortality rate. However, due to the efforts of many organizations, including Whittier and Dana-Farber, screening trends in Boston are changing. In fact, between 2005 and 2006 the percentage of black women in Boston receiving a mammogram within the past year increased 9% from 65% to 74%. While this indicates a promising trend, continued efforts are needed to ensure increased access to cancer resources for historically underserved populations.

While Boston residents live right next to some of the world's best hospitals, it is clear that some populations have better cancer education, access, and support when battling the disease. Whittier and Dana Farber have found that education, access, and support are especially crucial for Boston's most at-risk cancer patients as they transition from one stage of the battle to the next, traversing various institutions, care providers, emotions, and needs. Whittier and Dana-Farber's collaborative effort is designed to increase these support structures for both the patient and family to meet the clinical, social, and emotional needs of every cancer patient from screening to survival.

SURVIVORSHIP SERVICES AND PATIENT NAVIGATORS

With the assistance of Dana-Farber, Whittier has developed a system of compassionate, coordinated care to help cancer survivors address the long-term effects of cancer treatment and facilitate the transition of patients back into primary care after active treatment has concluded. This posttreatment service allows Whittier to meet the special health needs of cancer survivors. The initial results of this new endeavor are encouraging for survivors, and we are now working on a comprehensive patient navigation program to expand the support of patients while they are in treatment.

For many of Whittier's patients, familiarity and comfort with the health care system stops at Whittier. Whittier often stands as the first and only connection to the health care system and due to a multitude of reasons including fear, intimidation, distrust, a lack of transportation, and the stresses of poverty, many of Whittier's patients struggle to keep crucial appointments that require them to go to different institutions. The program provides critical patient navigation, case management, referral services, consultation, improved record transfers to the PCP, resource identification and evaluation, and education for patients who have abnormal results or ongoing critical health issues, including cancer diagnosis and treatment. Navigators continue their work with patients through survivorship.

Data from Whittier's electronic medical records indicate how patient navigation helps Whittier's patients facing abnormal screening results.

Colon Cancer Screening and Follow-Up for Abnormal Results

1. 479 of our age-appropriate active patients have had a colonoscopy.
2. 107 (22%) of those patients were diagnosed with either polyps or tubular adenoma and needed follow-up. We rely on the specialists to follow-up with patients needing further services.

Prostate Cancer Screening and Follow-Up for Abnormal Results

1. 444 age-appropriate men were screened in the last year.
2. 37 (8%) were referred to urologist for abnormal DRE or PSA.

Breast Cancer Screening and Follow-Up for Abnormal Results

1. 807 age-appropriate women were screened within the last 24 months.
2. 147 (18%) were diagnosed with breast abnormality (BIRADS 2 or greater) and were referred to the breast clinic for further evaluation.

Cervical Cancer Screening and Follow-Up for Abnormal Results

1. 1,857 age-appropriate women were screened within the last 24 months.
2. 150 (8%) had abnormal results. 135 (90%) of these patients had procedures (colposcopy and endometrial biopsy) done at Whittier and 15 (10%) were referred for surgical procedures in other facilities where they either had LEEP for persistent high-grade abnormality or hysterectomy for the diagnosis of cervical cancer.

The data show how the patient navigation program helped to significantly increase the numbers of low-income and minority patients access screenings, treatment, and evaluation. Based on the experiences of the success of this program, it was determined the Whittier cancer survivorship program would utilize the patient navigation model to engage survivors in care and support.

The flowchart below outlines how the patient navigators help our patients access the needed resources for diagnosis and treatment of cancer, while connecting them back to primary care and survivorship resources at Whittier once treatment has ended.

In 2008 when we implemented the cancer survivorship clinic, Whittier Street Health Center had 107 cancer survivors. Over 50% were diagnosed for breast and prostate cancer.

1. 67% of Whittier's cancer survivor patients had a visit with their primary care provider within the past year, meaning many were not accessing their PCP after cancer treatment.
2. Additionally, only 3% of those who had a visit with their provider had a complete physical exam.

WHITTIER STREET CANCER SURVIVORSHIP CLINIC

Many of Whittier's cancer survivor patients, once diagnosed with cancer, take their oncologist as their primary care provider and begin coming to Whittier for episodic care, for medication refills, or for other diseases, and not management of their cancer care plan, and other health needs. The primary goal of the survivorship program is to reestablish this connection back to primary care to ensure long-term management of the patient's needs.

During the clinic visit the needs of each patient are addressed through referrals to specialty providers, special services available in and out of the center, and community resource information. Case managers meet with each patient before the visit to explain what will be done during the visit and provide information about services available at the center. Patients receive comprehensive care by a multidisciplinary team consisting of physicians, nurses, and clinical case managers. This team assesses the patient, reviews the patient treatment summary, and creates a patient care plan. The visit is followed up by phone calls to ensure patients follow all recommendations related to further screenings, medication, and other parts of the care plan. If patients are unable to follow recommendations, case managers work with them to help them overcome barriers to accessing needed care and services.

Using the OncoLink summary/care plan tool (a website-based tool that summarizes patient treatment and creates treatment plans), clinicians and case managers prepare treatment summaries before the visit with patients. At the end of the visit patients receive a copy of the treatment plan with a second copy scanned in the electronic medical record.

TABLE 11.1 NUMBER OF PATIENTS SERVED AT THE INCEPTION OF THE CANCER SURVIVORSHIP CLINIC (2008) AND TYPE OF CANCER.

Breast	30	28%
Prostate	30	28%
Colon	14	13%
Uterine	9	8%
Cervical	6	6%
Esophageal	3	3%
Lung	3	3%
Ovarian	3	3%
Renal	3	3%
Others*	6	6%
Total	107	100%

*Others include skin, liver, fallopian tube, pancreas.
Source: Whittier Street Health Center Electronic Medical Records

In addition to clinical visits, learning sessions also occur at the clinic. Each session lasts approximately one and a half hours and includes the following subjects:

- A program overview and the screening of a documentary featuring cancer survivors and their testimonies
- Advice on how to manage the physical changes resulting from cancer survivorship
- Nutrition and its benefits during a cancer survivorship experience
- Pain management
- A discussion titled "Healthy Mind, Healthy Body"
- Intimacy and sexuality
- Rights as a cancer patient

A typical survivorship visit for a patient will include a meeting with their primary care provider for overall health needs and a review of progress toward the care plan, a meeting with a case manager and nurse for support in adhering to the care plan, and then a group information session, often led by their provider.

SURVIVORSHIP PROGRAM IMPLEMENTATION

The success of the implementation of the survivorship clinic was built on the expertise of Dana-Farber in providing cancer care and services, as well as the expertise of Whittier Street Health Center in providing medical care to a community that faces considerable barriers to accessing care and significant disparities in health outcomes. Several critical steps were needed to achieve this success, including the following:

- Developing a Clinical Advisory Committee to evaluate the elements of the electronic medical record system and how previous practices and protocols were arranged, and identify information technology innovations to improve the existing system, which is critical for patient navigation.
- Choosing a provider champion to support the implementation and sustainability of the program.
- Hiring patient navigators who are focused on addressing perceived barriers to care to help patients navigate through a complex and fragmented health care system.
- Hosting focus groups to solicit feedback from patients and cancer survivors so the program is tailored to meet their needs and is truly patient centered.
- Conducting significant outreach to the community to indentify cancer survivors who are not currently receiving care.

BARRIERS TO IMPLEMENTATION

During implementation of the program, Whittier and Dana-Farber worked to overcome several unforeseen barriers and adapted the program to ensure better patient engagement and improved results. The most formidable barrier was engaging cancer survivors in the program. During outreach to patients and the community, Whittier found that cancer survivors who finished treatment five or more years ago typically were not interested in the program because they felt that their cancer was "in the past" and did not see a need for further cancer programming. It was also found that those who very recently finished treatment were also not interested because cancer was such a large component of their lives and they were not willing to engage in more cancer-related programs. Those most willing to engage in the program were those who finished treatment 2–4 years prior to enrollment in the program. To overcome this barrier, Whittier case managers and outreach staff began referring to the program as a clinic visit, rather than a program, where the patient would be able to see their provider, refill medications, and address other health issues, while also receiving cancer survivorship specific services. This involved making the clinic provider specific. Instead of meeting with a case manager and nurse and then participating in the information sessions, participants now meet with their physician, and the case manager and nurse provide support in adherence to the treatment plan. After the provider visit, participants then meet as a group for information sessions, often led by their provider. By making these changes, program participants no longer feel like the survivorship program is an added program related to cancer; but rather the survivorship services are integrated into regular clinical visits with their trusted provider.

PROGRAM ACCOMPLISHMENTS

In 2008, when the program was implemented, Whittier had 108 cancer survivors, only 3% of which had received a physical exam with their primary care provider during that year, as many were only accessing care through their oncologist. For 2010, Whittier was the primary care provider for 155 cancer survivors and 121 accessed a well visit with their primary care provider in that year (78%). Along with the education and support provided to cancer survivors through the program, this reengagement in primary care is the most critical component of the program. Many of Whittier's patients present with multiple health care needs, in addition to survivorship services, and it is critical that they are engaged in comprehensive care and not just cancer management through their oncologist. Figure 11.1 shows current Whittier patients and their year of cancer diagnosis. One can see from the graph that many patients with a cancer diagnosis prior to 2003 have been lost to follow-up. The graph depicts active Whittier patients. Only four patients diagnosed with cancer between 1996 and 1999 currently access care at Whittier, implying that many started accessing care with their oncologist and were lost to follow-up. With the implementation of the program in 2008, Whittier has been more successful in keeping those recently diagnosed engaged in care.

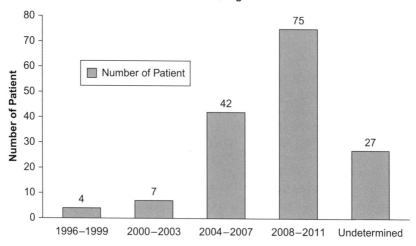

Figure 11.1. Patients served two years after implementation of the Cancer Survivorship Clinic (2010) and the year of their cancer diagnosis. Chart shows that patients are living longer and healthier lives with support of the Cancer Survivorship Clinic.

Source: Whittier Street Health Center Electronic Medical Records

THE FUTURE

Whittier and Dana-Farber continually evaluate and monitor the program to improve patient engagement and program outcomes. Additionally, the success of Whittier and Dana-Farber's survivorship services have led to new opportunities regarding cancer services for underserved populations. These areas of expansion and adaptation that Whittier and Dana-Farber are exploring include offering language-specific survivorship services for different populations (e.g., Spanish, Somali) and implementing an immigrant/refugee survivorship program. Due to a number of factors including cultural differences, a historical lack of health care in their country of origin, limited knowledge of American health care, documentation status, religious beliefs, chaos, post-traumatic stress disorder, stress, and unrest, recent immigrants and refugees often do not adequately access health care and are at greater risk for late-stage diagnosis of chronic diseases or for lapses in needed medical care.

Countries with limited health care resources tend to focus on the treatment of acute issues, rather than screening and prevention. We have found that many recent immigrants in our community believe you should only go to the doctor when you are sick. Furthermore, many recent immigrants and refugees believe American hospitals can cause sickness. Seemingly well when entering the hospital, they are confused when diagnosed with a disease such as cancer, believing it was caused by the hospital, not recognizing that it was evident, just undiagnosed while in their home country. As one Somali patient recently remarked, "Doctors are associated with the sick." The program will use the experiences and knowledge of cancer survivors who are immigrants and refugees to establish culturally appropriate care guidelines and a training curriculum for primary care doctors when working with these populations on survivorship.

In addition to survivorship services, Whittier and Dana-Farber are also working to bring other cancer services directly to the community. To streamline cancer care and services, Dana-Farber and Whittier will implement a Community Cancer Clinic within Whittier's facility. The clinic will include a consultation program, cancer education resources, a survivorship clinic, and fixed mammography, providing services directly within the community.

12

CANCER SURVIVORSHIP CARE PLANNING

CARRIE TOMPKINS STRICKER, PhD, RN, AOCN,
KENNETH MILLER, MD, AND LINDA A. JACOBS,
PhD, RN, AOCN

INTRODUCTION

There are currently estimated to be approximately 12 million cancer survivors living in the United States, and 20 million globally. These survivors are a diverse group in regards to age, sex, race, ethnicity, religion, and socioeconomic background (see Figure 12.1). The diversity of cancer diagnoses, stages of disease, and treatment modalities, which may range from surgery alone to complex combination therapy including surgery, radiation, chemotherapy, hormonal therapy, and targeted therapies, must also be considered. Following completion of initial treatment, over 50% of patients will be long-term cancer survivors, creating the potential for many years of healthy survivorship (see Figure 12.1).[1]

During the survivorship phase of care, defined as the phase of care following completion of primary treatment,[3] patients may have health care needs similar to the cancer-free population and require management of chronic conditions such as treatment for diabetes, hypertension, and hyperlipidemia. In addition, cancer survivors have unique needs and medical concerns including the risk of late and long-term effects of treatment and second and secondary malignancies, as well as psychosocial issues such as psychosocial distress that may impact their work and social relationships.[3,4]

CARING FOR CANCER SURVIVORS

As detailed in the 2006 Institute of Medicine (IOM) report, "From Cancer Patient to Cancer Survivor," the care of our nation's cancer survivors is characterized by poor communication and coordination, fragmented yet often duplicated services, under-emphasis on preventive care, and inadequate attention

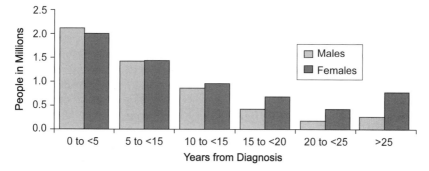

Figure 12.1. Estimated Number of Persons Alive in the U.S. Diagnosed with Cancer on January 1, 2007 by Time From Diagnosis and Gender (Invasive/1st Primary Cases Only, N = 11.7 M survivors).[2]

to long-term and late effects of cancer treatment.[3] The growing numbers of cancer survivors have begun to outstrip the capacity of cancer care systems, forcing survivors into the community where overburdened primary care providers (PCPs) face numerous competing demands and often are not adequately prepared to care for these survivors for many reasons, including a knowledge deficit regarding the individualized needs and surveillance plans for cancer survivors.[3,5–7] Several recent studies highlight these and other concerns related to survivorship care delivery.

In a study by Cheung et al.,[8] patients and physicians often had discordant expectations with respect to the roles of PCPs and oncologists in cancer survivorship care. Uncertainties around physician roles and responsibilities can lead to deficiencies in care, supporting the need to make explicit survivorship care planning a standard component in cancer management. There are a number of studies in the literature that highlight differences between PCPs and oncologists regarding cancer surveillance and routine follow-up care practices, as well as studies that examine patient and provider expectations for survivorship care and their influence on outcomes. For example, growing evidence points to suboptimal preventive and chronic non-cancer care in cancer survivors, as well as primary care physicians' underutilization of cancer-related surveillance in cancer survivors.[9–12] These and other studies highlight the importance of communication and care planning in helping to align expectations and ownership for the content and coordination of survivorship care, so as to improve alignment with guidelines for cancer survivorship care, and ultimately, patient outcomes.

Based on studies such as these, the IOM report[3] concluded that the consequences of cancer and its treatment are substantial, many of medical and psychosocial needs identified by cancer survivors during the survivorship phase of care remain unmet, and a carefully coordinated transition from active cancer treatment to cancer survivorship care was a luxury afforded to very few. To provide optimal care for all cancer survivors, the IOM recommended that quality survivorship care contain four essential elements:[3]

1. Prevention of recurrent and new cancers, and of other late effects;
2. Surveillance for cancer spread, recurrence, or secondary cancers; assessment of medical and psychosocial late effects;
3. Intervention for consequence of cancer and its treatment; and
4. Coordination between primary and specialty care to ensure that all of the survivor's health needs are met.

Providing Cancer Treatment Summaries and Survivorship Care Plans

In its report, the IOM also outlined 10 key recommendations for providing quality survivorship care and overcoming present deficits.[3] Recommendation number 2 advised that the provision of treatment summaries (TSs) and survivorship care plans (SCPs) be a part of a planned and coordinated transition to survivorship care. The dissemination of SCPs (the term that will include both TSs and SCPs in this chapter) was recommended by the President's Cancer Panel[13] and by the IOM committee[3] to help ensure that survivors' needs are more fully met and that opportunities for health promotion and management of persistent and delayed treatment effects (often called late effects) are optimized. The IOM called for a systematic dissemination of SCPs as a central strategy for facilitating transition to survivorship care. SCPs are intended to provide critical information regarding diagnoses, treatments, and potential late effects, as well as guidelines outlining recommended surveillance, preventive strategies, and education and referrals for management of other medical and psychosocial needs.

What Is an SCP?

The SCP includes a summary of the treatment a patient received as well as a plan for follow-up care.[14] The TS section of the SCP is a summary of a cancer survivor's diagnostic and treatment information including the type of cancer, size of the tumor, stage, and special characteristics such as hormone receptors or molecular testing. Key information regarding surgery, radiation, and/or chemotherapy should also be provided. This record can and should be shared with other medical care providers and provide contact information so that health care providers can communicate with the patient's permission.

The care planning section of the SCP details a follow-up plan for surveillance for cancer recurrence as well as recommendations for frequency of office visits, laboratory tests, and imaging studies. In addition, the SCP should provide key information regarding possible risk for late and long-term effects, as well as recommended screening. The IOM also recommends that the SCP also be a vehicle to recommend screening for other cancers and for promoting general preventive health care.[3] Additionally, the SCP should assist with coordination of care by outlining which providers are responsible for particular aspects of care and by recommending resources and individual referrals for ongoing issues related to cancer and its treatment.

Implementation of Survivorship Care Plans

Available Resources for Survivorship Care Planning

A number of TS and SCP care plan templates have been created and are available for application to practice. These include web-based documents created by professional and advocacy-based cancer organizations such as the American Society of Clinical Oncology (ASCO), as well as a variety of institutionally developed documents, several of which have been published or otherwise made publically available for use.

ASCO Cancer Treatment Plan and Summaries

The ASCO Chemotherapy Treatment Plan and Summary[15] was developed for cancer survivors and is intended to be a record of the patient's cancer treatment, as well as a brief outline of recommended follow up care (see Figure 12.2). The TS form includes details such as the stage and pathologic details of the cancer, the dose of chemotherapy, specific drugs used, number of cycles completed, and surgeries performed, as well as any additional treatment including radiation, targeted therapies, and/or hormonal therapy. The SCP form details recommended follow-up care, including a schedule of office visits, as well as surveillance testing, with space to indicate the provider responsible for performing each aspect of follow-up care. A sample SCP for breast cancer survivors is shown in figure 12.2. This, as well as treatment summary templates, are available at http://www.asco.org/ASCOv2/Practice+%26+Guidelines/Quality+Care/Quality+Measurement+%26+Improvement/Chemotherapy+Treatment+Plan+and+Summary. At present, disease-specific treatment summaries and ASCO survivorship care plans are available for breast cancer, colon cancer, lung cancer, and lymphoma. In addition, a generic form is available that can be applied for populations for which there is not a disease-specific template. ASCO's forms can be downloaded from the ASCO website in both Microsoft Word and Excel formats and are intended to be filled out by a member of the oncology care team.

Journey Forward

The Journey Forward plan was created through the collaborative efforts of the National Coalition for Cancer Survivorship, the UCLA Cancer Survivorship Center, WellPoint, Inc., and Genentech. Journey Forward is a free online program for cancer survivors that helps medical professionals create custom SCPs that are based on the ASCO Chemotherapy Treatment Summary templates and Surveillance Guidelines. Similar to the ASCO plans, Journey Forward is intended to be used by members of the oncology care team to generate detailed summaries of cancer treatments, as well as follow-up care plans that incorporate education regarding late effects, recommendations for cancer surveillance and other health care issues, and links to relevant resources for cancer survivors. This plan can be tailored for use by the patient, oncologist,

Patient Name:		Medical Oncologist Name:	
FOLLOW-UP CARE TEST	RECOMMENDATION		PROVIDER TO CONTACT
Medical history and physical (H&P) examination (see below)	Visit your doctor every three to six months for the first three years after the first treatment, every six to 12 months for years four and five, and every year thereafter.		
Post-treatment mammography (see below)	Schedule a mammogram one year after your first mammogram that led to diagnosis, but no earlier than six months after radiation therapy. Obtain a mammogram every six to 12 months thereafter.		
Breast self-examination	Preform a breast self-examination every month. This procedure is not a substitute for a mammogram.		
Pelvic examination	Continue to visit a gynecologist regularly, if you use tamoxifen, you have a greater risk for developing endometrial cancer (cancer of the lining of the uterus). Women taking tamoxifen should report any vaginal bleeding to their doctor.		
Coordination of care	About a year after diagnosis, you may continue to visit your oncologist or transfer your care to a primary care doctor. Women receiving hormone therapy should talk with their oncologist about how often to schedule follow-up visits for re-evaluation of their treatment.		
Genetic counseling referral	Tell your doctor if there is a history of cancer in your family. The following risk factors may indicate that breast cancer could run in the family - Ashkenazi Jewish heritage - Personal of family history of ovarian cancer - Any first-degree relative (mother, sister, daughter) diagnosed with breast cancer before age 50 - Two or more first-degree or second-degree relatives (grandparents, aunt, uncle) diagnosed with breast cancer - Personal or family history of breast cancer in both breasts - History of breast cancer in a male relative		
YEARLY BREAST CANCER FOLLOW-UP & MANAGEMENT SCHEDULE			

Visit Frequency for H&P Years 1-3	3 months	6 months	(circle one)
Years 4-5	6 months	12 months	(circle one)
Visit Frequency for Mammography	6 months	12 months	(circle one)

VISIT FREQUENCY	HISTORY AND PHYSICAL	MAMMOGRAPHY
3rd Month (if applicable)		
6th Month (if applicable)		
9th Month (if applicable)		
12th Month (if applicable)		
Notes:		

- Risk: You should continue to follow-up with your physician because the risk of breast cancer returning continues for more than 15 years after remission, and because, if you have not had bilateral mastectomies, you are at higher risk to develop a new, unrelated, breast cancer at some time in the future.

- Symptoms a Recurrence: Report these symptoms to your doctor: new lumps, bone pain, chest pain, shortness of breath or difficulty breathing, abdominal pain, or persistent headaches.

- Not Recommended: The following tests are not recommended for routine breast cancer follow-up: breast MRI, FDG-PET scans, complete blood cell counts, automated chemistry studies, chest x-rays, bone scans, liver ultrasound, and tumor markers (CA 15-3, CA 27,29 CEA). Talk with your doctor about reliable testing options.

Figure 12.2. ASCO Breast Cancer Follow-up Care Plan.[15]

and the primary care provider. At present, disease specific versions are available for breast cancer, colon cancer, and lymphoma, and a generic version is available for use with other cancer sites. These are available for download at http://journeyforward.org/.

Prescription for Living

The Cancer Survivor's Prescription for Living was developed by oncology nurses.[16] This paper document offers a TS template for recording cancer diagnostic and treatment details, as well as a follow-up care plan in a checklist

YOUR SUMMARY

You were treated for Breast Cancer

- mastectomy

- tamoxifen (nolvadex®)

- x-ray based radiation / don't know

- radiation treatment for breast cancer after mastectomy

All Survivors
Coordinating Your Care

As a survivor, it is important that you keep a journal or notebook of your care. Include your doctor's contact information, medications taken, therapies received and radiology testing you have had. (Visit the OncoPilot section for forms you can use to organize this material). While some survivors continue to see an oncologist, many return to a primary care provider or internist for care, many of whom are uncertain how to care for you. Developing the LIVE**STRONG** Survivorship Care Plan can help you and your primary care provider in understanding what effects to look for and how to handle them. If you are being seen only by a primary care practitioner, it is a good idea to be known to an oncologist or late effects clinic, should you need any guidance or referrals with regards to late effects. The Cancer Survivors Project maintains a list of late effects clinics, which will review the therapies you received, discuss risks with you and act as a consultant to your primary care team.

Risk of a second cancer

As a survivor, your chance of developing a second cancer is about twice that of a person of the same sex and age who has never had cancer. This may be a different type of cancer altogether, or a cancer in the same site as before, that is not related to the first cancer. While this sounds scary, it is important to be aware of this risk and be proactive in your own healthcare. It is not well understood why survivors have this risk, but having follow up care, cancer screening and a healthy lifestyle can decrease your risk. In some cases, a treatment (types of chemotherapy or radiation therapy) increases the risk of another cancer. These are called secondary cancers because they develop as a result of therapy. If you are at risk for a secondary cancer, it will be discussed further in your plan.

Figure 12.3. LIVE**STRONG** Care Plan.

format that allows the provider to individualize recommendations for follow up care and surveillance testing, preventive behaviors, and education regarding potential late effects. Its lack of availability as an electronic document limits it use. It can be downloaded from http://www.nursingcenter.com/library/static.asp?pageid=721732.

The LIVESTRONG Care Plan

The LIVE**STRONG** care plan (see Figure 3) is a product of a collaborative agreement between the University of Pennsylvania Abramson Cancer Center, OncoLink, and LIVE**STRONG**. (www.livestrongcareplan.org). In contrast to the ASCO care plans and Journey Forward, the LIVE**STRONG** care plan was developed to independently allow patients to create an SCP by inputting information regarding their cancer diagnosis, treatment, and present symptoms. The output from the tool typically has extensive textual information about survivorship issues that the patient is at risk for or presently experiencing. It is recommended that cancer survivors share their LIVE**STRONG** Care Plan with their oncology team, PCP, and other health care providers. The recommendations generated by the LIVE**STRONG** Care Plan are based on guidelines whenever available, such as those provided by the IOM, Children's Oncology Group (COG), the National Cancer Institute (NCI), and ASCO.

In addition to the publically available templates discussed above, many institutions have created their own SCP templates and documents for internal use. Several have published their SCP templates in part to make them available for external adaptation and use. A deidentified sample of the breast cancer follow-up care plan from the Abramson Cancer Center of the University of Pennsylvania is available (see Figure 4), which is provided to breast cancer survivors in addition to a detailed cancer treatment summary, a listing of relevant cancer survivorship resources, and a variety of educational materials. A number of centers have or are currently working toward SCP templates that interface with electronic medical records (EMR) systems, so as to improve both the efficiency of preparing, delivering, and sharing these documents with both patients and other providers.

IMPLEMENTING SURVIVORSHIP CARE PLANS

A number of issues must be considered when planning for the implementation of survivorship care plans, including structure, process, and timing of delivery, as well as content and scope of the treatment summary and care plan documents. To date, limited evidence is available to guide decision making, since research determining best approaches is in its infancy. Thus, clinical factors primarily influence selected approaches. Factors influencing decision making include characteristics of the patient population and of the setting for care plan delivery (e.g., institutional resources available), as well as determination of the intended audience for the SCP. Grant and colleagues[17] review both patient and setting characteristics that influence the delivery of survivorship care and propose a number of reflective questions that should be considered when developing survivorship programming, including the integration of SCPs into the survivorship phase of cancer care.

Structure and Process of Survivorship Care Plan Delivery

Although not well described in the literature, it appears that the provision of SCPs occurs most often within a formalized survivorship care program or clinic, rather than integrated into routine oncology follow-up care.[18,19] A number of models and systems for survivorship care have previously been well described.[17-20] Description of these models is beyond the scope of this chapter;

Recommended for you	General guidelines
History/physical examination - **Every 6 months, alternating between PCP & Breast Cancer Survivors Clinic**	Every 3 to 6 months for the first 3 years after primary therapy; Every 6 to 12 months for years 4 and 5; then, annually
Symptoms of recurrence - **Call Breast Cancer Survivors Clinic**	Breast cancer survivors should report to their physician or nurse the following symptoms: new lumps; persistent bone, chest, or abdominal pain, shortness of breath; persistent headaches.
Consider genetic counseling if you meet any of the following criteria: - **BRCA1/2 negative**	*Criteria include:* Ashkenazi Jewish heritage; history of ovarian cancer at any age in yourself or any first-or second-degree relatives; any first-degree relative with a history of breast cancer diagnosed before the age of 50 years; two or more first-or second-degree relatives diagnosed with breast cancer at any age; yourself or your relative with a diagnosis of breast cancer in both breasts; and a history of breast cancer in a male relative.
Breast self-examination - **Monthly**	Perform monthly breast self-examination
Mammography - **Annually in February, with PCP**	First post-treatment mammogram 1 year after the initial mammogram that led to your diagnosis; then, annually or as indicated for abnormal findings.
Cholesterol Check - **Every 5 years over age 34, by PCP**	Over age 34 should be checked every 5 years if within normal range. More frequently dependent upon family and personal history.
Blood Pressure - **Yearly**	Check BP yearly unless it is elevated and you are instructed otherwise.
Colonoscopy - **Beginning at age 50, by PCP**	Beginning at age 50, individuals with an average risk for developing colorectal cancer should have a colonoscopy every 10 years unless instructed otherwise.

Figure 12.4. Abramson Cancer Center Breast Cancer Survivorship Care Plan—Deidentified Sample.
Note: These recommendations are based on the American Society of Clinical Oncology (ASCO) 2006 Update of the Breast Cancer Follow-Up and Management Guidelines in the Adjuvant Setting. Accessed online on July 9, 2008 at http://www.asco.org/ASCO/Quality+Care+%26+Guidelines/Practice+Guidelines/Clinical+Practice+Guidelines/Breast+Cancer/American+Society+of+Clinical+Oncology+2006+Update+of+the+Breast+Cancer+Follow-up+and+Management+Guideline+in+the+Adjuvant+Setting.

however, for the purposes of understanding the placement of survivorship care planning within models of survivorship care delivery, a brief description is warranted. Landier[18] described different systems of survivorship care, including (1) the consultative system that involves single or multiple visits for assessment and management of survivorship concerns while the survivors maintains his/her usual cancer follow-up care; (2) the ongoing care system, consisting of ongoing care in long-term survivorship clinics or programs; and (3) the integrated care system, previously described as the integration of survivorship care into care provided by the primary cancer care team.[3,18,20,21] Exemplars of each of these systems of survivorship care have been published, for example, the consultative system,[22,23] the ongoing care system,[24] and the integrated care system.[21,25] Oeffinger and McCabe (2006) further described models of care that predominantly belong to the classification of ongoing care systems.[19] For example, "ongoing care" survivorship clinics and programs can be further classified as nurse-led, multidisciplinary, and shared care models of care, depending both on what provider(s) staff the programs and on the degree to which care is coordinated or "shared" with clinicians in other disciplines and in other settings, especially primary care. Provision of SCPs should be an integral component of each of these models of care, and the structure and process of their delivery will be influenced by the models of care and resources available. Across all models of care, nurses, including advanced practice nurses such as nurse practitioners, are increasingly critical to the implementation of survivorship care and care planning efforts.[17] Nurses' requisite education and skills in patient education, symptom assessment and management, and care planning optimally prepare them for principal roles in survivorship care, as myriad program exemplars attest.[3,17,20,23,25,26] Research is under way evaluating outcomes of a variety of models of survivorship care plan delivery, including a number of nurse-led models of care. In addition, novel approaches to survivorship care delivery, including telephone, Internet, mail-based, and peer-led interventions are currently being explored.[27] Results from both research and clinical endeavors will hold great significance for informing the development and dissemination of optimal models of survivorship care planning.

Timing

The best time-point for distribution of SCPs is unclear. Intuitively, it seems optimal to distribute SCPs around the time of completion of active treatment, as recommended within the American College of Surgeon's proposed Commission on Cancer (CoC) new standards.[28] If SCPs are provided by the patient's primary oncology provider(s) as the CoC advises, distribution at this time-point would ensure that the largest number of survivors receive SCPs, especially since some survivors are lost to oncology follow-up after the completion of active cancer treatment.[3] Additionally, much of the information contained in SCPs would intuitively be useful to patients at this juncture, since a primary goal of these documents is to provide a framework for follow-up care, including recommended surveillance and preventive strategies. Limited research on patient preferences supports distribution at this time-point. In one survey of 490 breast cancer survivors, 74.5% of women expressed a preference for receiving SCPs within three months of treatment completion.[29]

Finally, the literature has shown that the transition from active treatment is a time of great anxiety and uncertainty as patients transition from more frequent treatment visits to less frequent follow-up. Structured and supportive interventions surrounding this vulnerable time-point improve both psychosocial and quality of life outcomes.[30] Despite this, many centers have yet to integrate survivorship care planning at this time-point, especially given that the provision of SCPs is often linked to services provided within the context of a visit to specialized clinics for long-term survivors.[17,31] Integrated approaches[18,21] that engage the primary oncology treatment team in providing survivorship care may be the best approach to the provision of SCPs at the time of transition from cancer treatment to survivorship care, but this deserves study.

Content

Broadly speaking, the content of SCPs should be designed to comport with the IOM's four broad goals and components of survivorship care: (1) prevention and detection; (2) surveillance; (3) intervention for consequences of cancer and its treatment; and (4) coordination of care. As previously discussed, the IOM has defined specific elements that should be incorporated into SCPs in order to meet these goals.[3]

A checklist based on IOM recommendations for SCP content will soon be available to assist centers with designing SCPs and determining whether or not their documents comport with IOM recommended standards for content.[32] The actual content varies widely at present,[33] and there is no single gold standard for the information that should be included in an SCP. Thus, the specifics of actual content should be determined by a variety of factors, including the patient population served and availability of disease-specific survivorship guidelines, local survivorship resources available, and the intended audience for the SCP.

For example, content regarding the risk of late and long-term effects may vary widely depending on the population under consideration, given differential risk across different populations of cancer survivors. Risk for late effects can be stratified partially by looking at the cancer diagnosis and treatment.[3] For example, the risk of late and long-term effects for a woman treated for non-invasive breast cancer is less than for a man who underwent an allogeneic bone marrow transplant for acute myelogenous leukemia. Thus, individualized SCPs should reflect this variability in risk. In addition, different versions of the SCP may need to be produced for distribution to PCPs versus the patients. PCPs will likely desire greater detail on treatments received and surveillance recommendations, whereas patients may desire more information on resources and referrals for symptoms and late effects experienced. More research is needed to define and evaluate the optimal depth, breadth, and specifics for SCP content, and it is unlikely that a one-size-fits-all approach will be viable. Substantial individualization of content will likely be necessary to serve the needs of diverse survivor populations.

Overcoming Barriers to Survivorship Care Planning

Given the limited scope and reach of survivorship care planning across U.S. cancer care settings, an analysis of barriers becomes crucial, including identification of potential solutions. Barriers to the provision of SCPs are summarized in Table 12.1 and are largely extrapolated from the larger body of literature focused on barriers to survivorship care in general. Financial, time, and staffing constraints emerge as primary obstacles and are particularly difficult to overcome in community-based and ambulatory care settings.[17,26]

The preparation of detailed treatment summaries is often a time-consuming process, particularly in community settings where patients may be treated in many different settings, and thus their medical records are not centralized.[34] Further, reviewing the SCP with survivors is often time and resource intensive and requires the appropriation of staff to fulfill this responsibility. At present, no specific mechanism for reimbursement of survivorship care planning is available, although legislation in the form of the Comprehensive Cancer Care Improvement Act has been introduced to Congress and would accomplish this if passed. Community-based and ambulatory care settings, in particular,

TABLE 12.1 BARRIERS TO SURVIVORSHIP CARE PLANNING AND POTENTIAL SOLUTIONS

Barriers	Potential Solutions
Time intensity—development of survivorship care plans	Harnessing potential of EMRs to populate cancer treatment summaries
Time intensity—reviewing of survivorship care plans with patients	Group approaches Peer training based approaches Web, mail, internet-based approaches Dividing SCP review across multiple office visits/providers
Financial support Lack of reimbursement for survivorship care planning	Philanthropic and grant support Billing for office visits at which SCPs are provided
Lack of physician/provider support	Educational programs, online programs, Insurance mandated programs
Lack of institutional commitment	Insurance & accreditation mandates, philanthropy
Staffing issues	Grants support, philanthropy, tracking billing, downstream revenue, research

will suffer if this service is not reimbursed, since these settings will most likely prioritize staffing for reimbursable treatments, such as chemotherapy.[17]

A variety of approaches may be used to overcome these financial, time, and staffing constraints. Some centers have successfully secured grant and philanthropic funding to support survivorship program development, including the development and implementation of SCPs.[23,24] Harnessing the ability of electronic medical record (EMR) systems is one oft-quoted strategy for improving the efficiency of preparing cancer SCPs;[31,34] however, obstacles to this approach include an inability of many EMRs to easily translate cancer diagnostic and treatment data into an SCP template. For example, in 2007, ASCO convened the EMR Roundtable to encourage vendors to incorporate core elements of chemotherapy treatment plans and summaries into their EMR products,[35] and results have been disappointing (Ganz, personal communication). Nonetheless, case examples of successful EMR applications are growing,[23,25] and the increasing demand for SCPs should accelerate development. One promising example is the present collaboration between Journey Forward (a survivorship care planning tool) developers and major EMR vendor(s) to create an interface between EMR data and this web-based survivorship care planning tool. Other possible strategies for overcoming time and financial constraints include the use of template documents for SCPs, billing a high level follow-up visit (based on time or complexity of care) for the office visit at which the SCP is provided, and dividing review of the SCP across multiple, billable office visits to limit the time intensity of any one care planning session. Recently, the use of peer networks such as support groups, professional-led group-based survivorship care planning visits, and telephone, Internet, and mail-based survivorship care planning interventions are being explored as approaches to improve efficiency and decrease resource intensity of survivorship care planning.[27]

Another factor influencing the time and resource burden is the wide scope of content that SCPs are designed to address. IOM recommendations for content are both comprehensive and detailed, ranging from a summary of diagnostic and treatment details, through recommendations for surveillance, follow-up and preventive care, and identification of resources in a variety of domains (physical, psychosocial, financial), as well as implications for family members. For example, a checklist of IOM recommendations that can be used to evaluate SCP content was created for a study of breast cancer survivorship care planning across the LIVE**STRONG** COE Network. This resulted in an exhaustive checklist of 92 items by which SCPs could be evaluated for concordance with IOM recommendations.[32] As Salz and colleagues discovered in their analysis of survivorship care plans at NCI-designated cancer centers, this breadth and depth of scope was problematic for most centers.[33] No center's care plans addressed all of the IOM's recommendations, and most addressed only a small subset. Research is needed to define the most important elements of SCPs from a variety of stakeholder perspectives and to link specific elements of care plans to outcomes of interest. This will allow evidence-based refinement of the IOM framework and has the potential to improve both the feasibility and effectiveness of survivorship care planning efforts.

In the interim, a variety of strategies can be used to maximize ability to meet IOM standards for SCP content. Careful use of templates, available resources, and educational materials is one strategy. The various publically available resources for SCPs, such as Journey Forward, the ASCO Survivorship Care Plans, and the LIVESTRONG Care Plan, have different and complementary strengths. Several of these resources may be combined to create an SCP that is more comprehensive than would be possible with the use of any one document. For example, the LIVESTRONG Care Plan focuses heavily on education regarding potential toxicities and late effects of cancer treatment and is not intended to provide a detailed summary of cancer treatments received. Conversely, the ASCO, Journey Forward, and many institutionally developed templates offer detailed treatment summaries yet lack a detailed description of potential late effects. Thus, combining these resources would overcome deficiencies resulting from the use of only one. Further, a number of publically available cancer survivorship educational materials complement identified weaknesses of presently available SCPs. Salz and colleagues found that less than half of reviewed care plans from NCI-designated cancer centers addressed information and resources related to potential psychosocial effects of cancer, such as impact on relationships, sexual function, employment, and finances. However, many sites noted distributing additional materials to patients that were not formally a part of the SCP template. Some of these materials do address psychosocial topics that are often under-addressed by the templates themselves. The NCI *Facing Forward* brochure, for example, addresses the psychosocial effects and resources noted above. Careful review and integration of complementary, high-quality educational materials should improve Cancer Centers' ability to meet standards for survivorship care planning.

Other primary barriers to survivorship care especially relevant to survivorship care planning include lack of institutional commitment, limited provider buy-in, a dearth of guidelines for adult survivorship care, and patient factors such as the desire to stay with their present oncology providers rather than switch to a survivorship clinic. Patient reluctance to leave trusted oncology providers is being addressed by integrated models of survivorship care, where survivorship care is incorporated into services provided by the primary oncology team.[18,21] Other approaches include setting expectations early on in the cancer care trajectory that transition to a different survivorship care team will occur at a defined time-point. On the other hand, the dearth of available clinical practice guidelines for adult cancer survivorship is not as readily solved. For survivors of pediatric cancers, the Children's Oncology Group Survivorship Guidelines are integrated into survivorship care planning for this population (see Figure 12.3).[36] For adults, however, a plethora of research is needed to better define and stratify risk for late effects of cancer and cancer treatment and evaluate algorithms for surveillance and early intervention.[37] For now, the limited number of currently available guidelines should be incorporated into relevant SCPs, especially for populations such as breast and colorectal cancer and for individuals who receive mantle radiotherapy, for whom more data are available.[38-41]

Barriers related to a lack of provider support and institutional commitment are also not easily overcome and require multifaceted approaches that support gradual institutional culture change to ensure value for and sustainability of survivorship programming.[31] Advocacy efforts by survivors themselves, as well as increasing requirements by other external forces, including accrediting bodies,[28] should help to influence institutional culture changes toward greater valuing of survivorship care, including the distribution of SCPs. Pursuit and attainment of philanthropic and grant funding are also likely to accelerate progress.

More comprehensive data relevant to overcoming barriers to survivorship care planning will soon be available. A comprehensive analysis of barriers to the provision of SCPs is the focus of a mixed methods study across the LIVE**STRONG** COE Network that examines solutions to overcoming these barriers.[42] Data analysis is currently under way and will hopefully provide further insights into overcoming obstacles using creative approaches.

EXTERNAL FORCES INFLUENCING SURVIVORSHIP CARE PLANNING

For some time, a number of organizations have identified the provision of an SCP as a key component of quality cancer care. The Association of Community Cancer Centers adopted this process as a key characteristic of survivorship services in its 2008 Cancer Program Guidelines,[43] and the ASCO has included the provision of an SCP as a quality indicator in its Quality Oncology Practice Initiative (QOPI) program.[44] However, only recently is provision of these documents becoming tied to accreditation of cancer programs. The American College of Surgeon's Commission on Cancer has added a requirement for survivorship care planning into its working draft of its Cancer Program Standards 2012: Ensuring Patient-Centered Care, available online.[28] Proposed standard 3.3 states that institutional cancer committees must develop and implement a process to disseminate an SCP to patients as they are completing treatment. The standard identifies the principal provider(s) who coordinated cancer treatment for the patient as responsible for preparing this document, which should be based on minimum standards advocated by the IOM in its fact sheet on survivorship care planning. Given the large number of cancer centers that are accredited by the American College of Surgeons, this commission on cancer requirement should be a major catalyst for provision of SCPs across a large and heterogeneous number of cancer care settings.

SURVIVORSHIP CARE PLANNING—WHERE ARE WE?

Despite growing pressures to integrate survivorship care planning into routine oncology follow-up care, the distribution of SCPs is not yet standard practice in many cancer care settings, and even when it is, the content of these plans falls short of IOM recommendations. An understanding of survivorship care planning practices across a greater diversity of oncology practice settings is beginning to emerge.

In 2009, the Oncology Nursing Society (ONS) surveyed a random sample of its membership in order to assess survivorship care practices within members' work settings.[26] A sample of 399 eligible nurses responded, with respondent characteristics similar to those of the ONS membership as a whole. Overall, only 37% of nurses reported that an SCP was provided in their work environments. A greater proportion of nurses working in pediatric settings (70%) reported provision of this component of survivorship care compared to nurses working in adult settings (33%). The latter finding was not surprising given that the field of pediatric cancer survivorship has a much longer history than that of adult cancer survivorship.[31]

The most comprehensive data presently available on this topic results from Salz and colleagues' (2011) survey of survivorship care planning practices across the National Cancer Institute's (NCI) network of Cancer Centers.[33] Fifty-three NCI-designated Cancer Centers and Comprehensive Cancer Centers that treated adults as of July 2009 were contacted and asked if they provided SCPs to breast and colorectal patients. If so, they were asked to provide a copy of the plan(s) in use at the center and to answer several questions about scope of use. All 53 centers responded. Less than half (n = 23, 43%) of centers delivered SCPs to breast or colorectal cancer survivors, and the proportion that provided care plans to both populations was even lower at 7.5% (n = 4 centers). Care plans were more commonly provided to breast cancer (n = 21 centers) than colorectal cancer survivors (n = 6 centers). The impact of SCPs was further limited by the reach of care planning efforts. Fifty-two percent of institutions indicated that fewer than half of eligible survivors received SCPs, and an additional 25% of respondents were unable to estimate numbers served. Finally, the content of SCPs among this group fell short of IOM recommendations. No single center's care plan met 100% of the IOM's recommendations for care plans, and while approximately two-thirds of centers included a cancer treatment summary and 50% to 65% included information regarding cancer surveillance testing, only a third of care plans promoted coordination of care by identifying who was responsible for ordering such testing.

Other data support the limited uptake and scope of survivorship care planning across U.S. cancer care settings. An aforementioned study evaluated breast cancer survivorship care planning efforts across the eight academic member institutions of the LIVE**STRONG** Survivorship Centers of Excellence (COE) Network and their community-based affiliates.[42] Although all participating centers provided SCPs, findings are similar to those of Salz and colleagues in terms of both limited concordance with IOM recommendations and limited reach within institutions. Full results will be available in late 2011.

Conclusions and Future Directions

Caring for cancer survivors is complex and providing organization for this care is important. A growing number of organizations and individuals are calling for an SCP to be prepared for each cancer survivor so that survivors and their health care providers are made aware of the details of the cancer diagnosis and treatment, symptoms of concern, late and long-term risks, and special medical and psychosocial concerns, and so as to improve coordination of care and resultant outcomes.[3,28,45,46] Providing a written SCP is only the beginning of the process. It is equally or more important to translate this into a dynamic "living" document that is easy to access, read, understand, and follow. EMRs may contribute to the generation of these care plans and to their accessibility and dissemination within a given health care system. Ultimately, the hope is that survivorship care planning will positively influence cancer survivors' health and quality of life. Both research and clinical efforts are needed to accelerate the creation of comprehensive yet streamlined and efficient SCPs, as well as advance the science of defining best practices in the structure and process of their provision. A plethora of research is needed to examine the efficacy of survivorship care planning with respect to a wide variety of survivorship outcomes and to compare the effectiveness of various approaches to survivorship care planning. Such efforts hold great potential for improving the health care delivery and outcomes of our nation's 12 million and growing cancer survivors.

References

1. Altekruse SF, Kosary CL, Krapcho M, et al. SEER Cancer Statistics Review, 1975–2007. Bethesda, MD: National Cancer Institute,; 2010: http://seer.cancer.gov/csr/1975_2007/.

2. Ries L, Melbert D, Krapcho M, et al. SEER Cancer Statistics Review, 1975–2005. 2008; http://seer.cancer.gov/csr/1975_2005/. Accessed May 15, 2008.

3. Hewitt M, Greenfield S, Stovall E. *From Cancer Patient to Cancer Survivor: Lost in Transition.* Washington, D.C.: The National Academies Press; 2006.

4. Stricker CT, Jacobs LA. Physical late effects in adult cancer survivors. *Oncology: Nurse Edition.* 2008;22(8):33–41.

5. Shulman LN, Jacobs LA, Greenfield S, et al. Cancer care and cancer survivorship care in the United States: will we be able to care for these patients in the future? *Journal of Oncology Practice.* 2009;5(3):119–123.

6. Shulman LN. Challenges and opportunities in developing a cancer survivorship program in the context of current trends in oncology care. Paper presented at American Society of Clinical Oncology; June 7, 2010; Chicago, IL.

7. Grunfeld E, Earle CC. The Interface Between Primary and Oncology Specialty Care: Treatment Through Survivorship. *J Natl Cancer Inst Monogr.* 2010(40): 25–30.

8. Cheung WY, et al Comparisons of Patient and Physician Expectations for Cancer Survivorship Care. *J Clin Oncol.* 2009;27(15):2489–2495.

9. Snyder CF, Earle CC, Herbert RJ, Neville BA, Blackford AL, Frick KD. Preventive care for colorectal cancer survivors: a 5-year longitudinal study. *Journal of Clinical Oncology.* 2008;26(7):1073–1079.

10. Snyder CF, Earle CC, Herbert RJ, Neville BA, Blackford AL, Frick KD. Trends in follow-up and preventive care for colorectal cancer survivors. *Journal of General Internal Medicine.* Mar 2008;23(3):254–259.

11. Earle CC, Burstein HJ, Winer EP, Weeks JC. Quality of non-breast cancer health maintenance among elderly breast cancer survivors. *Journal of Clinical Oncology.* 2003;21(8):1447–1451.

12. Earle CC, Neville BA. Underuse of necessary care among cancer survivors. *Cancer.* 2004;101(8):1712–1719.

13. Presidents Cancer Panel, Living Beyond Cancer: Finding a New Balance. Bethesda, MD: National Cancer Institute; 2004.

14. Houlihan NG, Houlihan NG. Transitioning to cancer survivorship: plans of care. *Oncology (Williston Park).* 2009;23(8 Suppl):42–48.

15. American Society of Clinical Oncology. Chemotherapy Treatment Plan and Summary. http://www.asco.org/ASCOv2/Practice+%26+Guidelines/Quality+Care/ Quality+Measurement+%26+Improvement/Chemotherapy+Treatment+Plan+and +Summary. Accessed February 23, 2011.

16. Haylock PJ, Mitchell SA, Cox T, Temple SV, Curtiss CP. The cancer survivor's prescription for living: Nurses must take the lead in planning care for survivors. *American Journal of Nursing.* 2007;107(4):58–70.

17. Grant ME, Economou D, Ferrell BR. Oncology nurse participation in survivorship care. *Clinical Journal of Oncology Nursing.* 2010;14(6):709–715.

18. Landier W. Survivorship care: Essential components and models of delivery. *Oncology (Williston Park).* 2009;23(4 Suppl):46–53.

19. Oeffinger KC, McCabe MS. Models for delivering survivorship care. *Journal of Clinical Oncology.* 2006;24(32):5117–5124.

20. McCabe MS, Jacobs L. Survivorship care: models and programs. *Seminars in Oncology Nursing.* Aug 2008;24(3):202–207.

21. Survivorship: Integrated care model aims to cut costs, alleviate workload. *The Oncology Watch: News in Review.* February 2009.

22. Ganz PA, Hahn EE. Implementing a survivorship care plan for patients with breast cancer. *Journal of Clinical Oncology.* 2008;26(5):759–767.

23. Rosenberg CA. Living in the Future Cancer Survivorship Program. *Oncology Issues.* 2008;Supplement: ACCC's Comprehensive Survivorship Services: A Practical Guide:S12–S16.

24. Shapiro CL, McCabe MS, Syrjala KL, et al. The LIVESTRONG Center of Excellence Network. *Journal of Cancer Survivorship.* 2009;3(1):4–11.

25. Patton A.M.D. Anderson Breast Cancer Survivor Clinic. *Oncology Issues.* 2010; May/June:44–47.

26. Irwin M, Klemp JR, Glennon C, Frazier LM. Oncology nurses' perspectives on the state of cancer survivorship care: Current practice and barriers to implementation. *Oncology Nursing Forum.* 2011;38(1):E11–E19.

27. Oeffinger KC, Hudson MM, Mertens AC, et al. Increasing rates of breast cancer and cardiac surveillance among high-risk survivors of childhood Hodgkin lymphoma following a mailed, one-page survivorship care plan. *Pediatric Blood & Cancer.* 2010;[Epub ahead of print].

28. Commission on Cancer. Cancer Program Standards 2012: Ensuring Patient-Centered Care (v2). 2011; http://www.facs.org/cancer/coc/cps2012draft.pdf. Accessed February 20, 2011.

29. Mao JJ, Torradas JR, Xie SX, Scott C, Jacobs L. Assessing cancer knowledge and self-efficacy: the potential of treatment summaries in optimizing breast cancer survivorship. Paper presented at: 2010 Biennial Cancer Survivorship Research Conference; June 19, 2010; Washington, DC.

30. Stanton AL, Ganz PA, Kwan L, et al. Outcomes From the Moving Beyond Cancer Psychoeducational, Randomized, Controlled Trial With Breast Cancer Patients. *Journal of Clinical Oncology*. 2005;23(25):6009–6018.

31. Jacobs LA, Palmer SC, Schwartz LA, et al. Adult Cancer Survivorship: Evolution, Research, and Planning Care. *CA: A Cancer Journal for Clinicians*. 2009;59:391–410.

32. Stricker CT, Jacobs LA, Demichele A, Jones A, Risendal B, Palmer SC. Survivorship Care Plan Assessment Checklist (SCPAC): A tool to evaluate breast cancer survivorship care plans. Under review.

33. Salz T, Oeffinger KC, McCabe MS, Layne TM, Bach PB. Survivorship care plans for cancer survivors: Works in Progress. Under review.

34. Houlihan NG. Transitioning to cancer survivorship: Plans of care. *Oncology (Williston Park)*. 2009;23(8 Suppl):42–48.

35. ASCO Electronic Health Record Roundtable. Ensuring continuity of care through electronic health records. *Journal of Oncology Practice*. 2007;3(3):137–142.

36. CureSearch: Children's Oncology Group. Long-Term Follow-Up Guidelines for Survivors of Childhood, Adolescent, and Young Adult Cancers. Version 3.0. 2008; http://survivorshipguidelines.org/pdf/LTFUGuidelines.pdf. Accessed February 21, 2011.

37. Earle CC. Long term care planning for cancer survivors: a health services research agenda. *Journal of Cancer Survivorship*. 2007;1(1):64–74.

38. Hillner BE, Ingle JN, Chlebowski RT, et al. American Society of Clinical Oncology 2003 update on the role of bisphosphonates and bone health issues in women with breast cancer. *Journal of Clinical Oncology*. 2003;21(21):4042–4057.

39. Khatcheressian JL, Wolff AC, Smith TJ, et al. American Society of Clinical Oncology 2006 update of the breast cancer follow-up and management guidelines in the adjuvant setting. *Journal of Clinical Oncology*. 2006;24(31):5091–5097.

40. National Comprehensive Cancer Network (NCCN). NCCN Clinical Practice Guidelines in Oncology: Hodgkin's Lymphoma v.2.2010. 2010; http://www.nccn.org/professionals/physician_gls/pdf/hodgkins.pdf. Accessed February 23, 2011.

41. National Comprehensive Cancer Network (NCCN). NCCN Clinical Practice Guidelines in Oncology: Colon Cancer (v.2.2011). 2011; http://www.nccn.org/professionals/physician_gls/pdf/colon.pdf. Accessed February 23, 2011.

42. Stricker CT. Evaluating treatment summaries and survivorship care plans within the LIVESTRONG Survivorship Centers of Excellence Network: Project update. *Biannual meeting of the LIVESTRONG Survivorship Center of Excellence Network* Vol Austin, TX; 2010.

43. Association of Community Cancer Centers. ACCC's Cancer Program Guidelines 2008: Survivorship Services: Chapter 4, Section 16. *Oncology Issues*. 2008; Supplement: ACCC's Comprehensive Survivorship Services: A Practical Guide:S6.

44. American Society of Clinical Oncology. QOPI: The Quality Oncology Practice Initiative (QOPI) http://qopi.asco.org/. Accessed February 20, 2011.

45. Earle CC. Failing to plan is planning to fail: improving the quality of care with survivorship care plans. *J Clin Oncol.* Nov 10 2006;24(32):5112–5116.

46. Ganz PA, Casillas J, Hahn EE, Ganz PA, Casillas J, Hahn EE. Ensuring quality care for cancer survivors: implementing the survivorship care plan. *Seminars in Oncology Nursing.* Aug 2008;24(3):208–217.

13

CANCER SURVIVORSHIP AND THE ROLE OF REHABILITATION

JULIE K. SILVER, MD, AND LISA SCHULZ SLOWMAN, OTR

INTRODUCTION

Receiving the diagnosis of cancer, although frightening and with many consequences, no longer carries with it an expectation for certain death in a relatively short period of time. Surviving cancer is now the norm for many types of the disease. The five-year survival rate for cancer from 1999 to 2006 was 66%,[1] and with new and emerging diagnostic methods and treatments, those numbers will rise. The number of individuals diagnosed with cancer is also increasing, with an estimated 1.5 million new cases diagnosed in the United States in 2010.[2] Whether one is cured, in remission or living with cancer as a chronic condition, the treatments associated with most types of this multifaceted disease cause innumerable side effects that often have deleterious effects on both physical and emotional function. The decreases may be transient during the course of treatment or permanent—as a result of the cancer itself or the treatment. Regardless, they offer an opportunity for rehabilitation to be used to improve function and quality of life.

Certainly one reason for improved survival rates include the advances in the diagnosis and treatment of cancer. However, while cancer is being diagnosed and treated earlier, improving survival,[3] this is not necessarily morbidity. In fact, many new treatments cause an increase in morbidity. With these advances in treatment regimens come new side effects and potential for morbidity. For instance, targeted therapies, drugs or substances that interfere with the specific components of the cancer cells, are being developed and more widely used. However, the use of many (perhaps all) of these new treatments also bring about new and different side effects that negatively impact function.

For example, rehabilitation issues in breast cancer survivors have been well documented, including the use of aromatase inhibitors (AIs) in postmenopausal women that has led to an increased morbidity in some of these women with a relatively newly identified condition now called Arthralgia

Syndrome.[4] The relatively new use of AIs in the treatment of breast cancer is has led to a notable increase in pain and thus decrease in physical function for many women who take these drugs. AIs are drugs that interfere with estrogen's ability to promote the growth of estrogen receptor (ER) positive breast cancers. With the increased use of these drugs, women began suffering new side effects, including musculoskeletal pain and stiffness, particularly joint pain.[5] The onset of symptoms has been shown to usually occur within three months of beginning AI therapy; is inversely related to the time since cessation of menstrual function; and, the most frequently affected joints are the wrist/hands, ankles/feet, elbows, and knees.[6] Arthralgia syndrome is only one potential side effect of these drugs—there are many others, including increased risk of osteoporosis, which carries with it significant long-term and usually irreversible morbidity issues.

There are many examples of how these new treatments come with a physical functioning price. They may prolong lives, but not without significant side effects, increased morbidity, and decreased function and quality of life.

The combination of increased survival and development of new treatments, often with debilitating side effects, results in a larger survivor population living with cancer as a chronic condition and with more functional deficits. Survivors are often living with cancer as a chronic disease with deficits that can be improved through rehabilitation. The chronic side effects of treatments may be accepted by health care providers and patients as a price to pay for battling the cancer; both of which limit the referral of cancer survivors to rehabilitation to address these needs and improve functional outcomes.[7]

CANCER REHABILITATION AND SURVIVORSHIP CARE PLANS

In 2005, the Institute of Medicine (IOM) released a consensus report titled *From Cancer Patient to Cancer Survivor: Lost in Transition*.[8] This report documented the many unmet needs of cancer survivors and detailed 10 recommendations, including that survivorship should be developed as a distinct phase of cancer care. Cancer rehabilitation should play a major role in this phase of cancer care; it can be viewed as the missing piece and a key component in the survivorship puzzle. Before encouraging cancer survivors to accept a new normal, it is important to offer them cancer rehabilitation interventions—thereby helping them to optimally heal, regardless of their cancer type, stage, or prognosis.[9]

The widespread adoption of survivorship care plans is already taking place. This is an important initial step in developing survivorship as a distinct phase of care. However, the plan is just the beginning. A plan is not effective unless there are support resources developed and appropriate services available for survivors. Therefore, the obvious first step is to include cancer rehabilitation as part of the survivorship care plan, but that's not enough. Going beyond the first step means that medical professionals understand the rehabilitation needs of cancer survivors and how to implement services that will meet these needs.

REHABILITATION NEEDS OF CANCER SURVIVORS

The medical specialty of Physical Medicine and Rehabilitation (PM&R) was formed in large part because of World War II. Veterans who so bravely fought for our country deserved the best possible medical care to help them recover from their injuries. Today, when soldiers are injured, they are sent to rehab. The military has many highly trained physiatrists (doctors), physical, occupational and speech therapists and rehabilitation nurses who provide the rehabilitation care. Of course, once they are finished with rehabilitation, there are often other important interventions that may help with their recovery, including exercise classes. A similar paradigm should exist for cancer rehabilitation.

In the rehabilitation medicine setting, the most comprehensive care is offered by doctors (physiatrists) who work with a team of highly trained health care professionals such as physical, occupational, and speech therapists to address the patient's specific health (e.g., physical, cognitive, functional psychosocial) issues. It is these professionals who are the core providers of cancer rehabilitation along with nurses, mental health professionals, and dieticians. Recognition of the need for and referral to rehabilitation must be embraced by the entire oncology team including oncologists, primary care doctors and other physicians—anyone providing care to cancer survivors. Cancer rehabilitation seeks to reduce and possibly eliminate functional deficits associated with cancer and its treatment and cancer rehabilitation has become a recognized subspecialty.[10]

Cancer rehab should mirror stroke rehab and other types of rehabilitation that is offered to individuals who suffer from serious injuries and illnesses. For example, when cancer patients are finished with their acute treatment, sometimes they are referred to a group exercise class rather than more traditional rehabilitation services. On the other hand, if a patient has a stroke, a referral to an exercise class would usually not be the first (or only) rehab offered. Individualized rehabilitation interventions would typically be provided by physiatrists, physical/occupational/speech therapists, and rehabilitation nurses. Cancer survivors are often not afforded this level of care and instead of rehabilitation medical treatment—specifically designed to meet the patient's needs based on an extensive evaluation and provided one-to-one in multiple sessions over weeks to months—patients are often referred to a lower level of care that may or may not involve health care professionals. Although exercise classes (and individual sessions with a personal trainer or cancer exercise trainer) as well as other complementary services (e.g., yoga, massage, Reiki) have a role in helping cancer survivors, this is not ideal as a first or only step for many survivors.

Cancer and its treatment can result in deficits in many realms. These include physical, cognitive, and psychosocial function. Rehabilitation programs are appropriate to address these types of deficit areas. Physical deficits are the most easily understood as being amenable to rehabilitation, but these as well as problems in other areas need to be recognized in the cancer survivor, and identified as being deficits that can be improved through rehabilitation interventions.[11]

For example:

- A breast cancer survivor who has chemotherapy-induced peripheral neuropathy (CIPN) may be referred to physiatry for pain management as well as physical and occupational therapy for functional deficits.
- A lung cancer survivor who is reporting to his oncologist that he is feeling unsteady or even falling occasionally should be referred to physical therapy to assess, then address balance and gait issues.
- A melanoma survivor who has not been able to return to her pre-morbid level of function, has cancer-related fatigue, and requires some assistance with instrumental activities of daily living (IADLs) such as shopping and completing household chores, would benefit from referral to physical and occupational therapy for evaluation and to address these physical and functional deficits.
- A head and neck cancer survivor who has underwent surgical resection and radiation treatment and has limited cervical range of motion as well as difficulty with swallowing could benefit from a physiatry consultation that may include either trigger point or botulinum toxin injections as well as a referral to speech language pathology for dysphagia and an occupational or physical therapy consultation to address cervical range, posture, and upper-body strength.
- A brain tumor survivor with executive function deficits may benefit from occupational therapy or speech language pathology intervention to address high-level cognitive issues and develop a rehabilitation program to help him maximize his success in returning to his pre-cancer vocation as a sales executive.

Rehabilitation intervention may be appropriate throughout the continuum of care for cancer survivors. The key is to identify problems that can be addressed in rehabilitation.[12] There are some problems that are common to many cancer survivors:

- Difficulty returning to pre-morbid activities
- Difficulty with activities of daily living (ADLs) (e.g., bathing, dressing)
- Difficulty with IADLs (e.g., chores/shopping)
- Weakness
- Fatigue
- Balance and gait problems
- History of falls
- Musculoskeletal or neuropathic pain
- Adaptive equipment needs
- Durable medical equipment (DME) needs
- General deconditioning (need instruction on an appropriate exercise program)

Cancer survivors also have problems that are unique to specific types of cancer. Table 13.1 is a partial list of some of the areas that rehabilitation can address by cancer type.

TABLE 13.1 WHEN TO REFER TO PATIENTS FOR CANCER REHABILITATION

Type of Cancer	Referral to Rehabilitation to address*
Brain Tumor (rehabilitation needs will be dependent upon tumor location)	• Cognitive problems • Perceptual problems • Sensory deficits • Speech issues • Swallowing problems
Breast	• Scar adhesions (post surgical) • Shoulder problems • Lymphedema • Post-mastectomy Pain Syndrome (PMPS) • Brachial plexopathy (e.g., radiation-induced) • Cognitive problems • Sexual dysfunction • Chemotherapy-induced polyneuropathy (CIPN)
Lung	• Dyspnea on exertion • Scar adhesions (post surgical) • Shoulder problems • Brachial plexopathy (e.g., radiation-induced) • Cognitive problems • Chemotherapy-induced polyneuropathy (CIPN)
Melanoma	• Scar adhesions (post surgical) • Shoulder problems • Lymphedema • Cognitive problems
Head & Neck	• Scar adhesions (post surgical) • Swallowing issues • Speech problems • Shoulder problems • Headaches • Limited jaw excursion • Difficulty with cervical range of motion • Muscular asymmetry • Scapular winging • Cognitive problems • Chemotherapy-induced polyneuropathy (CIPN)
Metastatic Disease	• Scar adhesions (post surgical) • Compression neuropathy • Limited motion • Cognitive problems

(Continued)

TABLE 13.1 WHEN TO REFER TO PATIENTS FOR CANCER REHABILITATION (*Continued*)

Type of Cancer	Referral to Rehabilitation to address*
Lymphoma	• Scar adhesions (post surgical) • Cervical radiculopathy • Cervical dystonia • Lumbosacral plexopathy • Radiation fibrosis syndrome (e.g., spasticity, nerve root issues, myopathy) • Lymphedema • Cognitive problems • Chemotherapy-induced polyneuropathy (CIPN)
Ovarian	• Scar adhesions (post surgical) • Lumbosacral plexopathy • Urinary Incontinence • Lymphedema • Cognitive problems • Sexual dysfunction • Chemotherapy-induced polyneuropathy (CIPN)
Testicular	• Lumbosacral plexopathy • Scar adhesions (post surgical) • Cognitive problems • Sexual dysfunction • Chemotherapy-induced polyneuropathy (CIPN)
Colon	• Scar adhesions (post surgical) • Lumbosacral plexopathy • Compression neuropathy • Urinary incontinence • Cognitive problems • Sexual dysfunction • Chemotherapy-induced polyneuropathy (CIPN)
Prostate	• Compression neuropathy • Lymphedema • Urinary incontinence • Sexual dysfunction • Cognitive problems • Chemotherapy-induced polyneuropathy (CIPN)

*These are examples and this is not intended to be a comprehensive list
Source: Oncology Rehab Partners.

Rehabilitation services for cancer survivors can be provided in many settings including outpatient, acute care hospital, inpatient rehabilitation, and home care. Rehabilitation may even be appropriate prior to surgical intervention in some populations to provide patient education and a baseline assessment of function.[13] The key, regardless of the setting or stage of treatment, is to identify the survivor's rehabilitation needs and facilitate the referral to the appropriate rehabilitation clinician to address those needs. Cancer rehabilitation should be available to patients from the time of presentation through treatment and recovery or disease progression—throughout survivorship.[14]

REHABILITATION AND SURVIVORSHIP CARE

In order to help identify what rehabilitation can offer to cancer survivors and include that in every institution that offers care to cancer survivors, consider the following rehabilitation recommendations:

- Every institution that provides comprehensive cancer services should offer cancer rehabilitation.
- Cancer rehabilitation should be delivered by professionals who have health care degrees (e.g., MD, DO, PT, OT, SLP, RN), are highly skilled in the diagnosis and treatment of rehabilitation medical issues, including cancer-specific training, and are ideally reimbursed for their care by third party payers.
- Mental health services are an important part of cancer rehabilitation and social workers, psychologists and psychiatrists should be included in the multidisciplinary rehabilitation team.
- Exercise physiologists, trainers, and other experts in physical activity have an important role to play in helping people recover, and should be part of the referral process, usually after completion of formal cancer rehabilitation.
- Survivors should be referred first to the highest level of rehabilitation care that is covered by their health insurance and then transitioned to other providers and services when appropriate.

The current state of cancer rehabilitation is not ideal. There is a lack of understanding among many health care providers and hospital administrators about how rehabilitation interventions should fit into the survivorship puzzle. This is in part due to the lack of or incomplete education and training for clinicians in cancer rehabilitation. Therefore, many survivors who now have a post-acute treatment plan of care still do not receive rehabilitation services. The solution to the lack of including cancer rehabilitation services for survivors hinges on two things:

1. The education of clinicians and administrators about evidence-based cancer rehabilitation; and
2. The implementation of rehabilitation services in cancer centers, hospitals, and group and solo practices.

Indeed, too often survivors live with more pain, fatigue and disability than they need to. Cancer rehabilitation is the next frontier in survivorship care.

The American College of Surgeons' Commission on Cancer (CoC) is to be commended for requiring that cancer rehabilitation be provided by any program that is accredited by them.[15] Although rehabilitation is a requirement, there have yet to be established best practices as to what the rehabilitation should include or how a rehabilitation program should be implemented. While cancer rehabilitation is undeniably an important part of developing cancer survivorship as a distinct phase of care, hospitals and cancer centers need to work toward offering well executed, integrated, multidisciplinary cancer rehabilitation services.

Although the necessary resources to develop a multidisciplinary cancer rehab program are often available within an institution, the actual implementation of cancer rehab is fragmented. For example, the rehab may consist of referring patients to physical therapists who are part of the rehabilitation department that exists in a different location than the cancer center. These rehabilitation clinicians may have little or no contact with the oncology team. Going beyond simply offering rehabilitation services in a somewhat fragmented approach, a best practices model should have:

- Rehabilitation clinicians with expertise in treatment of cancer survivors who are up to date with evidenced-based care
- Oncologists who are aware of and understand the available rehabilitation needs of their patients and know how to refer them appropriately for services

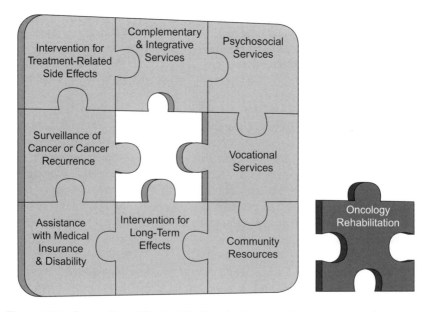

Figure 13.1. Cancer Rehabilitation Fits Into the Survivorship Care Puzzle. (Adapted from Oncology Rehab Partners.)

- Administrators who support the implementation of well coordinated, multi-disciplinary cancer rehab teams as an integrated component of the care provided to survivors
- Multidisciplinary teams that are ideally located in the same physical space or at least have a system to communicate regularly with each other in a programmatic manner

Barriers to developing a comprehensive cancer rehabilitation program may include a lack of understanding about how rehabilitation can positively impact survivor outcomes, poor communication between oncology and rehabilitation clinicians, perceived (or real) lack of identifiable rehabilitation services, perceived (or real) fear that rehabilitation professionals are not educated about how best to treat oncology patients, and discomfort (due to lack of training) of the rehabilitation clinicians in treating cancer survivors.

AN EXAMPLE OF A MODEL CANCER REHAB PROGRAM

The authors of this chapter have worked with many cancer centers and hospitals to help them develop and implement cancer rehabilitation services through the STAR (Survivorship Training and Rehab) certifications.[16] The STAR certifications were developed by the first author for institutions and individuals in order to quickly and effectively train clinicians and implement institutionally based cancer rehab programs with third party payer reimbursable services. The components of the STAR Program™, which is designed to help hospitals and cancer centers develop a cancer rehabilitation service line that is consistent with best practices, includes comprehensive training for clinicians that focuses on evidence-based care. Utilizing standardized tools that measure current physical deficits and can be used to track outcomes is an important part of all medical care. Developing not only individual clinician skill sets, but multidisciplinary team approaches (e.g., through in-service education, case presentations, communication strategies), is also part of providing excellent care. This shared knowledge and team participation helps to dissolve some of the barriers to cancer rehabilitation and promotes ongoing communication between the clinicians providing survivor care.

THE FUTURE OF CANCER REHABILITATION

In order to provide excellent survivorship care, which must include rehabilitation as a component, a commitment must be made to:

- Providing the best possible survivorship services
- Acknowledging that cancer rehabilitation should be the standard of care
- Offering every survivor the opportunity to heal as well as possible, even if living with cancer
- Bringing together two different medical disciplines—oncology and rehabilitation
- Training clinicians to become experts in cancer rehabilitation

- Develop multidisciplinary teams that provide comprehensive cancer rehab care
- Understand that cancer rehabilitation is typically reimbursable care
- Utilize evidence-based tools to identify deficits, track outcomes, and promote clinical research

It is hard to imagine a future where cancer rehabilitation is not the standard of care in all countries that offer excellent oncology treatment. The question remains then, not *if* it will become the standard of care, but *when*. Already, there are many progressive hospitals and cancer centers that have developed excellent cancer rehabilitation services for survivors. Their leadership understands that cancer rehab is a central part of the survivorship care puzzle and should be available to those who may benefit.

NOTES

1. National Cancer Institute: Survey and Epidemiology and End Results [SEER] Stat Facts Sheets: All Sites. Available at http://seer.cancer.gove/statfacts/huml/all.html. Accessed January 2011.

2. National Cancer Institute: Survey and Epidemiology and End Results [SEER] Stat Facts Sheets: All Sites. Available at http://seer.cancer.gove/statfacts/huml/all.html. Accessed January 2011.

3. International Association for the Study of Lung Cancer (2010, June 15). Lung cancer research concludes that early diagnosis is key to improving survival. ScienceDaily. Retrieved January 11, 2011, from http://www.sciencedaily.com/releas es/2010/06/100615112225.htm.

4. Silver JK. Rehabilitation in women with breast cancer. *Phys Med Rehabil Clin N Am.* 2007 Aug;18(3):521–537.

5. Burstein HJ, Winer EP. Aromatase inhibitors and arthralgias: a new frontier in symptom management for breast cancer survivors. *J Clin Oncol.* 2007;25(25):3797–3799.

6. Mao JJ, Stricker C, Bruner D, et al. Patterns and risk factors associated with aromatase inhibitor-related arthralgia among breast cancer survivors. *Cancer.* 2009 Aug 15;115(16):3631–3639.

7. Franklin D. Facing forward: meeting the rehabilitation needs of cancer survivors. ONCOLOGY *Nurse Edition.* 2010; 24(10):1–7.

8. Hewitt M et al. From Cancer Patient to Cancer Survivor: Lost in Transition. Washington, DC: National Academies Press, 2006.

9. Silver JK. Prescriptions for optimal healing. PM&R 2010; 2(2):94–100.

10. Franklin D. Facing forward: meeting the rehabilitation needs of cancer survivors. ONCOLOGY Nurse Edition. 2010; 24(10):1–7.

11. Silver JK, Gilchrist LS. Cancer rehabilitation with a focus on evidence-based outpatient physical and occupational therapy interventions. *Am J Phys Med Rehabil.* 2011;90(suppl 1).

12. Silver JK. Prescriptions for optimal healing. PMR. 2010 Feb;2(2):94–100.

13. Springer BA, Levy E, McGarvey C, et al. Pre-operative assessment enables early diagnosis and recovery of shoulder function in patients with breast cancer. *Breast Cancer Res Treat.* 2010;120(1):135–147.

14. Franklin D. Facing forward: meeting the rehabilitation needs of cancer survivors. ONCOLOGY Nurse Edition. 2010; 24(10):1–7.

15. Commission on Cancer. Cancer program accreditation. Available at http://www.facs.org/cancer/coc/whatis.html. Accessed January 2011.

16. Silver JK. A new frontier. Advance for physical therapy and rehab medicine. 2010 Sept;21(20):15–17.

14

TEACHING NUTRITION IN CANCER SURVIVORSHIP

STACY KENNEDY, MPH, RD, CSO, LDN, AND ABIGAIL HUEBER, DI

BACKGROUND AND RESEARCH

The understanding of nutrition's influence on cancer survivorship is a rapidly growing field. One of the most important things to encourage cancer survivorship is to eat a healthful diet, rich in fruits, vegetables, whole grains, lean protein sources, and omega-3 fatty acids. The vibrant colors of plant-based fruits and vegetables provide naturally occurring compounds called phytonutrients. Phytonutrients are known to contain anti-cancer properties and help support immune function. A diet rich in plant-based foods (fruits, vegetables, whole grains, spices, herbs, tea, nuts, seeds, and beans) provides essential vitamins, nutrients, and antioxidants that promote long-term health, weight management, and may reduce the risk of cancer recurrence.

Cancer survivorship is a relatively new field. Emerging research pertaining to nutrition-based interventions in cancer survivorship point to specific actions that can be taken to increase health; such as, consuming a largely plant-based diet and focus on weight management as well as an individualized supplemental regimen, which may include vitamin D and omega-3 fatty acids. The American Cancer Society publishes the Nutrition and Physical Activity Guidelines, which are updated every five years to maintain a standard for diet and physical activity patterns in Americans. These guidelines represent the most current scientific evidence related to diet, activity patterns, and cancer risk. The guidelines representing the most conclusive data on association with cancer risk are based around four main recommendations: (1) eat a variety of healthful foods, with an emphasis on plant sources, (2) adopt a physically active lifestyle, (3) maintain a healthful weight throughout life, and (4) if you drink alcoholic beverages, limit consumption. These four key recommendations represent a general overview of healthful lifestyle choices. The significance of these recommendations is highlighted by recent statistical findings published in a report by the American Institute for Cancer Research (AICR) along with the World Cancer Research Fund (WCRF). Through the analysis of over 7,000 scientific studies on food, nutrition, and physical activity in relation to cancer risk, they found that about one third of the cancers worldwide could be avoided through proper diet and physical activity.[1] The dietary recommendations for cancer prevention closely mirror those for cancer survivorship. Key recommendations emphasize dietary changes that promote overall health and highlight prevention of secondary cancer development. This chapter will focus on details of diet to promote cancer survivorship.

DIETARY RECOMMENDATIONS

Balanced Plate and Portion Sizes

A fundamental aspect of maintaining a healthful diet is to pay particular attention to consuming a balanced plate at each meal. Epidemiological studies have shown that populations whose diets are high in vegetables and fruits

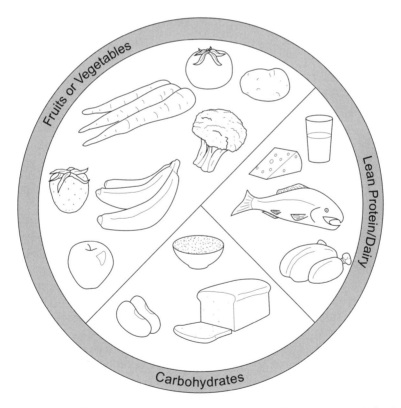

Figure 14.1. A well-balanced plate, divided into proper portion sizes for each food major food group. (Illustration by Lee Whale, Dana-Farber Cancer Institute.)

and low in animal fat, meat and/or calories have a reduced risk of most common types of cancer. It is recommended to consume whole foods and broad-based dietary patterns that encourage the incorporation of greater varieties of foods.[2] These findings support the importance of a balanced plate. A balanced plate consists of 50% fruits or vegetables, 25% carbohydrate such as a whole grain option and 25% lean protein such as wild fish. Figure 14.1 depicts a well-balanced plate, divided into proper portion sizes for each food major food group.

The portion sizes for each food group is another aspect that is fundamental in creating a balanced, healthy plate and maintaining a healthy weight. Knowing what constitutes a serving is very important, survivors are encouraged to read the nutrition labels of all food products to note what constitutes a serving for that item.

The goal is to aim for 5–10 servings of colorful fruits and vegetables every day.

What Counts as a Serving?

One serving = 1 cup leafy greens, berries or melon chunks
½ cup for all other fruits and vegetables
1 medium fruit/vegetable (e.g., apple, orange)
−¼ cup dried fruit
−¾ cup juice

Serving size for protein should be about three ounces of a lean protein source, such as chicken, fish, or tofu. To visualize this serving size, it is about the same size as a standard deck of cards. A serving size for whole grains should be also about two–three ounces; in general one ounce is equivalent to one slice of bread, one cup of ready-to-eat cereal or one-half cup cooked rice, pasta, or grain.

Plant-Based Diet

A large amount of evidence has put emphasis on consuming a largely plant-based diet for both optimal health as well as reduction in cancer risk and promotion of survivorship. Eating five or more servings of a variety of fruits and vegetables each day is recommended by the American Cancer Society. Trying to include a vegetable or fruit at every meal and as well as for snacks can facilitate reaching the recommended serving size. It is important to include a variety of different types and kinds of fruits and vegetables. Epidemiological studies done by the American Cancer Institute found that an increase in the consumption of fruits and vegetables has been associated with a lower risk of lung, oral, esophageal, stomach, and colon cancer.[3]

In order to gain the beneficial effects of fruits and vegetables it is recommended to consume the foods in their whole form rather than from isolated supplement sources. This is because a major part of total anticancer activity

these foods provide is from the combination of the different phytonutrients working together within the whole fruit or vegetable. Phytonutrients
are also known as phytochemicals; phytonutrients will be the term used
throughout the rest of the paper. Fruits and vegetables are complex foods
that can contain more than 100 potentially beneficial vitamins, minerals,
fiber, and other substances that may help prevent cancer. These foods also
contain specific phytonutrients such as carotenoids, flavinoids, terpenes, ste-
rols, indoles, and phenols that have all shown promise in having anti-cancer
abilities.[4] These powerful components in plant-derived foods work synergis-
tically together to provide a multifaceted defense strategy that shows much
greater promise than consumption of any individual single-component drug
or supplement.[5]

Phytonutrients

Phytonutrients are plant-based substances that are an innate part of the
plant—they function as the plants own immune system. Any plant-derived food
such as, fruits, vegetables, herbs, spices, and whole grains provides an endless
variety of phytonutrients with over 2,000 known types.[6] Research has deduced
four general mechanisms of actions for the cancer-reducing benefits of these
compounds: they (1) work largely as antioxidants that disrupt the activities of
carcinogens in the human body, (2) work as modulators for the metabolism of
toxic chemicals from environmental exposure, (3) suppress cellular proliferation which can lead to tumor formation, and (4) modulate tumor cell biology.
It is recommended to eat a variety of different colored fruits, vegetables, whole
grains, and spices because many of the phytonutrient compounds that provide
the health benefits are attributed to giving each fruit or vegetable its specific
color. Hundreds of phytonutrients exists within fruits and vegetables each ex-
hibiting individual health benefits and characteristics. A selection of the more
extensively studied phytonutrient food groups are outlined below.

Crucifers

Cruciferous vegetables contain a high amount of phytonutrients that have
been linked to cancer prevention and detoxification of cancer causing agents.
This family of vegetables includes broccoli, cabbage, cauliflower, Brussels
sprouts, bok choy, dark leafy greens, and watercress. These vegetables have
been shown to contain a phytonutrient known as Indol-3-Carbinol (I3C),
which has shown great promise in reducing the risk of breast cancer in women
as well as has shown to interfere with prostate cancer cell growth in both test-
tube and animal studies. Evidence has also been attributed to its effects against
the growth of tumors in lung and colon cancers. I3C as well as an additional
phytonutrient, sulforaphane, elicit active detoxification properties through acti-
vation of enzymes within the liver that work to convert cancer-causing chemicals to forms that can be excreted by the body.[7]

Flavonoids

Flavonoids are a family of phytonutrients found in berries, cherries, red and purple grapes, currants, pomegranates, walnuts, apples with skin, citrus, red onions, tomatoes, bell peppers, red wine, and grape juice. Research has highlighted the specific phytonutrient, ellagic acid, as a potent anti-cancer agent. In animal and test-tube studies, ellagic acid has shown to interfere with the steps that lead to uncontrolled cell growth and induce cell death of abnormal cells. It has also shown to stimulate detoxification enzymes in the liver. Other specific phytochemicals of this family include glucarate, resveratrol, quercetin, and anthocyanins. Research has shown glucarate to neutralize several cancer-causing compounds that arise from cooking proteins, such as poultry, at high temperatures. It has also shown promise in defense against estrogen-linked cancers, by preventing the reabsorption of estrogen from bile in the digestive tract; this may cause a reduction in the concentration of estrogen in the body. Anthocyanins, another subset of flavonoids, have shown promise in having anti-tumor activity and at the same time they inhibit enzymes in the liver that synthesize cholesterol.[8]

Carotenoids

There are over 600 compounds within the carotenoid family including the better known beta-carotene, along with lesser known alpha-carotene, crypoxanthin, lycopene, lutein, and zeaxanthin, which have each been linked to potential health benefits. Research has shown the carotenoid family to play a role in the prevention of colon, prostate, breast, and lung cancer. Two Harvard studies examining over 124,000 people, showed a 32% reduction in the risk of lung cancer in individuals that consumed a variety of high carotenoid-containing foods. However, the protective benefits were not examined in individuals taking carotenoid supplements; highlighting the importance of consuming the phytonutrients as part of the whole food.[9] Breast cancer studies have also showed promise in carotenoid intake. A longitudinal cohort study, conducted by the Women's Healthy Eating and Living Group, examined the relationship between 3,043 women diagnosed with early-stage breast cancer and blood levels of carotenoids in relation to cancer reoccurrence and survival. High biological exposure to carotenoids through dietary consumption of fruits and vegetables showed a significant likelihood of breast cancer-free survival over the six-year time frame.[10]

Another member of the carotenoid family that has received a great deal of attention for its anticancer abilities is lycopene. It is found primarily in deep red and orange plants, most specifically in tomatoes, and has been shown to act as an antioxidant as well as enhance cell-to-cell communication. It has shown particular promise in reducing the risk of prostate cancer; research has shown that those who consume cooked tomatoes four times per week had a 33% lower risk of prostate cancer that those who did not consume cooked tomatoes. Consuming cooked tomatoes prepared using a healthy fat such as olive oil has shown to be the most effective way to ensure absorption into the body, due to lycopene being a fat-soluble vitamin that requires this nutrient for absorption.[11] Carontenoids have also demonstrated great influence in eye health; in particular lutein and zeaxanthin protect the macula and retina of the eye from photo-damage. Research has shown that 10 mg of dietary lutein per day may reduce the risk of developing age-related macular degeneration and cataracts. A cup of cooked kale or spinach contains on average 30 mg, three times this recommended dose.

Terpenes

Terpenes are a group of phytonutrients that are found in citrus fruits; these compounds are found in the peel, membranes, seeds, flesh, and juice of the citrus fruit. More than 40 limonoid compounds exist, with specific compounds of interest including d-limonene, limonin, and nomilin. These compounds have been shown to elicit anti-cancer activities, as well as activate the detoxification enzymes in the liver to rid the body of cancer-causing agents.[12]

Nutrition Issues

Increasing the amount of fruits and vegetables one consumes has not only shown benefits for fighting cancer but also for aiding in the prevention of other disease conditions that pose a risk for cancer survivors. Two studies done at Harvard assessed risk for heart attack and stroke in 110,000 people who consumed 8 or more servings of fruits and vegetables a day versus those who consumed only 1.5 servings or less a day. The studies found that the group who consumed the 8 or more servings was 30% less likely to have a heart attack or stroke than the group consuming 1.5 or less.[13]

The consumption of flavonoid containing fruits and vegetables has been linked to a reduced risk of Type 2 diabetes. More specifically a Harvard study in 40,000 women found that the consumption of at least one apple with skin a day was found to reduce Type 2 diabetes risk by 28% compared with those that did not consume apples.[14] Flavonoid compounds resveratrol and quercetin have also been shown to provide protection against heart disease; working to reduce inflammation, preventing the clumping of blood platelets, and protecting against cholesterol from being converted to unsafe compounds that cause damage to the cardiovascular system.[15] Resveratrol is found largely in the skins of grapes and green tea; quercetin is found in the skins of apples.

Some phytonutrients are temperature sensitive and experience degradation with exposure to high heat, however, others become more bioavailable when eaten in cooked forms. Therefore, it is recommended to consume a variety of different kinds of fruits and vegetables in both cooked and raw forms. The vast array of phytonutrients and the numerous studies that exist supporting the specific health claims of each can be overwhelming. Therefore, if you aim to consume a variety of all types of fruits and vegetables you will be sure to get your fair share of each them! Make it a goal to consume a least two servings of fruit or vegetables by noon each day and retrain your thinking to create a meal around them. Be sure to fill half of your plate with fruits and vegetables in all colors and try adding orange and lemon zest to breads, casseroles, and desserts to spice up flavor and add a protective kick to those meals!

Plant-based diets have shown to aid in weight management as well as lower cholesterol, blood pressure, and blood sugar, all of which can contribute to many health concerns such as insulin resistance and hypertension. Increased intake has also shown to improve bowl regularity and colon health as well as reduce the risk of cataracts, macular degeneration, and vision loss and guard against development of many cancer types. The Women's Healthy Eating and Living study (WHEL) conducted an observational analysis that examined women who consumed a low-fat diet high in fruits and vegetables (more than five servings/day) and who exercised an amount equivalent to walking 30 minutes six days per week had a significant survival advantage. This advantage was only observed in women who engaged in both behaviors and not one or the other.[16] This study emphasizes the importance of maintaining a regular exercise regime as well as consuming a balanced diet to promote weight management and overall health.

Fats

It is highly recommended to limit the consumption of high-fat foods, particularly those from animal sources such as red meats and heavily processed, high-fat convenience foods. The Women's Intervention Nutrition Study observed breast cancer survivors relative cancer risk in conjunction with dietary fat consumption. It was found that survivors who had postmenopausal breast cancer and consumed a low-fat diet of 33 grams total fat per day, specifically low in animal fat sources, over a period of five years had a 24% reduction in risk of breast cancer recurrence. It is important to note that a typical diet consists on average of 51.3 grams total fat per day. These results showed even greater significance for women who experience estrogen receptor negative breast cancer.[17] This study suggests the benefit of limiting total fat intake; however, it is important to not only limit the total *amount* of dietary fat, but also focus on the *types* of fat consumed. Specifically, restricting the amount of saturated fats and Trans fat found primarily in animal sources and processed foods. However, monounsaturated fats and polyunsaturated fats found in oils and nuts are considered the heart-healthy fats and serve as a beneficial form of fat.[18] There has also been a large amount of evidence suggesting the beneficial role of omega-3 fatty acids or fish oils in preventing cardiovascular disease as well as other health benefits that will be discussed in greater detail later.

How to Eat Meat

It is recommended to choose wild fish, lean poultry, legumes, or beans as an alternative to beef, pork, and lamb in order to limit saturated fat and total fat consumption. When you do choose to consume meat, select lean cuts and have smaller portions and prepare by baking, broiling, or poaching rather than frying or charbroiling. According to a report done by the AICR, which compiled over 7,000 scientific studies over five years, found that high intakes of red and processed meats, particularly those preserved through smoking, curing, or salt such as bacon, sausage, bologna, ham, and salami, significantly increase the risk of colorectal cancer. It is recommended through this report to consume no more than 18 ounces of meat per week with very little to none being from processed meat sources.[19] By limiting the intake of high-fat foods from animal sources it will aid in efforts to limit saturated fat intake and help to lower the risk of cardiovascular disease and certain cancer types, such as colorectal.[20]

Whole Grains

It is recommended to choose whole grains in preference to processed refined grains and sugars. Whole grains including rice, quinoa, wheat berries, bulgur wheat, steel cut oats, barley, bread, pasta, and cereals are the best choices because they are higher in fiber as well as certain vitamins and minerals as opposed to processed refined flour products. They provide nutrients such as vitamin E, a powerful antioxidant, as well as magnesium and fiber. Increased consumption of whole grains has been shown to lower the risk for many difference cancer types, especially colorectal cancer.[21]

Benefits of Fiber

Fiber is found in plant foods such as fruits, vegetables, beans, nuts, seeds, and whole grains. Fiber serves many health-promoting benefits in the body such as aiding in digestion, helping to regulate blood sugar, promoting hunger management, and lowering the risk of heart disease.[22] It is recommended to get at least 25–35 grams of fiber a day depending on age and sex. The diet of early man provided on average 100 grams of fiber per day. Look for whole grain foods containing 5 grams or more of fiber per serving and increase consumption of plant-based foods to ensure adequate fiber intake. The average American eats only about 10–15 grams of fiber a day, well below the recommended amount.[23] Fiber has also been associated with lowering the risk for colorectal cancer, in a cohort study done by the European Prospective Investigation Into Cancer and Nutrition (EPIC) it was found that an increase in fiber was correlated with a significant decrease in colorectal cancer risk.[24] The benefits of increased fiber intake for cancer prevention have been associated with consumption of fiber-rich foods rather than supplemental sources.

Increased fiber intake has also been associated with weight management; the Nurses Health Study found that women who consumed a greater amount of whole grains and fiber consistently weighed less than women who consumed a lower amount.[25] These findings further support the intake of whole grains and fiber as a means to reduce cancer risk due to their direct beneficial effects as well as their influence on weight management.

Soy Intake

Soy consumption has been an area of controversy in the recent years; however, soy can offer a lean source of protein in place of meat products. Soy foods have been suggested to help prevent certain types of cancers such as, breast, colon, prostate, and bladder cancers as well as heart disease and osteoporosis. Soy compounds known as phytoestrogens, more specifically isoflavones, have a weak, estrogen-like effect in the body. These effects have been cited in some research to prevent the development of estrogen-dependent cancers, such as breast cancer, by blocking estrogens effects and may influence the body to create its own estrogen.[26] Estrogen receptor breast cancers survivors can safely consume three to four servings of natural whole soy, such as tofu, soy milk, soy nuts, tempeh, and edamame per week and may consume more if previously a lifelong eater. However, estrogen receptor survivors should avoid soy products that are made from concentrated sources of phytoestrogens such as soy protein powder, pills, soy sauce, concentrated soy protein in nutrition bars and vegan/veggie "meats." Many products contain soy lecithin as an emulsifying agent that is extracted from soybean oil. The amounts contained in foods are usually minute and don't contribute a substantial level of phytoestrogens to be of concern.

A Canadian study conducted in 2006 published in the *Journal of Nutrition* found a significant link between an increase in phytoestrogens consumed in the diet and a reduction in the risk of colon cancer. These phytoestrogens include isoflavones found in soy, but more substantially a group known as lignans. Lignans are chemoprotective agents found in food such as, ground flax seeds, sesame, pumpkin, sunflower, and poppy seeds; as well as whole grains such as rye, oats, barley, wheat, and oat bran. They are also found in kale, broccoli, cabbage, apricots, peaches, and berries. This study observed the diets of 1,095 people diagnosed with colon cancer and 1,890 people who were cancer free; food recall questionnaires and blood samples were collected from each subset of participants. The group that consumed the largest amount of lignan-rich foods experienced a 27% lower risk of colon cancer compared to those that consumed the least amount of lignans. Isoflavones also showed similar results, with a 29% risk reduction in colon cancer for participants who had the highest consumption of isoflavones versus those that consumed the least. It is significant to note that only a small amount of lignan or isoflavone rich foods are sufficient enough to produce beneficial effects, such as a glass of soy milk, two peaches, one-half multigrain bread or a pinch of ground flaxseed provide adequate amount of lignans.[27] Women who have had estrogen receptor positive breast cancer should consume lignan containing foods in moderation, similar to the limitations suggested for soy containing foods.

Cooking Methods

Various cooking methods have shown to have cancer-promoting properties. A review conducted in Lyon, France, in October 2006 suggests the influence of fumes produced from certain forms of frying to have a positive correlation with cancer risk. Animal and human studies conducted in China demonstrated that non-smoking women who frequently cook oils at high temperatures, such as stir-frying, pan-frying, or deep-frying have a significant increase in risk for developing lung cancer. This risk increased proportionately with the amount of exposure to these fumes produced; there was also no difference in cancer risk when varying oil types were used.[28]

Reading Nutrition Labels

It is important to pay attention to the nutrition labels on foods, selecting foods that are nutrient dense rather than calorie dense. Look for foods that contain protein and more than five grams of fiber per serving. Common examples of nutrient-dense foods are fruits, vegetables, beans, nuts, skim milk, warm liquids, and cooked grains such as oatmeal, breakfast cereals, and lean meats are all great options.

WEIGHT MANAGEMENT

It is recommended that cancer survivors work to lose weight if currently overweight or obese. Obesity has been linked to an increase risk of death in numerous cancer types, as illustrated from the ACS Cancer Prevention Study II. This study confirmed obesity to be a risk factor for death from various cancers, such as colon and prostate. Most significantly this study highlighted a 52% increase in risk of all cancer death for men who are severely obese (BMI > 40) compared to men who were of a normal weight (BMI of 18.5–24.9).[29] Overweight and obesity is a risk factor for at least six cancer types including colorectal, post-menopausal breast, pancreatic, kidney, and esophageal cancers.[30] Obesity, insulin, and inflammation are each related and have been associated with cancer development and progression. Excess body weight accounts for 20% on average of cancer-related deaths each year.[31] This evidence highlights the importance of maintaining a healthy weight throughout treatment and after.[32] Obesity is not only associated with an increase in other types of cancer but may predispose an individual to certain diseases such as cardiovascular disease, Type 2 diabetes, high blood pressure, dyslipidemia, kidney disease, hyerpinsulimeia, and sleep apnea. This increase in disease risk is a large concern among cancer survivors due to evidence suggesting that "cancer patients die of non-cancer causes at a higher rate than persons in the general population."[33]

Normal Weight Gain During Treatment

It has been demonstrated through research that excess weight loss or gain during and after cancer treatment can affect the risk of cancer recurrence or death. Therefore, it is recommended that cancer survivors aim to maintain a body mass index (BMI) between 20 and 25 to ensure a healthy weight for optimal health.[34] A small weight gain has been observed during the treatment of certain cancers most notably breast and prostate, with a weight gain recorded in 50–96% of women who undergo breast cancer treatment. Changes in body composition have also been observed, including fat gain and loss of lean tissue.[35] This emphasizes the importance of preventing additional weight gain after treatment. It has been shown that weight loss of 5–10% over 6–12 months reduces risk factors for disease, further emphasizing the significance of losing excess weight after the treatment process has concluded.[36]

Healthy Weight Loss

Weight loss in cancer survivors should be achieved in a very healthy manner in order to ensure that they are receiving the proper nutrients and calories to maintain normal body and metabolic processes. The same way of eating that will help a survivor to lose weight in a healthful way is the same way of eating that will promote immune function and anti-cancer properties. Six recommendations are outlined below that demonstrate basic lifestyle changes to aid in healthful weight loss.

1. Eat a plant-based diet: It is recommended to consume a largely plant-based diet, incorporating a wide variety of fruits, vegetables, whole grains, and spices. More detail is provided on consuming a plant-based diet in the above section.
2. Calorie intake: Balance calorie intake with calorie output. This is individual to each person depending on age, sex, and physical-activity level. It may be helpful to create a food and exercise journal to keep track of progress and make sure each survivor is finding a balance. It is important to limit excess intake of calories, but it is also just as important to ensure that you are getting a proper amount and type of calories each day.
3. Be physically active every day: This topic is covered in chapter 15 of this book.
4. Get more good quality sleep: It is important to get more undisturbed sleep; sleep disturbances have been correlated as a common side effect of cancer diagnosis and contribute to fatigue. Research has shown that not getting proper sleep can lead to weight gain by causing an elevated appetite for high-sugar and high-calorie foods. It has also been linked to cause nutritional metabolism impairment, which can promote the development of insulin resistance, diabetes, and high cholesterol.[37] Helpful ways to get a better sleep are to avoid watching

TV, reading, or eating in bed. Try to not go to bed until you feel tired and aim to wake up at the same time each day as well as avoid daytime naps. It is also recommended to get out of bed after 15 minutes of tossing and turning to try a relaxing activity such as deep breathing exercises, mindful meditation, or listening to calming imaginary CDs to prepare for sleep, while avoiding stimulating activities such as TV watching.

5. Mindfulness: Incorporating mindfulness into how we eat is an important tactic for being aware of what and how we are eating. Specific recommendations include eat slowly, take time to breathe deeply and sit up straight during meals, which may help to slow down eating. It is also important to eat in a relaxed environment; avoid other activities while eating such as driving, typing, reading, or watching TV; these activities may cause you to eat more and faster.

6. Address emotional eating: Cancer diagnosis and treatment can dramatically affect a person's life; it is common for many people to turn to food as a coping mechanism for emotional stress. It is important to look for support with a health psychologist who specializes in cancer to address emotional eating and embrace a more healthful approach to eating.[38]

SUPPLEMENTS

Supplements of all types have flooded the mainstream market, providing high concentrations of every compound imaginable. The huge variety of supplements can be overwhelming and make anyone feel like they need to be taking these in order to receive the claimed benefits. However, many of these supplements contain doses that are well above the recommended amount and are often unnecessary or unsafe if you are consuming a well-balanced plant-based diet. It is strongly recommended that high-dose vitamin, mineral and nutrient, supplements should be avoided in cancer survivors due to the lack of extensive research validating their safety and effectiveness.[39] It is recommended that survivors work to receive 100% of Dietary Reference Intake (DRI) for vitamins and minerals, largely though diet but also from supplements that fall within normative intake ranges, such as a multivitamin or specific supplements that will be discussed further in greater detail.[40] Check with your physician or registered dietitian for specific concerns or questions regarding intake of vitamins, minerals, or supplements.

Omega-3 Intake

Omega-3 fatty acids are a recommended supplement to take for cancer survivorship, if one does not regularly consume fatty fish sources at least two times per week. Omega-3 fatty acids are a highly recommended source of healthy fats. These fats play a large role in reducing the risk of heart disease, high blood pressure, prevention of blood clots, and promotion of healthy brain development in children. There has been research that suggests diets high in omega-3s have great potential in protecting against the development of cancer and its prognosis. The preventive characteristics of fish oil include reduction of inflammation, prevention of lean body mass loss associated with cancer treatment, and increase in the potency of certain chemotherapy drugs.[41] The main derivative of fish oil is alpha-linolenic acid (ALA), which is then further broken down into the more metabolically active compounds, eicosapentaenoic acid (EPA) and docosahexanioc acid (DHA).

It has been supported that individuals previously diagnosed with prostate cancer may decrease the risk of it returning through increasing their consumption of fatty fish. It is recommended to consume two or three servings of fatty fish a week; including, salmon, sardines in oil, Pollack, bluefish, lake trout, flounder, canned tuna, and herring. Increased intake may also work to slow the disease progression and decrease the risk of dying from prostate cancer.[42] Fish oil capsules are recommended as an effective and safe source of omega-3s if dietary intake of fatty fish is inconsistent or inadequate. Fish oil capsules should provide a least 500 mg of combined EPA/DHA per capsule. Fish free omega-3 capsules also exist for vegetarians that are sourced from sea algae. It is recommended to consult a physician or dietitian on the specific amount of omega-3 supplements.[43]

Vitamin D Supplementation/Assessment of Deficiency

Vitamin D has generated a great deal of interest in the research field over the past several years; it has been established that adequate blood levels of vitamin D have a strong correlation with cancer risk. Proposed mechanisms include vitamin D's control of abnormal cell grow by blocking a key phase in cell division, it hinders the growth of new blood vessels that feed tumors, triggers cell death of abnormal cells, and increases the development process of normal cells.[44] Adequate amounts of vitamin D have shown potential in certain cancer types, specifically decreasing the risk for colon, breast, prostate, ovarian, pancreatic, and digestive tract cancers.[45] Low-serum vitamin D levels have been associated with decreased breast cancer prognosis. Research has shown low levels of vitamin D to correlate with 1.94 times greater likelihood of breast cancer recurrence as well as correlate with 1.73 times more likely to die from the cancer.[46] The Health Professional Follow-Up Study followed up with 51,529 U.S. male health professionals, looking at the correlation between cancer risk and cancer death in relation to vitamin D levels. The study took into consideration skin pigmentation, body fat, geographical location, and physical activity in reference to vitamin D. The results of the study found that individuals with blood vitamin D levels of 25 ng/ml experienced a 17% reduction in the number of new cancer developments, a 29% reduction in the total number of cancer deaths and a 45% reduction in death from digestive systems cancers such as colorectal, pancreatic, and esophageal.[47] Evidence strongly suggests that maintaining adequate vitamin D serum levels is highly recommended to decrease ones risk of cancer recurrence or development of new cancers, especially considering evidence that suggests individuals with a higher pre-diagnosis serum vitamin D levels in colorectal cancer patients have a 50% greater chance of survival.[48]

Deficiency in serum vitamin D levels is marked below 20 ng/mL, insufficient levels are observed at 20–28.8 ng/mL, and adequate levels are observed above 28.8 ng/mL.[49] Check with your physician or registered dietitian to determine if a vitamin D supplement is necessary based on results of a blood test. The DRI for vitamin D is 600 IU for adults under 70 years of age and 800 IU for people over 70. However, some experts have recommended intakes of 1,000 IU per day.[50] People who live in the Northern part of the United States or areas of the country that experience less sun exposure as well as darker skin pigmentation are more prone to vitamin D deficiency.[51] It has also been shown that being overweight correlates with lower vitamin D blood levels because vitamin D is stored in body fat and becomes less available for use by the body. It is thus recommended to maintain a healthy body weight to ensure highest blood levels.

Vitamin D comes from several sources including sunshine, food, and supplements. The best source is sun exposure; however, several factors play a role in the efficiency of generating vitamin D from the sun such as time of year, intensity, sunscreen, and length of exposure. It is recommended to get 15 minutes of direct sun exposure without sunscreen a day to 50% of the body to boost vitamin D levels without increasing skin cancer.[52] Food is another source of receiving vitamin D. Foods high in vitamin D include:

- Salmon—3.5 ounces (360 IU)
- Mackerel—3.5 ounces (345 IU)
- Sardines—3.75 ounces (250 IU)
- Shrimp—4 ounces (162 IU)
- Milk, any type—8 fluid ounces (100 IU)
- Orange juice, D-fortified—8 fluid ounces (100 IU)
- Yogurt, vitamin D-fortified—6 to 8 ounces (40–80 IU)
- Fortified cereal—3/4 cup (40–50 IU).

However, obtaining enough vitamin D from diet alone is often difficult; therefore it may be recommended that certain survivors take a daily vitamin D supplement with their diet to ensure adequate intake.

Supplements are a great way to ensure that one is getting an adequate daily intake of vitamin D. A reasonable and safe starting dose is 1,000 IU of Vitamin D3 (cholecalciferol) per day, along with dietary food sources. This dose of Vitamin D3 increases blood levels by 10 ng/ml; some researchers therefore believe that it is safe to take 2,000 IU per day and some argue up to 4,000 IU per day. Consult with you doctor or dietitian before taking more than 1,000 IU per day.[53] Recent studies support that too much Vitamin D is also risky, which highlights the need for personalized supplementation recommendations by a qualified health care professional.

Key Things for Providers to Inform Their Patient

- Aim for 5–10 servings of fruit and vegetables a day, selecting an assortment of colors and types.
- Aim to consume 3–4 servings of whole grains a day, including a variety of sources such as brown rice, whole-wheat pasta, quinoa, barley, steel cut oats, and bulgur.
- Limit the consumption of red meat and avoid processed cured, smoked, and salted meats. Consume lean cuts of meats, focusing on lean poultry, fish, and natural soy foods (tofu, edamame) as the main sources.
- Weight management and/or weight loss if overweight or obese should be a priority. It is recommended to pay particular attention to portion sizes, avoiding excess sugars from processed and sweetened beverages as well as limiting processed foods that are high in fat and sugar.
- Discuss with your physician or registered dietitian if beginning a supplement regiment for omega-3 fatty acids and vitamin D is right for you.

Resources

- **Dana-Farber Cancer Institute www.dana-farber.org/nutrition**
- **American Cancer Society**
- **Nutrition for Cancer Patients**
- **American Institute for Cancer Research**
- **Center for Science in the Public Interest**
- **Fruits and Veggies, More Matters**
- **Harvard Medical School's Consumer Health Information Source**
- **Harvard School of Public Health**
- **National Cancer Institute**
- **Overview of Nutrition in Cancer Care**

Notes

1. http://www.dietandcancerreport.org/downloads/Policy_Report.pdf
2. ACS Guidelines, 2006
3. ACS guidelines, 2006
4. ACS guidelines, 2006
5. Lila, A M. (2007). From Bean to Berries and Beyond: Teamwork between plant chemicals for protection of optimal human health. *New York Academy of Sciences,* 1114, pp. 372–380.
6. Phytonutrients: revisiting these nutritional giants, Anne Chiavacci Brigham and Women's Hospital; http://www.intelihealth.com/IH/ihtIH/WSIHW000/35320/353 27/441606.html?d=dmtHMSContent.
7. Phytonutrients: revisting these nutritional giants, Anne Chiavacci Brigham and Womens Hospital; http://www.intelihealth.com/IH/ihtIH/WSIHW000/35320/353 27/441606.html?d=dmtHMSContent.
8. Phytonutrients: revisting these nutritional giants, Anne Chiavacci Brigham and Womens Hospital; http://www.intelihealth.com/IH/ihtIH/WSIHW000/35320/353 27/441606.html?d=dmtHMSContent.

9. Phytonutrients: revisting these nutritional giants, Anne Chiavacci Brigham and Womens Hospital; http://www.intelihealth.com/IH/ihtIH/WSIHW000/35320/353 27/441606.html?d=dmtHMSContent.

10. Al-Dekaimy et al. (2009). Longitudinal biological exposure to carotenoids is associated with breast cancer-free survival in the Women's Healthy Eating and Living Study. *Cancer Epidemiology*, 18 (2), pp. 486–494.

11. Sunshine, tea and tomatoes: can they prevent cancer? Stacy Kennedy, Brigham and Women's Hospital; http://www.intelihealth.com/IH/ihtIH/WSIHW000/35320/ 35327/456296.html?d=dmtHMSContent.

12. Phytonutrients: revisiting these nutritional giants, Anne Chiavacci Brigham and Women's Hospital; http://www.intelihealth.com/IH/ihtIH/WSIHW000/35320/353 27/441606.html?d=dmtHMSContent.

13. Phytonutrients: revisiting these nutritional giants, Anne Chiavacci Brigham and Women's Hospital; http://www.intelihealth.com/IH/ihtIH/WSIHW000/35320/353 27/441606.html?d=dmtHMSContent.

14. Phytonutrients: revisiting these nutritional giants, Anne Chiavacci Brigham and Women's Hospital; http://www.intelihealth.com/IH/ihtIH/WSIHW000/35320/353 27/441606.html?d=dmtHMSContent.

15. Phytonutrients: revisiting these nutritional giants, Anne Chiavacci Brigham and Women's Hospital; http://www.intelihealth.com/IH/ihtIH/WSIHW000/35320/353 27/441606.html?d=dmtHMSContent.

16. Ch 14; Pierce JP et al. (2010). Physical activity, diet, adiposity and female breast cancer prognosis: a review of the epidemiologic literature. *Maturitas* 66 (1), pp. 5–15.

17. http://www.dietandcancerreport.org/downloads/Policy_Report.pdf

18. Fiber. Healthy Lifestyle. Harvard Medical School. http://www.intelihealth.com/ IH/ihtIH?d=dmtContent&c=34043&p=~br,IHW|~st,35320|~r,WSIHW000|~b,*|

19. Redfern, J (2009). Fabulous Fiber. Brigham and Women's Hospital; http://www.intelihealth.com/IH/ihtIH?d=dmtHMSContent&c=480711&p=~br,IHW|~st,3 5320|~r,WSIHW000|~b,*|

20. Cancer Update: Two Studies Worth Heeding; Stacy Kennedy Brigham and Women's Hospital; http://www.intelihealth.com/IH/ihtIH/WSIHW000/35320/353 27/538275.html?d=dmtHMSContent.

21. Cancer Update: Two Studies Worth Heeding; Stacy Kennedy Brigham and Women's Hospital; http://www.intelihealth.com/IH/ihtIH/WSIHW000/35320/353 27/538275.html?d=dmtHMSContent.

22. Cancer Update: Two Studies Worth Heeding; Stacy Kennedy Brigham and Women's Hospital; http://www.intelihealth.com/IH/ihtIH/WSIHW000/35320/353 27/538275.html?d=dmtHMSContent.

23. Ch 14 Nutrition and cancer prevention

24. Losing Weigh Helps Promote Cancer Survivorship, Stacy Kennedy; Brigham and Women's Hospital; http://www.intelihealth.com/IH/ihtIH/WSIHW000/35320/353 27/724003.html?d=dmtHMSContent.

25. Losing Weight Helps Promote Cancer Survivorship, Stacy Kennedy; Brigham and Women's Hospital; http://www.intelihealth.com/IH/ihtIH/WSIHW000/35320/353 27/724003.html?d=dmtHMSContent.

26. World Cancer Research Fund, Global Report. Policy and Action for Cancer Prevention: Food, Nutrition, Physical Activity and the Prevention of Cancer: a Global Perspective, Washington DC: AICR, 2007 pp 322.

27. Brown BW., Brauner, C., Minnotte, MC. (1993). Noncancer Deaths in White Adult Cancer Patients. *Journal of the National Cancer Institute*, 85:979–997, 1993.

28. Does Diet Effect Cancer Recurrence: Stephanie Meyers Brigham and Women's Hospital; http://www.intelihealth.com/IH/ihtIH/WSIHW000/35320/35327/593215.html?d=dmtHMSContent.

29. Vance V., Mourtazakis, M., McCargar L., Hanning R. (2010) Weight gain in breast cancer survivors: prevalence, pattern and health consequences. *An Official Journal of the International Association for the Study of Obesity*, 12 (4) pp 282–294.

30. Diabetes Prevention Program, NIH 2008, http://diabetes.niddk.nih.gov/dm/pubs/preventionprogram/

31. Losing Weight Helps Promote Cancer Survivorship, Stacy Kennedy; Brigham and Women's Hospital; http://www.intelihealth.com/IH/ihtIH/WSIHW000/35320/35327/724003.html?d=dmtHMSContent.

32. Losing Weight Helps Promote Cancer Survivorship, Stacy Kennedy; Brigham and Women's Hospital; http://www.intelihealth.com/IH/ihtIH/WSIHW000/35320/35327/724003.html?d=dmtHMSContent.

33. Ch 14; www.dietandcancerreport.org

34. Abrams et al. (2009). Evidence-Based clinical practice guidelines for integrative oncology: complementary therapies and botanicals. *Journal of the Society for Integrative Oncology*, 7 (3), pp. 85–120.

35. www.danafarber.org/nutrition.

36. Does Diet Effect Cancer Recurrence: Stephanie Meyers Brigham and Women's Hospital; http://www.intelihealth.com/IH/ihtIH/WSIHW000/35320/35327/593215.html?d=dmtHMSContent.

37. www.danafarber.org/nutrition

38. The Cancer, Sunshine and Vitamin D connection, Anne Chiavacci Brigham and Women's Hospital; http://www.intelihealth.com/IH/ihtIH/WSIHW000/35320/35327/612393.html?d=dmtHMSContent

39. The Cancer, Sunshine and Vitamin D connection, Anne Chiavacci Brigham and Women's Hospital; http://www.intelihealth.com/IH/ihtIH/WSIHW000/35320/35327/612393.html?d=dmtHMSContent; Sunshine, tea and tomatoes: can they prevent cancer? Stacy Kennedy, Brigham and Women's Hospital; http://www.intelihealth.com/IH/ihtIH/WSIHW000/35320/35327/456296.html?d=dmtHMSContent.

40. Goodwin, P. (2009). Vitamin D in Cancer Patients: Above All, Do No Harm. *Journal of Clinical Oncology*. 27 (13) pp.2117–2119

41. The Cancer, Sunshine and Vitamin D connection, Anne Chiavacci Brigham and Women's Hospital; http://www.intelihealth.com/IH/ihtIH/WSIHW000/35320/35327/612393.html?d=dmtHMSContent

42. Dietary Supplement Fact Sheet: Vitamin D; NIH; http://ods.od.nih.gov/factsheets/VitaminD-HealthProfessional/

43. Binkley N, Ramamurthy R, Krueger D. (2010). Low vitamin D status: definition, prevalence, consequences, and correction. *Endocrinology And Metabolism Clinics Of North America* 39 (2), p. 287. Available from http://web.ebscohost.com/ehost/detail?vid=25&hid=15&sid=aa63fcad-a1df-4be3-91fe-4569c3f8db3b%40sessionmgr4&bdata=JnNpdGU9ZWhvc3QtbGl2ZQ%3d%3d#db=cmedm&AN=20511052 Ipswich, MA. Accessed February 7, 2011.

44. Dietary Supplement Fact Sheet: Vitamin D; NIH; http://ods.od.nih.gov/factsheets/VitaminD-HealthProfessional/

45. Sunshine, tea and tomatoes: can they prevent cancer? Stacy Kennedy, Brigham and Women's Hospital; http://www.intelihealth.com/IH/ihtIH/WSIHW000/35320/35327/456296.html?d=dmtHMSContent.

46. The Cancer, Sunshine and Vitamin D connection, Anne Chiavacci Brigham and Women's Hospital; http://www.intelihealth.com/IH/ihtIH/WSIHW000/35320/35327/612393.html?d=dmtHMSContent.

47. The Cancer, Sunshine and Vitamin D connection, Anne Chiavacci Brigham and Women's Hospital; http://www.intelihealth.com/IH/ihtIH/WSIHW000/35320/35327/612393.html?d=dmtHMSContent.

REFERENCES

McCann S, Ambrosone C, Graham S, et al. Intakes of selected nutrients, foods, and phytochemicals and prostate cancer risk in western New York. *Nutrition and Cancer* [serial online]. 2005;53(1):33–41. Available from: MEDLINE, Ipswich, MA. Accessed January 29, 2011.

Pierce JP et al. (2010). Physical activity, diet, adiposity and female breast cancer prognosis: a review of the epidemiologic literature. *Maturitas* 66(1), pp. 5–15

The Cancer, Sunshine, and Vitamin D connection, Anne Chiavacci Brigham and Womens' Hospital; http://www.intelihealth.com/IH/ihtIH/WSIHW000/35320/35327/612393.html?d=dmtHMSContent.

Dietary Supplement Fact Sheet: Vitamin D; NIH; http://ods.od.nih.gov/factsheets/VitaminD-HealthProfessional/.

Sunshine, tea and tomatoes: can they prevent cancer? Stacy Kennedy, Brigham and Women's Hospital; http://www.intelihealth.com/IH/ihtIH/WSIHW000/35320/35327/456296.html?d=dmtHMSContent.

Goodwin, P. (2009). Vitamin D in Cancer Patients: Above All, Do No Harm. *Journal of Clinical Oncology.* 27(13) pp. 2117–2119.

Dana-Farber Cancer Insitute website www.danafarber.org/nutrition

Does Diet Effect Cancer Recurrence: Stephanie Meyers Brigham and Women's Hospital; http://www.intelihealth.com/IH/ihtIH/WSIHW000/35320/35327/593215.html?d=dmtHMSContent.

Losing Weight Helps Promote Cancer Survivorship, Stacy Kennedy; Brigham and Women's Hospital; http://www.intelihealth.com/IH/ihtIH/WSIHW000/35320/35327/724003.html?d=dmtHMSContent.

www.dietandcancerreport.org/recommendations

Abrams et al., (2009) Evidence-Based clinical practice guidelines for integrative oncology: complementary therapies and botanicals. *Journal of the Society for Integrative Oncology,* Vol.7 (3) pp. 85–120.

Brown BW., Brauner, C., Minnotte, MC. (1993). Noncancer Deaths in White Adult Cancer Patients. *Journal of the National Cancer Institute,* 85:979–997, 1993.

Does Diet Effect Cancer Recurrence: Stephanie Meyers Brigham and Women's Hospital; http://www.intelihealth.com/IH/ihtIH/WSIHW000/35320/35327/593215.html?d=dmtHMSContent.

Cancer Update: Two Studies Worth Heeding; Stacy Kennedy Brigham and Womens. http://www.intelihealth.com/IH/ihtIH/WSIHW000/35320/35327/538275.html?d=dmtHMSContent.

World Cancer Research Fund, Global Report 2007. AICR (2007). World Cancer Research Fund/American Institute for Cancer Research. Policy and Action for Cancer

Prevention: Food, Nutrition, Physical Activity and the Prevention of Cancer: a Global Perspective, Washington DC: AICR, 2007 pp 322.

Redfern, Julie (2009). Fabulous Fiber. Brigham and Womens Hospital. http://www.intelihealth.com/IH/ihtIH?d=dmtHMSContent&c=480711&p=~br,IHW|~st,353 20|~r,WSIHW000|~b,*|.

AICR (2009). World Cancer Research Fund/American Institute for Cancer Research. Policy and Action for Cancer Prevention: Food, Nutrition and Physical Activity: a Global Perspective, Washington DC: AICR, 2009 pp iv. http://www.dietandcancer report.org/downloads/Policy_Report.pdf

Fiber. Healthy Lifestyle. Harvard Medical School. http://www.intelihealth.com/IH/ihtI H?d=dmtContent&c=34043&p=~br,IHW|~st,35320|~r,WSIHW000|~b,*|.

Pierce JP et al. (2010). Physical activity, diet, adiposity and female breast cancer prognosis: a review of the epidemiologic literature. Maturitas. 66 (1) pp. 5–15.

Phytonutrients: revisiting these nutritional giants, Anne Chiavacci Brigham and Womens' Hospital http://www.intelihealth.com/IH/ihtIH/WSIHW000/35320/35327/441606.html?d=dmtHMSContent

Al-Dekaimy et al., (2009) Longitudinal biological exposure to carotenoids is associated with breast cancer-free survival in the Women's Healthy Eating and Living Study. Cancer Epidemiology, 18 (2) pp. 486–494.

Ambrosone CB et al., (2005) Intakes of selected nutrient, food and phytochemicals and prostate cancer risk in western New York. Nutrition and Cancer, 53 (1) pp. 33–41.

Kushi, LH., Byers, T., Doyle, C., Bendera, EV., McCullough, M., Gansler, T., Andrews, KS., Thun, MJ. (2006). American Cancer Society Guidelines on Nutrition and Physical Activity for Cancer Prevention: Reducing the Risk of Colon Cancer with Health Food Choices and Physical Activity. CA A Cancer Journal for Clinicians, 56, pp 264

Lila, A M. (2007) From Bean to Berries and Beyond: Teamwork between plant chemicals for protection of optimal human health. New York Academy of Sciences, 1114 pp. 372–380.

Vance V, Mourtzakis M. McCorgar L, Hanning R. (2010) Weight gain in breast cancer survivors: prevalence, pattern and health consequences. Obes Rev.

Diabetes Prevention Program, NIH 2008; http://diabetes.niddk.nih.gov/dm/pubs/pre ventionprogram/.

Binkley N, Ramamurthy R, Krueger D. Low vitamin D status: definition, prevalence, consequences, and correction. *Endocrinology And Metabolism Clinics Of North America* [serial online]. June 2010;39(2):287. Available from: http://web.ebscohost. com/ehost/detail?vid=25&hid=15&sid=aa63fcad-a1df-4be3-91fe-4569c3f8db3 b%40sessionmgr4&bdata=JnNpdGU9ZWhvc3QtbGl2ZQ%3d%3d#db=cmedm& AN=20511052. Accessed February 7, 2011.

15

EXERCISE AND SURVIVORSHIP

NANCY CAMPBELL, MS

BACKGROUND AND RESEARCH

Recent research has continued to reinforce the benefits of physical activity for cancer survivors. The majority of the research has been focused on breast, colorectal, and prostate cancer, but much of the data is applicable to all cancer survivors. In 2010, the American College of Sports Medicine (ACSM) and the American Cancer Society (ACS) developed exercise guidelines for cancer survivors.[1] The bottom line of the research is that exercise is safe both during and after cancer treatment and avoiding inactivity is very important.

One of the largest prospective observational studies has been with the Nurses' Health Study. The investigators examined a cohort of 2,987 women that had been diagnosed with stage 1–111a breast cancer and showed that the women who participated in nine MET-hours/week of exercise, which is equivalent to walking at an average pace for three hours/week, had a 50% lower risk of breast cancer recurrence and all cause mortality than women who were inactive.[2]

In breast cancer studies alone, more than 10,000 survivors have participated in exercise-based research. The studies have examined multiple time points, including during adjuvant therapy, immediately after completion of therapy, and several years later. There are even a small number of studies that looked at the benefits of exercise in the metastatic setting. The majority of these studies have shown that survivors who engage in moderate amounts of exercise have improved, disease free and overall survival, in comparison to their inactive counterpart.

In spite of all this evidence, the majority of cancer survivors do not accumulate the recommended levels of activity. In fact, the Health, Eating, Activity, and Lifestyle study found that breast cancer survivors decreased their total physical activity by almost two hours per week from pre-diagnosis to post-diagnosis.[3] Therefore, the ultimate question is, how do we motivate cancer survivors to incorporate physical activity into their lifestyle?

CARDIAC REHABILITATION MODEL

One place we can look to for answers is by examining the cardiac rehabilitation model. If someone had a heart attack in the 1920s, they stayed in the hospital for at least six weeks and were told to limit their physical exertion. In the 1940s, chair exercises were introduced and clinicians began to realize that exercise was beneficial, but needed to be supervised. Fortunately, by the 1950s, the concept of progressive supervised activity via cardiac rehabilitation was presented and has been adopted worldwide. The World Health Organization has defined cardiac rehabilitation in this way:

> The rehabilitation of cardiac patients is the sum of activities required to influence favorably the underlying cause of the disease, as well as the best possible physical, mental and social conditions, so that they may by their own efforts, preserve or resume when lost, as normal a place as possible in the society. Rehabilitation cannot be regarded as an isolated form of therapy but must be integrated within the entire treatment.

This model is very helpful and can be referenced in the design of a cancer rehabilitation program. Many insurance companies will pay for all or a portion of cardiac rehabilitation, and this would be ideal for the design of a cancer rehabilitation program. Most cardiac rehabilitation programs have three phases. The Phase 1 portion occurs inpatient at a hospital and generally involves assisted range of motion exercises. Phase 2 involves medical supervision with exercise, counseling, and education about stress management, smoking cessation, nutrition, and weight loss. The final phase is maintenance and it is typically not supervised, but the goal is to promote and maintain the habits learned. This schema could easily be tailored to a cancer rehabilitation program in the future.

The Physical Activity Component of a Cancer Survivorship Clinic

Until a cancer rehabilitation program is designed and implemented, a cancer survivorship clinic can teach many of the skills needed for survivors to begin and maintain an exercise program. It is important to do an initial assessment of the survivors' current and past exercise history. Once you have a clear picture, the next consideration is medical history. An exercise prescription will be influenced by a myriad of items including surgical history, medications, and type of cancer treatment. Some of the most important considerations will be discussed in detail below, including fatigue, weight gain, cardiovascular issues, osteoporosis, lymphedema, and neuropathy.

Fatigue

The most prevalent side effect of cancer and its treatment is fatigue. Previously, people were told to rest if they were fatigued, but recent research is encouraging the opposite. A recent Cochrane review of 28 studies found that exercise can help to reduce fatigue both during and after treatment.[4] The fatigue can affect people physically, emotionally, and mentally, while lasting months to even years. Starting with small doses of 10 minutes of walking most days can help to get survivors into a routine. Once they have mastered the 10 minutes, encourage them to slowly increasing activity by 3% to 5% each week.

Weight Gain

Traditionally, cancer treatment is associated with weight loss, but surely that isn't always the outcome. Currently, many survivors enter treatment already being overweight or obese. Partridge et al. found that at least half of women receiving adjuvant chemotherapy for breast cancer gained between 5 and 11 pounds.[5] The exact cause of the weight gain is unknown, but is certainly multifactorial. Some potential causes of weight gain are the use of steroids during cancer treatments, a potential decrease in metabolism from certain chemotherapies, a decrease in activity levels, or the triggering of premature menopause in women.

Another issue that leads to weight gain is sarcopenia, which is the loss of lean body mass and strength. Recently, there has been more interest in examining the relationship between body composition and cancer outcomes.[6] Investigators reported that being overweight or obese was linked with poorer functional status and was an independent predictor of survival. A moderate intensity, progressive exercise program will help address the issues that lead to weight gain and sarcopenia. Being overweight also increases the chance that some cancers, such as prostate, colorectal, and breast cancers will return, and exercise helps control weight gain.

Cardiovascular Concerns

Many of the current cancer treatments, such as chemotherapy and radiation, can lead to cardiovascular issues. For example, cardiovascular disease is the second leading cause of death in long term survivors of Hodgkin's disease after second malignancies.[7] Certain drugs, such as Adriamycin and Herceptin, can lead to cardiomyopathy, congestive heart failure, or stroke. Fortunately, a simple walking program can help reduce the risk of cardiovascular problems. Exercise is also helpful in reducing other cardiovascular risk factors, such as high blood pressure and cholesterol.

Osteoporosis

As cancer survivors are living longer, the side effects from treatment are growing. For example, women who undergo treatment for breast cancer may have a higher risk of osteoporosis. The chemotherapy and/or surgery may result in a loss of ovarian function and therefore a decrease in estrogen levels. Since estrogen has a protective effect on bone, the reduction in estrogen levels leads to a higher risk of osteoporosis. Even if a woman is premenopausal prior to her diagnosis, she is likely to enter menopause at an earlier age. One of the classes of medications that contributes to the increased risk of osteoporosis are aromatase inhibitors. These drugs significantly reduce the amount of circulating estrogen and are widely prescribed to postmenopausal women. Aromatase inhibitors certainly decrease the risk of breast cancer recurrence, but greatly increase the risk of osteoporosis and bone fracture. In 2008, Chapman et al. examined the competing causes of death in postmenopausal women taking an aromatase inhibitor. The diagnosis of osteoporosis was the second highest cause of statistically significant increased risk of death, after cardiovascular disease.[8]

Osteoporosis is also common in survivors who have undergone a bone marrow transplant, had exposure to high doses of steroids, or men who undergo androgen deprivation therapy for prostate cancer. Since the risk of osteoporosis is so high, it is important for survivors to incorporate weight bearing activities and strength training into their lifestyle. A moderate intensity strength training program should emphasize certain muscle groups (e.g., spinal extensor muscles, hip abductors and extensors, knee extensors and flexors) as well as those related to gait and balance (such as ankle plantar flexors and dorsiflexors and hip abductors). There are also certain exercises that should be avoided if a survivor has osteoporosis, such as running, jumping rope, high impact aerobics, or any exercise that causes bending forward at the waist (for example, touching your toes, doing sit-ups, and certain yoga poses). It is important for cancer survivors to seek assistance in designing an exercise routine from a certified professional who has experience. Later in this chapter there will be a list of resources.

Lymphedema

The ACS defines lymphedema as a build-up of lymph fluid in the fatty tissues just under your skin. This build-up causes swelling, most often seen in the arms or legs, though the face, neck, abdomen (belly), and genitals can also be affected. According to the National Cancer Institute, lymphedema is one of the most poorly understood, relatively underestimated, and least researched complications of cancer or its treatment. In 2006, The Institute of Medicine published a report recommending a "survivorship care plan" for cancer patients that incorporates information about late effects of treatment, one of which is lymphedema. Even years after completion of cancer treatment, the risk of lymphedema still exists, with a higher risk if a survivor undergoes a full lymph node dissection and/or radiation to the axilla or groin.

Many cancer survivors are told that lifting more than 10 pounds with the effected limb could induce lymphedema, and for years, strength training was contraindicated because of this. Recent research by Schmitz et al. reported on

141 women with breast-cancer associated lymphedema, who followed a slow, progressive strength training routine. This exercise training had no significant effect on limb swelling and in fact there were a decreased incidence of exacerbations of lymphedema and reduced symptoms.[9] All of the women in this study wore compression sleeves and started with little-to-no resistance with the strength training. There is no consensus as to how long after a strength training session to leave the sleeve on. There are six other randomized control trials that have all shown that upper body exercise does not contribute to the onset or worsening of lymphedema.

Neuropathy

Another potentially debilitating side effect of cancer treatment is peripheral neuropathy. Certain chemotherapies can have adverse effects on the nervous system, such as paclitaxel and cisplatin. Symptoms can vary from mild tingling in the toes and fingers to numbness, or burning, all the way up to excruciating pain. These side effects may disappear after the completion of treatment, but other people suffer from persistent pain and numbness. Generally, low-impact exercise is recommended because it is less strenuous on joints and feet. Some examples are walking, water aerobics, recumbent biking, and the elliptical trainer. Many people will also have issues with their balance, so it will be important to incorporate exercises to address this.

Exercise Prescriptions

Cardiovascular exercise will help ameliorate some of the fatigue and weight gain that may have occurred during cancer treatment. The ACS and the ACSM have both developed exercise guidelines for cancer survivors. Generally, it is recommended to aim for three to five days per week of cardiovascular activity for 20 to 60 minutes. However, the exercise can be broken down into 10-minute increments accumulated throughout the day. During the exercise assessment, it is important to determine what activities are best for the patient, based on their past experience, current limitations, and goals. For an inexperienced exerciser the intensity level should be mild, and it is more important to focus on frequency and duration of exercise. It is also imperative to take into account the following factors: age, medication related side effects, other health issues, and or any cardiac limitations. Lastly, teaching survivors how to gradually progress their cardiovascular exercise will keep them from doing too much too soon, while helping them reach their goals. Some days/weeks will be harder and a modifiable program will be crucial.

Strength training will assist in many ways, such as increasing lean body mass and decreasing the risk of osteoporosis. A basic strength training program does not require a gym membership, usually a small set of dumbbells will be sufficient. But, it does require proper instruction from a certified personal trainer, physical therapist, or other medical professional with prior experience working with cancer survivors. It is best to start with one or two non-consecutive days per week. Depending on the type of surgery and/or radiation, certain modifications will be necessary.

A flexibility and/or relaxation routine will help balance out an exercise prescription. The recent ACSM guidelines conclude that there is a research gap regarding the safety and efficacy of yoga and Pilates. Most of the research with yoga has been with breast cancer survivors and seems safe as long as arm and shoulder morbidities are taken into consideration.

Helpful Tools

There are some simple, inexpensive tools that can enhance the exercise portion of a survivorship clinic. One example is a pedometer, which can help with awareness and motivation to exercise. It is common for people to overestimate the amount of activity they do and a pedometer can help to quantify and compare activity over time. A good pedometer should have a stride adjustment on it, this will increase the accuracy. But, certain activities such as biking and lateral movements are not always captured by a pedometer. In 2007, Vallance et al.[10] found that simply giving cancer survivors a pedometer and written material about exercise helped increase their physical activity and quality of life.

Another helpful tool is providing a journal for people to log their activity, daily steps, and/or heart rate. These journals do not need to be fancy; the main goal is to increase awareness of activity levels. Some people find it helpful if there is a place for notes regarding how they were feeling that day, how much sleep they got, or any other relevant information.

When the patient walks out the door, they need to have a concrete plan in place for how to start or maintain their exercise plan. Help them to put together a schedule of progression over 8 to 12 weeks. Recommend that they look at their schedule for the upcoming week and plan certain days and times where exercise will fit. Pencil it into the schedule and make sure that it is treated with the same importance as a doctor's appointment. If the patient has never exercised before, they need to start slowly and progress in a step-wise manner.

The final component to help increase success is goal setting. Properly set goals can be incredibly motivating, and as people get into the habit of setting and achieving goals, they will find that their self-confidence grows. There are a few basic concepts that should encompass any goal to increase the chances of success. A goal should be SMART, which stands for Smart, Measurable, Attainable, Realistic, and Time Sensitive. It's also important to recognize and have rewards for all that has been accomplished as people strive to reach their goal.

Resources

In 2008, the ACSM and the ACS collaborated to design a certification program, the Cancer Certified Exercise Trainer. There is a list of certified professionals available on ACSM's website with contact information.

Recently, the Lance Armstrong Foundation partnered with the YMCA to offer exercise classes for cancer survivors. Certain YMCAs across the country offer a 12-week program that helps cancer survivors build muscle mass and muscle strength, increase flexibility, and endurance and improve functional ability.

The Wellness Community is also a resource for professionally led support groups, educational workshops, nutrition and exercise programs, and stress-reduction classes. There are locations all over the country that offer resources specifically designed for cancer survivors.

References

1. Schmitz, K., et al. *ACSM roundtable on exercise guidelines for cancer survivors.* MSSE, 2010.

2. Holmes, M., et al. *Physical activity and survival after breast cancer diagnosis.* JAMA, 2005. 293(20): p. 2479–86.

3. Irwin, M., et al. *Physical activity levels before and after a diagnosis of breast carcinoma. The health, eating, activity, and lifestyle (HEAL) study.* Cancer, 2003. 97: p. 1746–57.

4. Cramp, F. and J. Daniel, *Exercise for the management of cancer-related fatigue in adults.* Cochrane 2009.

5. Partridge, A.H. and E.P. Winer, *Long-Term Complications of Adjuvant Chemotherapy for Early Stage Breast Cancer.* Breast Disease, 2004. 21(1): p. 55–64.

6. Prado, C., et al. *Sarcopenia as a Determinant of Chemotherapy Toxicity and Time to Tumor Progression in Metastatic Breast Cancer Patients Receiving Capecitabine Treatment.* Clin Canc Res, 2009. 15(8): p. 2920–26.

7. Henry-Amar, M. and R. Somers, *Survival outcome after Hodgkin's disease: a report from the international data base on Hodgkin's disease.* Seminars in Onc, 1990. 17: p. 758–68.

8. Chapman, J., et al. *Competing Causes of Death From a Randomized Trial of Extended Adjuvant Endocrine Therapy for Breast Cancer.* JNCI, 2008. 100(4): p. 252.

9. Schmitz, K., et al. *Weight lifting in women with breast-cancer–related lymphedema.* NEJM, 2009. 361: p. 664–73.

10. Vallance, J., et al. *Randomized controlled trial of the effects of print materials and step pedometers on physical activity and quality of life in breast cancer survivors.* JCO, 2007. 25(17): p. 2352–59.

16

PSYCHOSOCIAL ISSUES
OF SURVIVORSHIP

HESTER HILL SCHNIPPER, LICSW, OSW–C

It is often an unhappy surprise to cancer survivors that a range of psychosocial issues persist long after the completion of active treatment. During the months of active treatment, most people are forced to concentrate on the basics: how to manage the side effects of chemotherapy or radiation, how to allocate their reduced energy, and how to maintain as active and normal a life as possible. Once treatment has ended, there is time and emotional space to recognize what has happened and to begin to contend with the many changes wrought by the diagnosis and treatment of a life-threatening illness.

An important rule of thumb is that it takes at least as long as the total duration of treatment to feel fully physically and psychologically recovered. This extended recovery is much longer than most patients expect and very much longer than the assumptions of family, friends, and work colleagues. It is vital that providers warn their patients of this likely timeline and support their efforts to thoughtfully plan the transition back to health.

During the early months of recovery, when the individual is balanced somewhere between sickness and health, there is a unique opportunity for reflection and movement towards a new normal that better reflects one's priorities. The months of active treatment are generally a time of a forced slower schedule, and survivors should be encouraged to resume their usual obligations carefully and thoughtfully. After some months of a reduced work and social routine, there is a rare opportunity to consider the relative importance of each obligation and relationship. Most people race through their busy days with little time for reflection, and this period of recovery can be used to make choices and changes that will support lifelong physical and mental health.

For most people, the most intense issues are emotional. It is normal to be anxious and to be sad after cancer. Almost everyone who has received a cancer diagnosis, regardless of the type of stage of the disease, has worried that she will die. This dramatic reminder of mortality is the primary issue for almost all cancer survivors, especially during the early months and years after diagnosis. Younger people may experience this distress even more intensely as these fears may be completely out of sync with their stage of life. However, even older cancer survivors may not have truly grappled with mortality until faced with this diagnosis. For everyone, the challenge is clear: one must learn to live as if the disease will not recur. Whether it does or whether it does not, living "as if" will enable the survivor to enjoy a rich and satisfying life. The alternative, living always in fear of a recurrence, will certainly damage quality of life and may result in a chronic state of low-level depression and generalized anxiety.

It is not helpful to minimize these normal fears or to reassure a cancer survivor that good health is certain. False promises only result in diminished trust. It is helpful to encourage survivors to express their worries, to normalize the fears and provide reality testing, and to support the legitimate hope that accompanies recovery.

It is estimated that approximately 25% of cancer patients and survivors struggle with depression. The incidence of anxiety is similar, and both should be evaluated and addressed when working with this population. There are differences between a clinical depression that will likely respond to medication and a normal reaction to a difficult and stressful situation. Except for people who have extraordinary denial, an adjustment reaction with mixed feelings is almost a given. Remember that sadness and worry are not signs of a psychiatric disorder. Neither do emotional liability and a shorter than usual temper mean that a patient needs psychopharmacological assistance. It is difficult to tease out symptoms of major depression from those normally associated with cancer treatment and recovery. The usual symptom list, including difficulties with sleep and appetite, fatigue, reduced interest in usual activities and relationships, difficulty with concentration, and a sense of being out of control, is just as relevant for normal reactions to cancer treatment as it is for depression.

It is often most helpful to ask if the individual thinks that he is depressed. It is always helpful to normalize these feelings, reassure the survivor that everyone has an emotional as well as a physical recovery, and to suggest talking with a therapist if the feelings have persisted for more than a few months after active treatment. Do remember the importance of working with a therapist who is experienced with oncology issues. Ideally, any survivorship program will either have such clinicians on staff or will maintain relationships with therapists in the community who can be readily available.

It may be useful to frame survivors' psychological concerns as PTSD. A cancer diagnosis and treatment are traumatic, and the feelings fit this profile. Some survivors will feel less threatened by a PTSD diagnosis than one of depression or anxiety, and this normal human reaction to a crisis is common and treatable.

It takes time for most survivors to feel comfortable with future thinking and making plans. Many live in three or six month increments, counting their lives off between scans or doctor visits. There is no way to hasten the return to a longer perspective, and it would be counter-productive to pressure a survivor to do so. With the safe passage of time, most people slowly adapt to a more normal calendar and view, although some never regain comfort with planning for a distant future.

Many cancer survivors feel vulnerable. It takes time to rebuild trust in a body that has seemingly betrayed you, and it may seem that all manner of bad things may now happen. Accompanied by physical and psychological exhaustion, this emotional fragility should be anticipated and respected. Again, it is helpful for providers to provide reassurance that such feelings are normal, that time will help, and that one is no more likely to experience additional catastrophes than anyone else in the world who has not had cancer.

Body issues and self-esteem are concerns for many people in this situation. There may have been permanent changes, likely not positive, from cancer surgeries, and there may be other temporary changes like alopecia and weight gain. The reality is that the cancer survivor will have to adapt to her new physical self, and this takes time. Given the emphasis on youth and good looks in our culture, it is painful to feel that both have been lost through the course of illness and treatment. The first flush of euphoria about completing treatment and being alive fades quickly, and the survivor is left with a body and looks that often seem unfamiliar and dystonic. Gained weight can usually be lost through a disciplined program of diet and exercise, and it is helpful to encourage these efforts. It is also important to remind the survivor that the pounds may hang on tenaciously, and that the more important goals are fitness and improved energy.

Cognitive issues are a concern for many survivors. Chemobrain has been well documented and may continue well beyond the completion of treatment. Survivors who feel that they are intellectually diminished will likely have related issues about self-esteem and confidence. Most people find ways to compensate for any troubles with memory, word-finding, or general blunting of mental acuity, but some will have major challenges with their work or engagement with the world. It may be helpful to refer such a patient for neuro-psych testing; this referral will both reflect appreciation of the serious nature of the complaint and may result in the development of positive coping strategies.

Cancer affects the whole family. Cancer also affects the patient's close friends and work colleagues. All important relationships are impacted by the diagnosis, and there likely will be changes and stresses in the survivorship period. If they are parents, most cancer patients worry the most about their children. If the children are small or if there are family circumstances that are especially worrisome (e.g., the cancer patient is a single parent or married to someone with a serious disability), these concerns may be overwhelming. It is helpful to explore these worries, give reassurance when it is appropriate, and help the patient problem solve as needed. If there are issues around care or guardianship of children, it is important to help think them through and make sure that the necessary plans and safeguards are in place. Although it may seem that this conversation could be upsetting, the opposite is much more likely to be true. There is real relief in sharing these serious concerns and having some direction towards solutions.

Cancer is hard on the patient's spouse or partner, too. Although a few relationships are fractured by this experience, most survive the stress and, over time, may even be enriched. As in the case in all situations, communication and mutual support are key in maintaining a strong relationship. It may go without saying that that the spouse has been scared and sad, too, but the fact that it may indeed have been unsaid should be corrected. Studies have suggested that cancer patients' spouses are also vulnerable to depression, and they probably have not received the same kinds of family and community support that have benefited the partner with the illness. Asking about the spouse, expressing empathy towards his experience while always acknowledging the primary problem as belonging to the patient, likely will support and encourage this primary tie.

One big issue for many couples through and after cancer is intimacy. Having cancer is never a sexual aide, and virtually all physical relationships endure at least a period of diminished vitality and satisfaction. Again, it is very helpful to normalize this experience by commenting that all couples find that their sexual relationship is affected by the illness, and that it may take time to re-establish a positive connection. Both libido and responsiveness are impacted by cancer treatment, and men and women worry alike about these changes. Women who have experienced a surgical or chemical menopause probably are dealing with vaginal dryness, or even pain, in addition to lessened libido. Some surgical or hormonal treatments for men directly damage potency. Since sexuality is highly influenced by thoughts and feelings, these physical changes may quickly add additional negative stress. Providers can offer education and information about sexual techniques and aides or can make a referral to a therapist with expertise in this area.

Younger cancer patients may be very distressed about infertility. Although this is not always the case, there are instances when cancer treatment has taken away the choice of a natural pregnancy. The impact of this loss cannot be over-emphasized, and survivors may need to grieve the loss of this dream. It is fortunate that there are other avenues to parenthood, both those involving surrogates or IVF and adoption. However, these possibilities do not lessen the sadness and anger, and it would be a mistake to assume otherwise.

Most cancer survivors report changes in some friendships. It is common to find that some so-called good friends vanish and some acquaintances become marvelous supporters and confidantes. During the period of survivorship, there may be further changes in these relationships. Especially if some friends' behaviors have been hurtful, survivors will have to decide if it is worth trying to repair the damage. This falls into the larger category of changing perspectives, but changing social connections and social support are a likely accompaniment to recovery. Many survivors participate in support groups, advocacy programs, cancer fundraisers, or other opportunities to be with others who have been through a similar experience. These activities may result in very strong personal ties and help with adjustment to the post-acute period.

Professional and workplace issues are another common area of concern. Many people undergoing active cancer treatment reduce their work hours or take a medical/sick leave for the duration. Deciding when and how to return to work can be complicated, and many survivors are ambivalent about resuming their old work schedules too quickly. If possible, it is often most helpful to return to work part-time, perhaps working fewer hours each day rather than fewer days per week. Returning to work also means having to interact with managers and colleagues who may or may not have been fully supportive during the months of illness. It is not unusual for survivors to return to a mixed scenario of warm welcomes and resentment about additional workloads during their absence. Although it is illegal to discriminate against someone because of a medical illness or disability, it is practically impossible to prove that a missed promotion or raise is due to the diagnosis. Job lock and lay offs and discrimination do happen, and a cancer survivor is well advised to be aware of these unfortunate possibilities while maintaining a positive outlook about their own work situation.

Some cancer survivors, as part of their new outlook on life, decide that a professional change is in order. It is wise to take time to consider these possibilities, to explore options, and to understand the benefits and risks associated with a major career move. It may be tempting to make a quick decision about professional direction and priorities, but it is always wiser to take time to settle back into life first.

Financial issues are a major problem for many cancer survivors and their families. During the illness, there may have been reduced income due to leaves or reduced hours, and there certainly were additional expenses both directly and indirectly related to cancer treatment. There are dramatic and terrible stories about people who were forced to sell their homes or deplete their retirement accounts to pay for their care. More often, there are big bills and debts to be faced.

The economic impact of cancer on a person's ability to find and keep a good job is significant. It can be hard to explain a large gap in a resume or to decide when and if to mention a cancer history to a potential employer. Although it is never wise to lie, it is often smarter to say little and to be prepared to explain long absences. Providers sometimes feel pressured to continue to support disability applications long after it seems that the survivor is well enough to return to work. In this instance, it is better to have a frank discussion and try to offer strategies that may be helpful to a job seeker. For example, a job applicant can say something like this in an interview: "You may notice that I have not worked for a couple of years. There were some health problems in my family, but everything is now fine."

Insurance is frequently an issue after cancer or any other major illness. Until medical insurance is universally available and affordable, there will be survivors who cannot purchase a policy because of pre-existing conditions and/or very high premium costs. It may be impossible for a cancer survivor to purchase disability, long-term care, or life insurance for a very long time, and some people are never able to identify available policies unless they are benefits of employment. These insurance gaps can easily harm a whole family's economic security and can be a major source of stress and concern.

Cancer, no matter what the eventual medical outcome, is a major life crisis for both the identified patient and her family. There are always significant psychosocial issues related to recovery, and the most valuable intervention begins with understanding and reassurance that these problems and feelings are normal and will gradually improve. Although there may never be a silver lining associated with a cancer diagnosis, many people go on to believe that there is a rusty tin lining related to a gradual shifting of perspective and appreciation of life.

17

"WAITING FOR THE OTHER SHOE TO DROP": COPING WITH FEAR OF RECURRENCE AFTER CANCER TREATMENT

AMY GROSE, MSW, LICSW

Completing cancer treatment is a goal that patients look forward to throughout the rigors of chemotherapy, surgery, and radiation. And yet, many are not prepared for the surprising emotional challenges that can arise as they seek ways to live their lives post-treatment. As Hester Hill Schnipper described in the chapter on psychosocial issues of survivorship, it is normal to feel sad, anxious, and vulnerable after cancer. And one of the most ubiquitous and enduring emotional adjustments patients face is the fear that cancer might return.

The fear that comes after cancer has often been referred to as the *Damocles Syndrome,* referring to the Greek legend about living with uncertainty. The legend tells of Damocles, a courtier in the fourth century court of his King Dionysius II, who spoke often about how fortunate Dionysius was to live with such wealth and power. Dionysius, upon hearing of the courtier's envy, offered to switch places with him for a day. Damocles eagerly accepted and greatly enjoyed being waited on like a king, filling his belly at a lush banquet given in his honor that evening. When, at the end of the meal, he looked up to see a long, sharp-edged sword hanging directly over his head, held only by a single horse hair, he suddenly lost all delight in the food and company. Dionysius had given Damocles the chance to experience first-hand the constant fear that comes with never knowing when danger might come.

The Damocles legend communicates the sense of feeling vulnerable to future threat from some awaiting danger that many cancer patients experience. When the activity of treatment ends, patients often feel that they are no longer doing something to keep cancer at bay and instead are waiting for the other shoe to drop. Fear that cancer might return (or a new diagnosis might be found) is a common concern of the patients seen in survivorship clinics. One breast cancer patient seen at a survivorship visit voiced the challenge very succinctly by explaining that, "fear of cancer is worse than having cancer."

It is important to note that while it is a common and central issue for many patients, there are some that have a different perspective such as the patient who had been treated for Hodgkin's disease who said, "I don't think of the cancer coming back. I feel that time is too precious and I want to focus on being alive." As was true with diagnosis and treatment, the experience after treatment is unique to each person who is going through it.

What is fear of recurrence? How is it experienced and by whom? And what can providers do to help patients cope with its impact? And if one questions if this is really a subject that warrants attention, consider how the journalist and cancer survivor John Diamond describes this challenge: "Living in the time after cancer is similar to being on death row." This sentiment coming at a time when much of the outside world expects the patient to be celebrating with delight at being done with treatment can be confusing and distressing for many (Hodges & Humphris, 2009). Providers can play an essential role in helping patients verbalize, understand, and cope with these emotions and fears.

Worrying about cancer returning is a normal reaction to having gone through the emotional and physical trauma of being diagnosed with and treated for a life-threatening illness. While the literature recognizes fear of recurrence as being a central and lingering concern for many cancer patients, there is little consensus on the best way to define and measure it. One definition offered is that fear of recurrence is "the degree of concern reported by subjects about the chances of cancer returning at a future time" (Northouse, 1981). There is a variety of ideas as to the prevalence, causes, and effective interventions to decrease fear of recurrence. Some studies have shown there is a decrease in fear of recurrence the further out from diagnosis a patient gets while other studies have found no change in fear of recurrence even 10–20 years out from treatment.

Younger age at diagnosis has been found to be a predictor of higher levels of fear of recurrence with significant decrease in fear seen in older patients. In breast cancer patients, pain levels were a strong predictor of fear of recurrence but education and income levels had no predictive value. Studies have shown inconsistency of the correlation between fear of recurrence and diagnosis, stage and/or treatment. There is also a wide range of reported percentage of patients reporting fear of recurrence ranging from 5% to 89% of survivors (Lee-Jones, Humphris, Dixon, & Hatcher, 1997; Mellon, Kershaw, & Northouse, 2007). Some of the disease sites found to have the most frequent *moderate to high levels* of worry about cancer relapse/new diagnosis are Breast: 31–70%; Head and neck: 72–80%; Gynecological: 22–64%; Colorectal: 27–33%; Testicular: 24–31% (Mehnert, Berg, Henrich, & Herschbach, 2009; Humphris, 2003; Skaali, Fossa, Bremnes, & Dahl, 2009).

Whatever the cause, high levels of fear of recurrence obviously indicate increased emotional distress and difficulty adjusting to post-treatment life. Patients report lower quality of life with more worry, inability to plan for the future, lower energy, more intrusive thinking, and overall lower quality of life. There can also be an avoidance of medical follow-up or the converse, an increase of visits to providers due to higher level of vigilance and body monitoring for symptoms indicating cancer's return. Some patients have a more positive response of making changes in health behaviors such as increasing exercise, eating a healthier diet, and managing stress (Mellon, Kershaw, & Northouse, 2007).

Patients often report that fear of recurrence is a consistent concern but one that is generally manageable and not intrusive the majority of time. However, there are times when the fear "rises like a wave or like the highest point of the roller coaster ride right before your stomach drops and you can't catch your breath," as one person treated for sarcoma aptly described. These are the times when fear of cancer's return moves from the background into the foreground and causes what Annette Stanton and colleagues call "islands of disruption" (Stanton, Ganz, Rowland, Meyerowitz, Krupnick, & Sears, 2005). Some of these increases of worry occur around events such as: anniversaries of diagnosis, surgery, or end of treatment; follow-up scans; body aches/pains; hearing of family, friends or celebrities being diagnosed or relapsing; learning of the death of a cancer survivor; finding out about new treatments that hadn't been available; and/or having to make decisions about future plans such as retirement. One support group coined the term scanaphobia when talking about the heightened level of fear that caused some of its members to lose sleep weeks or days, before and sometimes after, follow-up scans. Normalizing these spikes of worry are important as often patients report feeling crazy or that they may not be as positive as they are supposed to be. Reassurance and education about these reactions can be especially helpful to patients experiencing these responses.

It is also important to recognize that it isn't *just* the patients who worry about cancer coming back. It is well known that cancer impacts many people around the patient and that partners, family members, friends, and colleagues also have to adjust emotionally after treatment ends. Some studies have shown that family care partners have significantly *more* fear of recurrence than survivors and can also have lower quality of life as a result. In a study exploring survivors and family caregivers' level of fear of recurrence, Mellon, Kershaw, and Northouse (2007) found that those who reported more family stress had more fear of recurrence. They also learned that as one family member's fear of recurrence increased so did the other family member's. Thus, it is important to be aware that it is not just the patient who will benefit from education and normalization around coping with fear of cancer coming back, partners and other family members are also in need of this support.

How then to provide this education and needed support to patients and their family members? The "don't worry, be happy you are alive" approach that is sometimes offered may let the person saying it feel better but overall it is not effective. Patients report feeling more isolated and anxious when well-meaning providers encourage them to not be concerned about cancer returning. Yet, it is also not useful for patients to feel overwhelmed and paralyzed by fear or as one patient voiced, "not risk moving forward because the next bomb might fall."

Providing some basic education for patients that encourage them to focus on what they *can* do, rather than what they cannot, is a good beginning. Moving from there, patients and families can be given suggestions for developing a wellness plan with part of it focusing on ways to manage the fear which is a normal part of adjusting to life after cancer. Anne Coscarelli, PhD, a psychologist at Simms/Mann UCLA Center for Integrative Oncology, specializes in helping patients cope effectively with fear of recurrence. She suggests the following components be included in a patient's Fear Management plan:

- Talk with medical team about what symptoms to pay attention to and when to contact the team
- Develop cognitive approaches/phrases to replace automatic thoughts
- Make a list of who you can talk to about your fears
- Explore creative outlets, such as writing, art, and music
- Seek counseling (and medication if needed)
- Develop a list of distraction techniques
- Exercise, be as active as possible, find activity you like to do
- Engage in pleasurable activities
- Avoid Internet surfing
- Ask for support from families and friends
- Utilize mind-body approaches such as meditation, acupuncture, yoga, massage . . .
- Contact survivorship support resources
- Develop helpful "self-talk" such as:
  - It is unlikely this is cancer, I was screened __ months ago and things were fine.
  - If I have this pain in two weeks I will go see my doctor, but I can call sooner if I need to.
  - There are things I enjoy doing and I can focus on one of those.
  - I can write about this in my journal and leave it.

Medical providers can also offer some statements that patients (and family members) can repeat to themselves when fear of recurrence increases. Most patients, and especially those who had lengthy diagnostic work-ups with lack of clarity and timely treatment, may be especially vulnerable to feeling they must be hypervigilant about watching for any symptoms or signs of recurrence. It can be very reassuring to them to be reminded that they are not alone in monitoring their health, that they are known to the oncology team, and that they have been given specifics about the schedule for screening and monitoring for any signs of cancer. It is also very helpful, if it is true, to remind the patient that they have received the best treatment possible and that they do not have active cancer at this time. Dr. Coscarelli also encourages providers to let patients know that fear is a normal part of the process, that it can be managed, and that if worry is high to come to speak with the providers. It is also helpful to normalize the usefulness of meeting with a counselor and to refer patients and family members to appropriate clinicians for support and education on coping strategies after treatment ends, as this is a new phase in the cancer experience and new skills are required (Coscarelli, April 4, 2009).

Sometimes distraction, self-talk, thought-suppression, journaling, and other strategies work well and no other approaches are needed. But sometimes these techniques may only be effective for a period of time. The message to not think about it, to live as if there is nothing to fear, may work—but more often, worry continues to arise, despite efforts to try to eliminate it. In fact, sometimes trying not to think about something can have a different outcome than expected.

Think for a moment about a giraffe, imagine it with all of its spots being different colors of the rainbow. Visualize it in your mind's eye for a few moments, seeing the long neck covered with bright colored spots, the big ears, dark eyes, perhaps chewing its cud as it looks at you. Shut your eyes to give yourself a bit of time to really see this unexpected sight. Then, open your eyes, now, take a breath and stop thinking about the polka dotted giraffe for 20 seconds. Don't imagine any of the colors, the movement, the length of the neck . . . really, just clear you mind.

What did you notice? How successful were you?

For many people, when asked to not think about something, it actually has the opposite effect. In fact, the more that people try to resist thinking about something, it becomes a more insistent focus. As Dr. Wegner found in his work on the paradoxical effects of thought suppression, the more that effort is expended to stop thinking about something, the more repetition of remembering occurs as attempts are made to stop thinking! Suppression of thought, as many studies have shown, may be the starting point of obsession, rather than the other way around. As a result, doubts, worries, and fears that have been tried to be erased end up persisting more strongly than ever (Wegner, Schneider, Carter, & White, 1987). What does this mean for people worrying about cancer coming back?

For some patients and their families, trying *not* to think about the fear is simply adding strength of focus to their worry. A different approach, which can appear paradoxical at first, is to turn toward the fear, to learn to accept that fear is a companion in the survivorship journey. This is a mindfulness approach, a way of being present with what is here right now. It is helpful to remind patients that allowing oneself to feel fear does not mean not being hopeful, it is simply recognizing that one is imagining an undesired future rather than imagining a hoped for future.

A powerful antidote to worry is to remain in the present moment, to see what is happening at this moment in time. In a mindfulness approach, patients are encouraged to turn toward the feeling of fear and to learn more of how it is experienced by their body, mind, spirit, and emotion, bringing a sense of curiosity to the experience without judgment. What can be discovered is that fear is a thought, a feeling, it is not a truth nor is it constant. Helping patients to learn to ride the waves of the fear of cancer recurrence can bring a sense of mastery and relief as they learn to live with and through the experience as it arises, peaks, and passes through.

Mindfulness-based psychotherapy has been found to be a successful approach to helping patients cope with anxiety and fear of recurrence. Christopher Germer, Ron Siegel, and Paul Fulton, in their book *Mindfulness and Psychotherapy* (2005), offer some suggestions about coping with anxiety. These are strategies that some cancer survivors have found helpful to remember and incorporate into their coping strategies:

- Anxiety is a fact of life, it protects us from danger.
- We cannot control what we think.
- Trying to control or avoid our experience is futile and often makes it worse.
- The brain makes mistakes.
- Problems occur when we believe in the reactions of the body to a false alarm by the brain
- Panic is never permanent. It has a beginning, middle, and end.
- Treatment for anxiety is the gradual process of redirecting attention toward the fear, exploring it in detail as it arises, and befriending it.
- Freedom from anxiety entails becoming disillusioned with our fear. Worries become ordinary mental events occurring in the brain. (Germer, Siegel, & Fulton, 2005)

It is important to acknowledge that there is a continuum of anxiety and fear of recurrence and that a range of approaches and strategies are needed to provide the tools for each person's coping needs. Assessment by a psychosocial oncology clinician is also a very important resource to utilize if symptoms are disruptive or don't decrease to a manageable level over time. It is important to provide referrals to therapists in the cancer center or therapists in the community with oncology experience for patients and/or partner or family members when needed. Because fear of recurrence is normal, it is important that patients have the opportunity to learn new coping strategies to deal with this emotional challenge effectively.

In summary, fear of recurrence is a central challenge for cancer survivors and its intensity can ebb and flow over time. It is important to recognize that providers have an essential role in educating cancer survivors that fear of recurrence is a normal part of the post-treatment experience and that there are many effective ways to deal with this fear. A mindfulness approach, including a willingness to recognize and accept fear, can be a helpful strategy to decrease distress around fear of recurrence. Providers have an essential role in providing education to help patients better understand their physical and emotional post-treatment recovery and in offering support to patients and family as they move forward in their lives.

Jon Kabat-Zinn, nationally recognized for his work in mindfulness, stress reduction, health care and research, offers the following perspective of viewing the future (Kabat-Zinn, 2007). It can be a useful reminder for patients, family members, and providers alike:

We do not know what will happen next.
If we wish to take care of the future,
the only way we can do that is to be present to each moment.

REFERENCES

Coscarelli, A. (April 4, 2009). The Challenges of Cancer Survivorship: Psychological Understandings and Strategies. UCLA Cancer Survivorship Education Day.

Germer, C., Siegel, R., & Fulton, P. (2005). *Mindfulness and Psychotherapy.* New York: Guilford Press.

Hodges, L., & Humphris, G. (2009). Fear of recurrence and psychological distress in head and neck cancer patients and their carers. *Psycho-oncology, 18,* 841–848.

Humphris, G. R.-J. (2003). Fear of recurrence and possible cases of anxiety and depression in orofacialcancer patients. *International Journal of Oral Maxillofacial Surgery, 32,* 486–491.

Lee-Jones, C., Humphris, G., Dixon, R., & Hatcher, B. (1997). Fear of Cancer Recurrence— A Literature review and proposed cognitive formulation to explain exacerbation of recurrence fears. *Psycho-Oncology, 6,* 95–105.

Mehnert, A., Berg, P., Henrich, G., & Herschbach, P. (2009). Fear of cancer progression and cancer-related intrusive cognitions in breast cancer survivors. *Psycho-Oncology.*

Mellon, S., Kershaw, T., & Northouse, L. F.-G. (2007). A family-based model to predict fear of recurrence for cancer survivors and their caregivers. *Psycho-Oncology, 16,* 214–223.

Northouse, L. (1981). Mastectomy Patients and the fear of cancer recurrence. *Cancer Nurse, 13,* 213–220.

Skaali, T., Fossa, S., Bremnes, R., & Dahl, O. H. (2009). Fear of recurrence in long-term testicular cancer survivors. *Psycho-Oncology, 18,* 580–588.

Stanton, A., Ganz, P., Rowland, J., Meyerowitz, B., Krupnick, J., & Sears, S. (2005). Promoting adjustment after treatment for cancer. *Cancer, 104,* 2608–2613.

Wegner, D. M., Schneider, D., Carter, S., & White, T. (1987). Paradoxical effects of thought suppression. *J Pers Soc Psychol, 53*(1): 5–13.

18

Co-Survivors, Family, and Friends

Ashley Varner, MSW, MBA, LCSW-C

In recent years, a new term has been coined in cancer survivorship: *co-survivor*. Co-survivors, also sometimes known as *informal caregivers* or simply *caregivers*, are family, friends, and colleagues who offer support to survivors from diagnosis through treatment and beyond. Historically, the experiences and challenges of co-survivors have not received much attention in health care or research communities. More recently, researchers are exploring the experience of co-survivors and interventions to mediate negative repercussions during diagnosis and treatment (Alfano & Rowland, 2006; Bucher et al., 2001; Northouse, 2005). Nonetheless, the experience of co-survivors once their loved one's treatment is complete continues to be largely unexplored (Northouse, Mellon, Harden J., & Schafenacker, 2009). This chapter will provide background information about cancer co-survivors, and discuss the social, emotional, physical, and spiritual or existential issues that co-survivors may confront once their loved one's treatment is complete. It will also offer concrete suggestions for ways health care providers can help co-survivors during their co-survivorship journeys.

Who Are the Co-Survivors?

The number of cancer co-survivors quoted in the literature ranges from around 3.5 million to more than 12 million. This range is due to differences in definitions of co-survivor and caregiver, as well as various research limitations.

Some estimate that every cancer survivor has at least one co-survivor. Since there are currently an estimated 12.5 million cancer survivors (National Cancer Institute, 2010), 12.5 million is often quoted for the number of cancer caregivers or co-survivors.

On the other end of the spectrum, the National Alliance for Caregiving and the American Association of Retired Persons completed a telephone survey of more than 6,000 individuals in 2004, and identified slightly less than 1,250 caregivers caring for adults with a variety of illnesses. Extrapolating these results, researchers estimated that at the time of the survey there were approximately 44.4 million unpaid caregivers in the United States. Of the caregivers identified in this study, 8% reported caring for someone with cancer (National Alliance for Caregiving & American Association of Retired Persons, 2004). This would equal approximately 3.6 million cancer caregivers, a daunting number when one recognizes that for the purposes of this study the definition of caregiver was quite narrow: anyone 18 years of age or older providing care for an adult who needed help with at least one activity of daily living such as bathing or dressing. The emotional burden for those who care about someone with cancer can be high, even if no physical assistance is needed (Kim & Schultz, 2008).

Among cancer co-survivors, more than half are the spouse of the survivor (Mellon, Northouse, & Weiss, 2006). Another estimated 20% are adult children (Mosher & Weiss, 2010). Other co-survivors include siblings, friends, neighbors, and work colleagues (Case, 2006). Co-survivors are the primary source of support for cancer survivors, particularly during long-term survivorship when visits with the health care team dwindle. It is crucial, then, for health care providers to have a strong understanding of the experience of co-survivors in order to support them and the survivor.

EMOTIONAL CHALLENGES

The emotional experience of cancer co-survivors has received more attention than any other aspect of long-term cancer co-survivorship (Lewis & Hammond, 1992; Northouse et al., 2009). In short, like survivors, co-survivors are frequently surprised to experience issues of emotional adjustment when their loved one's treatment is done (Ell, Nishimoto, Mantell, & Hamovitch, 1988; Northouse, 1988). Longitudinal studies are few and far between, so the duration of co-survivor's emotional distress is unclear. It is clear, however, that emotional sequelae for some co-survivors can continue for years, even after the survivor has ceased to have evidence of disease (Gritz, Wellisch, Siau, & Wang, 1990; Zahlis & Shands, 1993).

Co-survivors experience many of the same long-term emotional challenges as cancer survivors, including fear of recurrence (Matthews, Baker, & Spillers, 2003), worry (Northouse, 2005), and uncertainty (Kim et al., 2008; Walker, 1997). However, at the time that treatment is done, co-survivors are often ready to get back to normal, whereas survivors may be trying to come to terms with all that has happened during the months of treatment (Lethborg, Kissane, & Burns, 2003). This difference in focus between survivors and co-survivors can cause additional emotional distress for both survivors and co-survivors. Moreover, the normal after cancer for both survivors and co-survivors is often a new normal rather than the normal that survivors and their loved ones experienced pre-cancer.

The emotional well-being of survivors and co-survivors is also interdependent (Baider & Kaplan De-Nour, 1988; Gritz et al., 1990; Northouse, Mood, Templin, Mellon, & George, 2000). When co-survivors are struggling with emotional issues, survivors are more likely to struggle and vice versa.

Not all co-survivors experience high levels of emotional distress. A subgroup of about 20% of co-survivors appears to experience high levels of distress in response to cancer (Edwards & Clarke, 2004). Given the interdependence of familial emotional well-being and a one-in-five chance that a co-survivor will experience high distress, psychosocial screening of both survivors and co-survivors could be most effective in improving quality of life for all affected.

Co-Survivors Will Benefit If Health Care Providers Will

- Educate co-survivors that the emotional impact of cancer continues even after treatment is done, for both the co-survivor and the survivor.
- Teach co-survivors and their loved ones that survivors may take a year or more to return to normal, and that normal may be a new normal.
- Screen for emotional distress among both survivors and co-survivors.
- Address fears of recurrence and feelings of worry and uncertainty with both survivors and co-survivors.
- Help co-survivors and survivors to understand that their emotional well-being is interdependent. Addressing emotional health will benefit both members of the dyad.

SOCIAL CHALLENGES

Social challenges during long-term cancer co-survivorship include relationship, communication, financial, and social role issues. To date, in the area of social changes secondary to cancer, researchers have primarily focused on the marital relationship. Cancer does stress the marital relationship, but research shows that separation and divorce are not common consequences of a cancer diagnosis (Northouse et al., 2009). On the contrary, studies have shown increased intimacy over time in relationships where one partner has been diagnosed with cancer (Gritz et al., 1990; Lewis & Hammond, 1992).

Researchers have found that differences in communication styles and lack of communication about cancer can be one source of strain in marital relationships post cancer treatment. Typically, the female would like more discussion of cancer, the experience of treatment, and how to make sense of it in her life, and the male usually is more reticent. More open styles of communication have been found to correlate positively with better adaptation post-treatment (Edwards & Clarke, 2004; B. B. Germino, Fife, & Funk, 1995).

Most recently, more attention has been given to the financial impact of cancer on both survivors and co-survivors. In a recent study completed by the Cancer Support Community, survivors and co-survivors reported levels of trauma from trying to manage the financial aspects of cancer that were greater than those reported by individuals who were in Manhattan on September 11, 2001, and equal to those of African Americans who were in New Orleans during Hurricane Katrina. This financial distress often lasts long after treatment is complete. The co-survivor is often impacted by the financial stress of cancer just as much as the survivor.

A final social challenge for co-survivors during long-term survivorship is role identification and role confusion. Co-survivors often do not identify with the role of co-survivor or caregiver. Although they are fulfilling the duties of a co-survivor, they do not identify with the title, and therefore do not recognize that support is available for them. The roles of the survivor and co-survivor are also likely to be renegotiated once treatment is done and in an ongoing way as survivorship continues. These renegotiations can be stressful.

Co-Survivors Will Benefit if Health Care Providers Will

- Prepare survivors and co-survivors in committed relationships to understand that cancer can strain the relationship, but also inform couples that, long-term, many couples report an increase in intimacy after cancer.
- Teach survivors and co-survivors open styles of communication.
- Screen for financial distress and connect individuals with resources to help them cope with the cost of care.
- Address role identification and role confusion. Teach co-survivors the word "co-survivor" and refer them to resources for additional support.

PHYSICAL CHALLENGES

Little is known about the long-term physical effects of cancer on caregivers of survivors with no evidence of disease. One study does suggest that cancer can serve as a wake-up call to co-survivors to take better care of their own health (Mellon, 2002). Cancer co-survivors have been shown to have a variety of health concerns during the treatment period, including increased incidence of disturbed sleep (Carter & Acton, 2006), anxiety and depression (Carter & Acton, 2006; Pitceathly, Maguire, Haddad, & Fletcher, 2004), fatigue (Jensen & Given, 1993), and poor health (Borg & Hallberg, 2006) compared to their non-caregiving counterparts.

Research with family caregivers of people with chronic illness indicates that caregivers who experience increased role strain may have an increased mortality risk. Strained caregivers were not as likely to participate in preventive wellness practices and also less likely to seek help for themselves for symptoms or illness (Schultz & Beach, 1999). While this study was done with caregivers of individuals with cardiovascular disease, cancer co-survivors experiencing high levels of strain may have similar experiences.

Sexuality and fertility issues also may arise in relationships between co-survivors and survivors. In one study, 66% of long-term survivors of prostate cancer reported that their partners had at least one sexual concern that interfered with their sexual relationship (Schover, Fouladi, et al., 2002). Sexuality issues may come up no matter what the age of the couple. Fertility issues are most common with younger couples. Survivors and co-survivors will benefit from more research in this area.

> ## Co-Survivors Will Benefit if Health Care Providers Will
>
> - Encourage co-survivors to attend to their own health care and wellness needs.
> - Teach survivors and co-survivors healthy survivorship behaviors including exercise, nutrition, and follow-up care.
> - Refer survivors and co-survivors to behavior change programs such as *Cancer Transitions Online* (www.cancertransitionsonline.org) that assist individuals with developing healthy habits.
> - Address issues of sexuality and fertility throughout the survivorship journey.

SPIRITUAL/EXISTENTIAL CHALLENGES

The chief existential challenge for cancer co-survivors is making meaning or sense out of their loved one's cancer diagnosis. Cancer can be a transformative experience, causing some families to reconsider priorities. Families reported a greater appreciation of everyday life as they reflected on the past and thought about ways to make the most of the present and future (Mellon, 2002). Family members who associate a more positive meaning with their cancer have a more positive emotional response to the cancer (B.B. Germino et al., 1995; B.B. Germino & O'Rourke, 1996).

> ## Co-Survivors Will Benefit if Health Care Providers Will
>
> - Acknowledge spiritual well-being as an important aspect of quality of life.
> - Provide resources such as pastoral care, social work, or other counseling to discuss meaning making with co-survivors.

CONCLUSION

Co-survivors are a primary source of support for cancer survivors, particularly during long-term survivorship when visits with the health care team dwindle. It is crucial for health care providers to have a strong understanding of the experience of co-survivors in order to support them and the survivor. Co-survivors face very real emotional, social, physical, and existential challenges secondary to their loved one's cancer. This chapter details these challenges as well as providing concrete suggestions for ways health care providers can assist co-survivors on their journeys.

REFERENCES

Alfano, C.M., & Rowland, J.H. (2006). Recovery issues in cancer survivorship: A new challenge for supportive care. *The Cancer Journal*, (12), 432–443.

Baider, L., & Kaplan De-Nour, A. (1988). Adjustment to cancer: Who is the patient—the husband or the wife?. *Israel Journal of Medical Sciences, 24*(9–10), 631–636.

Borg, C., & Hallberg, I.R. (2006). Life satisfaction among informal caregivers in comparison with non-caregivers. *Scandinavian Journal of Caring Sciences, 20*(4), 427–438. doi:10.1111/j.1471–6712.2006.00424.x

Bucher, J.A., Loscalzo, M., Zabora, J., Houts, P.S., Hooker, C., & BrintzenhofSzoc, K. (2001). Problem-solving cancer care education for patients and caregivers. *Cancer Practice, 9*(2), 66–70.

Carter, P.A., & Acton, G.J. (2006). Personality and coping: Predictors of depression and sleep problems among caregivers of individuals who have cancer. *Journal of Gerontological Nursing, 32*(2), 45–53.

Case, P. (2006). Social opportunity in the face of cancer: Understanding the burden of the extended caregiver network. *Illness, Crisis & Loss, 14*(4), 299–318.

Edwards, B., & Clarke, V. (2004). The psychological impact of a cancer diagnosis on families: The influence of family functioning and patients' illness characteristics on depression and anxiety. *Psycho-Oncology, 13*(8), 562–576.

Ell, K., Nishimoto, R., Mantell, J., & Hamovitch, M. (1988). Longitudinal analysis of psychological adaptation among family members of patients with cancer. *Journal of Psychosomatic Research, 32*(4–5), 429–438.

Germino, B.B., Fife, B.L., & Funk, S.G. (1995). Cancer and the partner relationship: What is the meaning? *Seminars in Oncology Nursing, 11*(1), 43–50.

Germino, B.B., & O'Rourke, M.E. (1996). Cancer and the family. In R. McCorkle, M. Grant, M. Frank-Stromborg & S.B. Baird (Eds.), *Cancer nursing: A comprehensive textbook* (pp. 81–92). Philadelphia, PA: W.B. Saunders Company.

Gritz, E.R., Wellisch, D.K., Siau, J., & Wang, H.J. (1990). Lon-term effects of testicular cancer on marital relationships. *Psychosomatics, 31,* 301–312.

Jensen, S., & Given, B. (1993). Fatigue affecting family caregivers of cancer patients. *Supportive Care in Cancer, 1*(6), 321–325.

Kim, Y., & Schultz, R. (2008). Family caregivers' strains: Comparative analysis of cancer caregiving with dementia, diabetes, and frail elderly caregiving. *Journal of Aging and Health, 20*(5), 483–503.

Kim, Y., Kashy, D.A., Wellisch, D.K., Spillers, R.L., Kaw, C.K., & Smith, T.G. (2008). Quality of life of couples dealing with cancer: Dyadic and individual adjustment among breast and prostate cancer survivors and their spousal caregivers. *Annals of Behavioral Medicine, 35*(2), 230–238.

Lethborg, C.E., Kissane, D., & Burns, W.I. (2003). 'It's not the easy part': The experience of significant others of women with early stage breast cancer, at treatment completion. *Social Work in Health Care, 37*(1), 63–85.

Lewis, F.M., & Hammond, M.A. (1992). Psychosocial adjustment of the family to breast cancer: A longitudinal analysis. *Journal of the American Medical Womens Association, 47*(5), 194–200.

Matthews, B.A., Baker, F., & Spillers, R.L. (2003). Family caregivers and indicators of cancer-related distress. *Psychology, Health & Medicine, 8*(1), 45–56.

Mellon, S. (2002). Comparisons between cancer survivors and family members on meaning of the illness and family quality of life. *Oncology Nursing Forum, 29*(7), 1117–1125.

Mellon, S., Northouse, L.L., & Weiss, L.K. (2006). A population-based study of the quality of life of cancer survivors and their family caregivers. *Cancer Nursing, 29,* 120–131.

Mosher, C.E., & Weiss, T.R. (2010). Psychosocial research and practice with adult children of cancer patients. In J.C. Holland, W.S. Breitbart, P.B. Jacobsen, M.S. Lederberg, M.J. Loscalzo, & R. McCorkle (Ed.), *Psycho-oncology* (2nd ed., pp. 532–535). New York, NY: Oxford.

National Alliance for Caregiving, & American Association of Retired Persons. (2004). *Caregiving in the U.S.* Washington, DC: National Alliance for Caregiving.

National Cancer Institute. (2010). *Cancer trends progress report—2009/2010 update.* Washington, DC: National Cancer Institute.

Northouse, L.L., Mellon, S., Harden J., & Schafenacker, A. (2009). Long-term effects of cancer on families of adult cancer survivors. In S.M. Miller, D.J. Bowen, R.T. Croyle & J.H. Rowland (Ed.), *Handbook of cancer control and behavioral science: A resource for researchers, practitioners, and policymakers* (pp. 467–485). Washington, DC: American Psychological Association.

Northouse, L.L. (1988). Social support in patients' and husbands' adjustment to breast cancer. *NURS RES, 37,* 91–95.

Northouse, L.L. (2005). Helping families of patients with cancer. *Oncology Nursing Forum, 32*(4), 743–750.

Northouse, L.L., Mood, D., Templin, T., Mellon, S., & George, T. (2000). Couples' patterns of adjustment to colon cancer. *Social Science & Medicine, 50*(2), 271–284.

Northouse, L.L., Rosset, T., Phillips, L., Mood, D., Schafenacker, A., & Kershaw, T. (2006). Research with families facing cancer: The challenges of accrual and retention. *Research in Nursing & Health, 29*(3), 199–211.

Pitceathly, C., Maguire, P., Haddad, P., & Fletcher, I. (2004). Prevalence of and markers for affective disorders among cancer patients' caregivers. *Journal of Psychosocial Oncology, 22*(3), 45–68. doi:10.1300/J077v22n03•03.

Schultz, R., & Beach, S.R. (1999). Caregiving as a risk factor for mortality: The caregiver health effects study. *Journal of the American Medical Association, 282*(23).

Walker, B.L. (1997). Adjustment of husbands and wives to breast cancer. *Cancer Practice, 5*(2), 92–98.

Zahlis, E.H., & Shands, M.E. (1993). The impact of breast cancer on the partner 18 months after diagnosis. *Seminars in Oncology Nursing, 9,* 83–97.

19

CANCER FATIGUE: MECHANISMS AND MANAGEMENT IN PATIENTS AND SURVIVORS

FURHA COSSOR, MD, AND
KENNETH B. MILLER, MD

INTRODUCTION

Cancer-related fatigue is defined as "a distressing persistent, subjective sense of physical, emotional and/or cognitive tiredness or exhaustion related to cancer or cancer treatment that is not proportional to recent activity and interferes with usual functioning."[1] It is present in 70–100% of oncology patients during active treatment, with an even higher prevalence in patients with metastatic disease.[1] Patients have reported fatigue to be a more distressing side effect of treatment than pain, nausea, or vomiting (Figure 19.1). Cancer-related fatigue (CRF) often lasts months to years after treatment ends, and is an under-reported, under-diagnosed, and under-treated condition in oncology patients.

With treatment regimens in all subtypes of cancer becoming more effective, the population of cancer survivors is increasing. As of January 2007, in the United States about 11.7 million individuals are alive with a previous diagnosis of cancer.[2] Approximately 66% of people diagnosed with cancer are now expected to survive at least five years after diagnosis. Considering the prevalence of CRF in survivors, knowledge of the causative mechanisms, diagnostic criteria, and treatment of this condition is needed. In this chapter we review the proposed pathophysiology, diagnosis, treatment options and recommendations, as well as current areas of research in CRF.

PATHOPHYSIOLOGY

CRF can be induced by the physiologic and psychological stresses associated with cancer, treatment of the disease, or the malignancy itself.[3] The biologic mechanisms underlying CRF are unclear and no single definitive

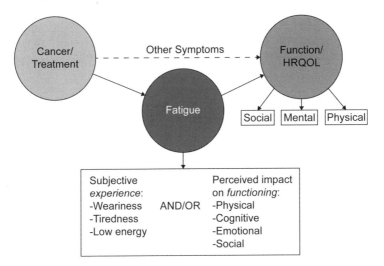

Figure 19.1. ICD-10 Criteria for the diagnosis of cancer-related fatigue

mechanism has been found in most patients. Several proposed mechanisms include serotonin dysregulation, endocrine dysfunction including abnormalities of the hypothalamic-pituitary-adrenal axis, circadian rhythm disruption, and cytokine dysregulation (Table 19.1).[4]

The dysregulation of serotonin (5-HT), either via increased levels of 5-HT in the brain,[5,6] or via altered function of 5-HT receptors in the hypothalamus,[7,8] may play a role in the etiology of CRF. Studies in animal models have shown that sustained exercise increases 5-HT levels in the hypothalamus and brain stem, and fatigue correlated with higher concentrations of 5-HT.[9,10] Regarding 5-HT receptor activity, early studies using indirect measures of 5-HT function found evidence of both upregulation and possible hypersensitivity of 5-HT receptors in patients suffering from chronic fatigue syndrome.[7,11] A more recent study, however using PET scan imaging techniques failed to demonstrate either decreased 5-HT receptor number or affinity in individuals with CRF. Two randomized, prospective, placebo-controlled studies in breast cancer patients on active treatment examined the effect of paroxetine, a selective serotonin reuptake inhibitor, on CRF. Both studies failed to find a significant improvement associated with the use of paroxetine.[12,13]

Another possible etiology of CRF is hypothalamic-pituitary-adrenal (HPA) axis dysfunction. Cancer and/or its treatment alters homeostasis of the HPA axis, which can result in endocrine changes that cause or contribute to fatigue.[4] The HPA axis controls the release of cortisol in response to physical or psychological stress, and also influences the development of immune cells and cytokine production. Low levels of cortisol, a key hormone in the axis, have been associated with fatigue and may result from direct suppression or decreased stimulation of the HPA axis.[14] In a study of 27 breast cancer survivors, the

TABLE 19.1 ISSUES CONTRIBUTING TO CANCER-RELATED FATIGUE

Symptoms burden
  Pain
  Anxiety
  Depression
  Sleep dysfunction
    Obstructive sleep apnea
    Restless leg syndrome
    Narcolepsy
    Insomnia
Nutritional imbalances
  Weight changes
  Changes in caloric intake
  Fluid and electrolyte imbalances
  Motility disorders
Physical function
  Decreased physical activity
  Deconditioning
Medical Issues
  Anemia
  Other comorbidities
    Infection
    Cardiac disease
    Connective tissue diseases
    Pulmonary dysfunction
    Renal dysfunction
    Hepatic dysfunction
    Neurologic dysfunction
    Endocrine dysfunction
      Hypothyroidism
      Hypogonadism
      Diabetes Mellitus
      Adrenal Insufficiency
Medications
  Sedating agents (hypnotics, narcotics, neuropathic agents, etc.)
  Beta-blockers
  Supplements (homeopathic agents)

(Continued)

TABLE 19.1 (*Continued*)

Cancer treatment effects

   Chemotherapy

   Radiation therapy

   Surgery

   Bone marrow transplant

   Biologic response modifiers

   Hormonal treatment

Adapted from Escalante, C. and E. Manzullo. "Cancer-Related Fatigue: The Approach and Treatment." *J Gen Intern Med* 2009; 24(S2): 412–416.

fatigued cohort had significantly blunted cortisol response after exposure to a stressor as compared to the non-fatigued cohort.[15] Though the study was small, it indicated that abnormalities in the HPA axis may play a role in CRF. In addition abnormalities of thyroid function, gonadotropin hormones either related to the cancer or its treatment may contribute to the development of CRF.

Disruption of circadian rhythms may also play a role in CRF. Circadian rhythms describe a group of biochemical, physiologic, and behavior patterns that are regulated by the suprachiasmatic nuclei in the anterior hypothalamus according to a 24-hour period. They are regulated by both environmental and psychological factors via neuroanatomic pathways, cytokines, and hormones.[16] In patients with cancer, alterations in several circadian functions have been found, including changes in cortisol, melatonin, and prolactin secretion, temperature and circulating protein levels, levels of circulating leukocytes and neutrophils, and rest-activity patterns.[4] The biologic basics of these alterations, however, are not well defined.

Increased plasma levels of proinflammatory cytokines are associated with cancer and its treatment and may be important mediators in CRF. The tumor micro-environments contain pro-inflammatory cytokines such as IL-1, IL-2, IL-6, and TNF-α.[17] Moreover, cancer and its treatments, including chemotherapy, surgery, radiation, and biologic therapies are associated with increased plasma levels of TNF-α, IL-1β, and IL-6.[18–20] Genome-wide expression microarrays have shown that pro-inflammatory transcription factors, particularly NF-κB, may also play a role in CRF.[21] Increased cytokine levels can in turn contribute to anemia, cachexia, muscle wasting, anorexia, fever, infection and depression, all of which can exacerbate fatigue.[22]

In addition to one or all of the above possible etiologies, comorbid conditions such as anemia, cachexia, depression, and sleep disorders, which independently can cause fatigue, are also common in cancer patients. The difficulty in determining the cause of cancer related fatigue is the multitude of contributing factors, both physiologic and psychologic, which can coexist in the same patient (Figure 19.2).

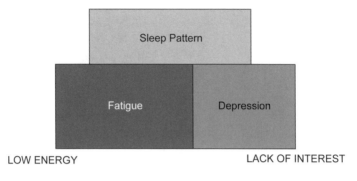

Conceptually Different

Figure 19.2. Multifactorial Model of Cancer-Related Fatigue.

DIAGNOSIS

National Comprehensive Cancer Network (NCCN) guidelines recommend screening for cancer-related fatigue at a patient's initial visit, at regular intervals during and following cancer treatment, and as clinically indicated.[1] The guidelines suggest the following screening question: "How would you rate your fatigue on a scale of 0–10 [0 = no fatigue and 10 = worst fatigue imaginable] over the past 7 days?" A score of 0–3 is mild fatigue, 4–6 is moderate fatigue, and 7–10 is severe fatigue, and the scale was shown to be approximately 70% sensitive and 70% specific for the diagnosis of fatigue.[23] If fatigue is absent or mild, patients and caregivers should be educated on common management strategies for fatigue. If, however, fatigue is moderate or severe, a more in-depth assessment is usually required.

A cancer patient that scores above a 4 on the screening scale for fatigue generally requires a more detailed evaluation. Details regarding onset, duration, patterns, and changes in severity of fatigue should be noted. While disease progression may cause the new onset of moderate to severe fatigue in survivors, other causes including medications and the timing of medications should be considered. A detailed review of all medications, including supplements, is important. In addition, associated or alleviating factors as well as the degree to which fatigue impacts functional status are important. A diagnosis of cancer-related fatigue also requires assessment of any possible contributing factors. These include pain, depression, anemia, sleep disturbances, changes in appetite, medication effects, substance abuse, or any of a number of comorbid diseases (see Table 19.1). It is important to evaluate and treat any comorbidities, as this could reduce or alleviate fatigue and improve the patient's quality of life.

To meet diagnostic criteria for the International Classification of Diseases, 10th revision (ICD-10), the diagnosis of CRF must include documentation of the following four criteria: indicators of symptom presence (ex, score ≥ 4 on

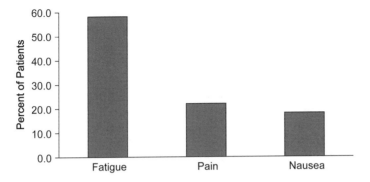

Figure 19.3. Fatigue Is the Most Common Symptom Associated with Cancer Survivorship. (Adapted from Stone P, Richardson A, Ream E et al. Cancer-related fatigues: Inevitable, unimportant, and untreatable? Results of a multi-centre patient survey. *Annals Onc.* 2000; 11: 971–975.)

fatigue screening question), distress or impairment due to fatigue, etiology related to cancer or cancer treatment, and absence of psychiatric disorder.[24]

TREATMENT

Though treatment of cancer-related fatigue does not impact survival, it can positively impact quality of life, which is an equally important and clinically relevant endpoint. In a study of 597 solid tumor patients on active treatment, 326 patients reported a score of 4 or greater on a 0–10 scale of fatigue and 82% of patients reported fatigue relief would significantly improve their quality of life.[23] Considering the increasing population of cancer patients and survivors there is a growing need for effective strategies to address and treat CRF.

Treatment of CRF can be subdivided into two categories: pharmacologic and non-pharmacologic treatments. Pharmacologic agents that have been studied for CRF include stimulants, antidepressants, steroids, and a cholinesterase inhibitor, donepezil. Multiple non-pharmacologic methods have been studied, including psychosocial methods, exercise training, sleep therapy, yoga, and acupuncture. Before treating CRF with any of these modalities, however, the NCCN stresses the importance of treating contributing conditions first.[1]

Treatment of Comorbid Conditions

Studies have shown that in cancer patients, fatigue most commonly occurs with sleep disturbances, emotional distress, and pain.[25,26] In addition to these, the NCCN includes anemia, nutrition, activity level, medication side effects, and alcohol or substance abuse as other common treatable factors in patients with CRF.[1]

Sleep disturbances can range from hypersomnia to insomnia, and are present in 30 to 75% of patients with cancer and survivors. Many of the same mechanisms thought to induce CRF have also been implicated in sleep disturbances, including disrupted circadian rhythms and alterations in the HPA axis. As part of the assessment of sleep disturbances, one should rule out obstructive sleep apnea, thyroid abnormalities, or changes in hormone status (estrogen, testosterone). Screening for depression is also important, as sleep disturbances are a common manifestation of depression. Treatment strategies include cognitive behavioral therapy, complimentary therapy (relaxation techniques, meditation, yoga), education, and exercise.[27]

Depression and anxiety are also common comorbid conditions in cancer patients. If they occur along with fatigue, it is difficult to determine the true etiology of either condition. Therefore treatment of both the emotional distress of cancer and any related fatigue is important for improving patients' quality of life. Traditional methods of treatment for depression are warranted, including psychotherapy or drug therapy with SSRIs, SNRIs, or other anti-depressants.

Pain, anemia, nutritional status, and activity level can also contribute to fatigue. Anemia can be treated with erythopoetin-stimulating agents or transfusions and may be helpful in alleviating fatigue. In all patients, nutritional status should be evaluated with careful attention paid to changes in weight, caloric intake, impediments to nutritional intake, and fluid and electrolyte imbalances. Consultation with a nutritionist is recommended in cases where weight loss, anorexia, or a decrease in oral intake is noted. Activity level should be assessed as fatigue is often associated with deconditioning and muscle wasting. This is also important before recommending exercise programs for the treatment of fatigue. Exercise may improve many of the symptoms associated with fatigure.[28] Structured, supervised exercise improves muscle fatigue, mood, and perception of fatigue. Exercise is a important component of cognitive behavioral therapy and is part of improving sleep hygiene. The other contributing factors discussed in the most recent NCCN guidelines on treatment of CRF were medication side effects and alcohol or substance abuse. Many prescription and non-prescription drugs can contribute to CRF, including beta-blockers, narcotics, anti-depressants, anti-emetics, and antihistamines. Titrating these medications to treat the patient's other symptoms without causing excess fatigue can be challenging. Clinicians should also screen for alcohol or substance abuse, as these habits can exacerbate sleep disturbances and worsen fatigue-inducing comorbidities.[1]

Pharmacologic Agents

Multiple agents have been studied in CRF, but the most frequently studied are the stimulants methylphenidate and modafinil. Methylphenidate is a sympathomimetic agent that stimulates CNS activity by blocking the reuptake and increasing the release of norepinephrine and dopamine in the extraneuronal space. The drug was initially marketed for treatment of attention-deficit hyperactivity disorder in children, however, was found to successfully treat several conditions in cancer patients, including opioid-induced sedation,[29] cognitive failure associated with brain tumors, and depression.[30] Methylphenidate has been formally tested for management of cancer fatigue in several studies. In a pilot study of 14 patients with interferon-induced fatigue, the combination of methylphenidate and an exercise program provided modest symptom improvement. Methylphenidate was then studied in a cohort of 41 metastatic cancer patients and was found to improve self-reported fatigue scores including overall, functional, and physical well-being on standardized fatigue-specific questionnaires.[30] However, when methylphenidate and its long-acting formulation were studied in two randomized trials no significant differences between the treatment and placebo arms were found in either study.[31,32] Dexmethylphenidate, the d-isomer of methylphenidate, has also been studied for treatment of cancer-related fatigue. In a randomized, placebo-controlled trial comparing dexmethylphenidate[33] to placebo in patients recently treated for malignancy, there was a statistically significant improvement in self-reported fatigue scores in the dexmethylphenidate group.[34] The dose of methylphenidate most commonly used in these studies was 5–10 mg by mouth once to twice daily, usually given in the morning and/or mid-day. Side effects that limit use of this drug include headache, insomnia, tremor, and anorexia. Current NCCN guidelines recommend considering treatment with methylphenidate, but caution that comorbid conditions should be sought out and treated first.[1]

A second agent, modafinil, has also been investigated for use in CRF. Modafinil is a wakefulness promoting agent that is currently FDA approved for narcolepsy, obstructive sleep apnea, shift work sleep disorders, and multiple sclerosis–related fatigue. Modafinil selectively enhances catecholaminergic signaling in the central nervous system, primarily in the anterior hypothalamus, an area specifically involved in sleep regulation. Thus, modafinil acts more selectively on the sleep-wake centers of the brain to promote wakefulness, which is in contrast to amphetamine derivatives, which act throughout the striatum and cortex to produce generalized excitation. This could explain modafinil's lower incidence of side effects and abuse potential.[33,35] Several pilot studies examined the use of modafinil for fatigue in different patient populations: lung cancer patients, breast cancer survivors, cancer patients on active treatment with opioids for pain, and a mixed group of patients with any past or current history of cancer.[35–38] These studies showed significant improvements in fatigue severity, cognitive performance, daytime sleepiness, and depression/anxiety when patients were treated with 100–200 mg/day of modafinil. Randomized studies examining the effects of modafinil, however, have produced mixed results. modafinil at 200 mg daily improved psychomotor speed and information processing, depression, and drowsiness.[33] In a multicenter, randomized, placebo-controlled trial of 631 cancer patients undergoing chemotherapy, modafinil at 200 mg per day was shown to significantly reduce fatigue for those patients who had a high level of baseline fatigue, which consisted of more than 70% of patients in the study. It showed no benefit over placebo in those who had mild or moderate fatigue.[39] Further randomized trials are ongoing, testing not only modafinil but also the long-acting version of modafinil (armodafinil) for the treatment of cancer related fatigue.

Non-Pharmacologic Therapies

For all cancer patients, regardless of disease stage or status (active treatment, post-treatment, or end of life), education and counseling are important regarding fatigue.[1] It is critical to educate survivors and patients who are on active treatment that fatigue is not necessarily a sign of disease recurrence, progression, or of treatment failure. It can be a side effect of therapy, and patients should be encouraged to discuss symptoms of fatigue with the medical team. After completion of cancer treatment, most patients will experience a gradual return of normal energy levels, though a large subset will continue to experience fatigue that interferes with normal daily activity. At the end of life, fatigue often occurs in combination with pain, weakness, anorexia, weight loss, and dyspnea. Patients and caregivers should be educated on how to best manage these conditions.

The NCCN recommends counseling all cancer patients who report fatigue on energy conservation strategies. Energy conservation is the deliberate, planned management of an individual's personal energy resources to prevent their depletion and is an important part of cognitive behavioral therapy.[40] The objective of energy conservation is to balance rest and activity during times of high fatigue so that valued activities and goals can be maintained. Energy conservation strategies include taking additional rest periods, priority setting, delegation, pacing oneself, and planning high-energy activities at times of peak energy.[40]

Beyond education and counseling, there are a number of non-pharmacologic treatments with proven efficacy in treatment of CRF. Exercise therapy, massage therapy, acupuncture, cognitive behavioral therapy, psycho-educational therapies, nutrition consultation, and sleep therapy have all been studied for CRF. The techniques with the strongest supporting data are exercise therapy, the psychosocial therapies, and sleep therapies.

In 2008, a Cochrane analysis compiled data from 28 randomized controlled trials to examine the effect of exercise on CRF. The majority of these studies were done in breast cancer patients (16 of 28 studies, 1,172 out of 2,083 participants), and there was significant variability in exercise regimens used, ranging from unsupervised home-based exercise programs to supervised, institutionalized exercise programs.[28] Examples of exercises used for CRF include walking, stationary cycling, resistance training, flexibility training, and yoga.[41] The overall meta-analysis showed that exercise programs were statistically more effective than controls in decreasing CRF.[28] Based on this data, it is clear that physical activity in some form can help reduce CRF, and efficacy does not seem to change with type of exercise regimen used.

Psychosocial therapies such as cognitive behavioral therapy, educational therapy, and supportive expressive therapies have been studied in the treatment of CRF. These therapies include a wide range of psychological tech-niques for coping with fatigue, including support groups, individual counseling, comprehensive coping strategy training, stress management training, individu-alized behavioral interventions, listening to guided imagery soundtracks, and encouraging discussion of how fatigue has affected lifestyles and emotional well-being.[41] Several meta-analyses have combined the data from studies done in this field,[42-44] and they each concluded that these interventions can have a modest effect on reducing CRF. One analysis pointed out that five studies that included individual sessions provided by oncology nurses that focused specifi-cally on fatigue education, self-care or coping techniques, or learned activity management were most effective in reducing fatigue.[43]

Sleep disturbances in cancer patients can range from insomnia to hyper-somnia, and several types of non-pharmacologic methods have been designed to optimize sleep quality. Cognitive behavioral techniques focus on stimulus control, sleep restriction, and sleep hygiene. Stimulus control involves going to bed when sleepy and not remaining in bed for more than 20 minutes if not sleeping. Sleep restriction includes avoiding long or late afternoon naps and limiting total time in bed.[1] Sleep hygiene is defined as a set of sleep-related behaviors that expose persons to activities and cues that prepare them for and promote appropriately timed and effective sleep.[45] Techniques include ensur-ing a warm, dark, quiet space for sleeping, having a regular sleep/wake sched-ule, using a consistent routine before going to bed, and avoiding exercise, large meals, or caffeine in the hours preceding sleep. A recent study tested the effect of a behavioral therapy plan including stimulus control, modified sleep restriction, relaxation therapy, and sleep hygiene on cancer related fatigue in 219 women receiving adjuvant chemotherapy for breast cancer.[46] The behav-ioral therapy group, on average, experienced significant improvement in sleep quality, as measured by a patient survey, over the control group.

SUMMARY

Cancer-related fatigue is a complex, multifactorial problem, with both physi-ologic and psychologic factors contributing to its etiology. Continued research into the basic mechanisms of fatigue at the cellular and molecular level are ongo-ing, as are studies examining the efficacy of new treatments for fatigue. Looking forward, oncology practitioners should strive to create interdisciplinary teams that will be able to tailor interventions to the needs of the individual patient.

REFERENCES

1. Mock V, Atkinson A, Barsevick A, Cella D, Cimprich B, Cleeland C *et al.* NCCN Practice Guidelines for Cancer-Related Fatigue. *Oncology (Williston Park, NY)* 2010.

2. Altekruse SF KC, Krapcho M, Neyman N, Aminou R, Waldron W, Ruhl J, How-lader N, Tatalovich Z, Cho H, Mariotto A, Eisner MP, Lewis DR, Cronin K, Chen HS, Feuer EJ, Stinchcomb DG, Edwards BK (eds). SEER Cancer Statistics Review, 1975–2007. In. Bethesda, MD: National Cancer Institute, 2010.

3. Gutstein HB. The biologic basis of fatigue. *Cancer* 2001; 92(6 Suppl): 1678–1683.

4. Ryan JL, Carroll JK, Ryan EP, Mustian KM, Fiscella K, Morrow G. Mechanisms of cancer-related fatigue. *Oncologist* 2007; 12 Suppl 1: 22–34.

5. Davis JM, Bailey SP. Possible mechanisms of central nervous system fatigue during exercise. *Med Sci Sports Exerc* 1997; 29(1): 45–57.

6. Fernstrom JD, Fernstrom MH. Exercise, serum free tryptophan, and central fatigue. *J Nutr* 2006; 136(2): 553S–559S.

7. Bakheit AM, Behan PO, Dinan TG, Gray CE, O'Keane V. Possible upregulation of hypothalamic 5-hydroxytryptamine receptors in patients with postviral fatigue syndrome. *BMJ* 1992; 304(6833): 1010–1012.

8. Sharpe M, Hawton K, Clements A, Cowen PJ. Increased brain serotonin function in men with chronic fatigue syndrome. *BMJ* 1997; 315(7101): 164–165.

9. Blomstrand E, Perrett D, Parry-Billings M, Newsholme EA. Effect of sustained exercise on plasma amino acid concentrations and on 5-hydroxytryptamine metabolism in six different brain regions in the rat. *Acta Physiol Scand* 1989; 136(3): 473–481.

10. Bailey SP, Davis JM, Ahlborn EN. Neuroendocrine and substrate responses to altered brain 5-HT activity during prolonged exercise to fatigue. *J Appl Physiol* 1993; 74(6): 3006–3012.

11. Cleare AJ, Bearn J, Allain T, McGregor A, Wessely S, Murray RM *et al.* Contrasting neuroendocrine responses in depression and chronic fatigue syndrome. *J Affect Disord* 1995; 34(4): 283–289.

12. Roscoe JA, Morrow GR, Hickok JT, Mustian KM, Griggs JJ, Matteson SE et al. Effect of paroxetine hydrochloride (Paxil) on fatigue and depression in breast cancer patients receiving chemotherapy. *Breast Cancer Res Treat* 2005; 89(3): 243–249.

13. Morrow GR, Hickok JT, Roscoe JA, Raubertas RF, Andrews PL, Flynn PJ et al. Differential effects of paroxetine on fatigue and depression: a randomized, double-blind trial from the University of Rochester Cancer Center Community Clinical Oncology Program. *J Clin Oncol* 2003; 21(24): 4635–4641.

14. Barsevick A, Frost M, Zwinderman A, Hall P, Halyard M. I'm so tired: biological and genetic mechanisms of cancer-related fatigue. *Qual Life Res* 2010; 19(10): 1419–1427.

15. Bower JE, Ganz PA, Aziz N. Altered cortisol response to psychologic stress in breast cancer survivors with persistent fatigue. *Psychosom Med* 2005; 67(2): 277–280.

16. Innominato PF, Focan C, Gorlia T, Moreau T, Garufi C, Waterhouse J et al. Circadian rhythm in rest and activity: a biological correlate of quality of life and a predictor of survival in patients with metastatic colorectal cancer. *Cancer Res* 2009; 69(11): 4700–4707.

17. Seruga B, Zhang H, Bernstein LJ, Tannock IF. Cytokines and their relationship to the symptoms and outcome of cancer. *Nat Rev Cancer* 2008; 8(11): 887–899.

18. Bianco JA, Appelbaum FR, Nemunaitis J, Almgren J, Andrews F, Kettner P et al. Phase I–II trial of pentoxifylline for the prevention of transplant-related toxicities following bone marrow transplantation. *Blood* 1991; 78(5): 1205–1211.

19. Greenberg DB, Gray JL, Mannix CM, Eisenthal S, Carey M. Treatment-related fatigue and serum interleukin-1 levels in patients during external beam irradiation for prostate cancer. *J Pain Symptom Manage* 1993; 8(4): 196–200.

20. Hong JH, Chiang CS, Campbell IL, Sun JR, Withers HR, McBride WH. Induction of acute phase gene expression by brain irradiation. *Int J Radiat Oncol Biol Phys* 1995; 33(3): 619–626.

21. Bower JE, Ganz PA, Irwin MR, Arevalo JM, Cole SW. Fatigue and gene expression in human leukocytes: Increased NF-kappaB and decreased glucocorticoid signaling in breast cancer survivors with persistent fatigue. *Brain Behav Immun* 2010.

22. Kurzrock R, The role of cytokines in cancer-related fatigue. *Cancer* 2001; 92(6 Suppl): 1684–1688.

23. Butt Z, Wagner LI, Beaumont JL, Paice JA, Peterman AH, Shevrin D *et al.* Use of a single-item screening tool to detect clinically significant fatigue, pain, distress, and anorexia in ambulatory cancer practice. *J Pain Symptom Manage* 2008; 35(1): 20–30.

24. Barsevick A, Cleeland C, Manning D, O'mara A, Reeve B, Scott J *et al.* ASCPRO Recommendations for the Assessment of Fatigue as an Outcome in Clinical Trials. *Journal of Pain and Symptom Management* 2010; 39(6): 1086–1099.

25. Jacobsen PB, Hann DM, Azzarello LM, Horton J, Balducci L, Lyman GH. Fatigue in women receiving adjuvant chemotherapy for breast cancer: characteristics, course, and correlates. *J Pain Symptom Manage* 1999; 18(4): 233–242.

26. Dodd MJ, Miaskowski C, Paul SM. Symptom clusters and their effect on the functional status of patients with cancer. *Oncol Nurs Forum* 2001; 28(3): 465–470.

27. Berger AM. Update on the state of the science: sleep-wake disturbances in adult patients with cancer. *Oncol Nurs Forum* 2009; 36(4): E165–177.

28. Cramp F, Daniel J. Exercise for the management of cancer-related fatigue in adults. *Cochrane Database Syst Rev* 2008; (2): CD006145.

29. Bruera E, Chadwick S, Brenneis C, Hanson J, MacDonald RN. Methylphenidate associated with narcotics for the treatment of cancer pain. *Cancer Treat Rep* 1987; 71(1): 67–70.

30. Bruera E, Driver L, Barnes EA, Willey J, Shen L, Palmer JL *et al.* Patient-controlled methylphenidate for the management of fatigue in patients with advanced cancer: a preliminary report. *J Clin Oncol* 2003; 21(23): 4439–4443.

31. Bruera E, Valero V, Driver L, Shen L, Willey J, Zhang T et al. Patient-controlled methylphenidate for cancer fatigue: a double-blind, randomized, placebo-controlled trial. *J Clin Oncol* 2006; 24(13): 2073–2078.

32. Moraska A, Sood A, Dakhil S, Sloan J, Barton D, Atherton P et al. Phase III, Randomized, Double-Blind, Placebo-Controlled Study of Long-Acting Methylphenidate for Cancer-Related Fatigue: North Central Cancer Treatment Group NCCTG-N05C7 Trial. *Journal of Clinical Oncology* 2010; 28(23): 3673–3679.

33. Lundorff LE, Jonsson BH, Sjogren P. Modafinil for attentional and psychomotor dysfunction in advanced cancer: a double-blind, randomized, cross-over trial. *Palliat Med* 2009; 23(8): 731–738.

34. Lower EE, Fleishman S, Cooper A, Zeldis J, Faleck H, Yu Z *et al.* Efficacy of dexmethylphenidate for the treatment of fatigue after cancer chemotherapy: a randomized clinical trial. *J Pain Symptom Manage* 2009; 38(5): 650–662.

35. Blackhall L, Petroni G, Shu J, Baum L, Farace E. A pilot study evaluating the safety and efficacy of Modafinil for cancer-related fatigue. *J Palliat Med* 2009; 12(5): 433–439.

36. Spathis A, Dhillan R, Booden D, Forbes K, Vrotsou K, Fife K. Modafinil for the treatment of fatigue in lung cancer: a pilot study. *Palliat Med* 2009; 23(4): 325–331.

37. Kohli S, Fisher SG, Tra Y, Adams MJ, Mapstone ME, Wesnes KA et al. The effect of modafinil on cognitive function in breast cancer survivors. *Cancer* 2009; 115(12): 2605–16.

38. Wirz S, Nadstawek J, Kuhn KU, Vater S, Junker U, Wartenberg HC. [Modafinil for the treatment of cancer-related fatigue: An intervention study.]. *Schmerz* 2010; 24(6): 587–595.

39. Jean-Pierre P, Morrow G, Roscoe J, Heckler C, Mohile S, Janelsins M et al. A phase 3 randomized, placebo-controlled, double-blind, clinical trial of the effect of modafinil on cancer-related fatigue among 631 patients receiving chemotherapy. *Cancer* 2010; 116(14): 3513–3520.

40. Barsevick AM, Dudley W, Beck S, Sweeney C, Whitmer K, Nail L. A randomized clinical trial of energy conservation for patients with cancer-related fatigue. *Cancer* 2004; 100(6): 1302–1310.

41. Escalante C, Manzullo E. Cancer-Related Fatigue: The Approach and Treatment. *J GEN INTERN MED* 2009; 24(S2): 412–416.

42. Kangas M, Bovbjerg DH, Montgomery GH. Cancer-related fatigue: a systematic and meta-analytic review of non-pharmacological therapies for cancer patients. *Psychol Bull* 2008; 134(5): 700–741.

43. Goedendorp MM, Gielissen MF, Verhagen CA, Bleijenberg G. Psychosocial interventions for reducing fatigue during cancer treatment in adults. *Cochrane Database Syst Rev* 2009; (1): CD006953.

44. Jacobsen PB, Donovan KA, Vadaparampil ST, Small BJ. Systematic review and meta-analysis of psychological and activity-based interventions for cancer-related fatigue. *Health Psychol* 2007; 26(6): 660–667.

45. Jan JE, Owens JA, Weiss MD, Johnson KP, Wasdell MB, Freeman RD et al. Sleep hygiene for children with neurodevelopmental disabilities. *Pediatrics* 2008; 122(6): 1343–1350.

46. Berger A, Kuhn B, Farr L, Von Essen S, Chamberlain J, Lynch J et al. One-Year Outcomes of a Behavioral Therapy Intervention Trial on Sleep Quality and Cancer-Related Fatigue. *Journal of Clinical Oncology* 2009; 27(35): 6033–6040.

47. Portenoy RK, Itri LM. Cancer-related fatigue: guidelines for evaluation and management. *Oncologist* 1999; 4(1): 1–10.

20

SEXUALITY AND INTIMACY AFTER CANCER

JENNIFER POTTER, MD

As noted in previous chapters, cancer and its treatment have far-reaching effects that impact psychological, interpersonal, physiological, and spiritual realms. Many women experience changes that adversely affect their intimate relationships and sexual function. This is a huge challenge, as emotional closeness and sexual gratification provide needed physical comfort, relaxation, stress relief, sleep assistance, pleasure, and relief from pain, all of which are especially beneficial when people are working through the trauma of cancer. Clinicians can provide invaluable assistance by learning to ask routinely about and effectively address concerns about intimacy and sexuality.

Research shows that clinicians initiate discussions in these areas infrequently, in large part because of lack of comfort regarding what to ask and how to respond.[1] This chapter provides a general overview that will enable clinicians to identify intimacy and sexuality issues promptly, to provide basic education and information about lifestyle and behavioral interventions, and to make appropriate referrals for additional evaluation when indicated. Readers who desire an in-depth review of the physiology of female sexual difficulties after cancer and/or detailed evidence to support or refute use of various pharmacological interventions are referred to a recent, comprehensive review on this topic,[2] from which this chapter is heavily excerpted.

A large proportion of women experience sexual difficulties after reproductive cancers (50% of women with breast cancer and 80% of women with gynecological cancers), especially during the first 12–18 months after treatment.[3,4] In addition, dramatic changes in sexual function are also common among women whose cancers affect sites far distant from the breasts and genitalia. In one comparative review, the prevalence of sexual difficulties was nearly the same in women with non-reproductive (76%) versus reproductive (84%) cancer locations.[5] This fact underscores the importance of asking *all* women about their sexual function, regardless of cancer type.

Table **20.1** Domains of Female Sexual Function and Their Neurobiological Correlates[1]

Domain	Key Anatomy Involved	Modulating Influences
Desire (libido)	• Central nervous system	Enhanced by dopamine, oxytocin, testosterone; inhibited by prolactin, serotonin
Arousal (excitement)	• Central nervous system (subjective appreciation of arousal- pleasure)	Enhanced by dopamine, norepinephrine, oxytocin; inhibited by prolactin, serotonin
	• Genital structures (objective evidence of physical arousal)	Enhanced by estrogen, testosterone; inhibited by prolactin, serotonin
	⁻ Nerves (sensation)	
	⁻ Blood vessels (vasocongestion, lubrication)	Enhanced by vascular mediators such as nitric oxide; inhibited by vasoconstricting substances
	⁻ Muscles (contraction during arousal and orgasm)	Enhanced by cholinergic agonists; inhibited by anticholinergics and muscle relaxants
Orgasm (climax)	• Central nervous system (subjective appreciation of orgasm- pleasure)	Enhanced by dopamine, norepinephrine, oxytocin; inhibited by prolactin, serotonin
	• Genital structures (objective evidence of orgasmic event)	Enhanced by cholinergic agonists; inhibited by anticholinergics and muscle relaxants

[1]This information is oversimplified, but included to help the reader understand the effect of various modulating influences (neurotransmitters, hormones, vasoactive substances) on key anatomical sites (CNS, genital structures) involved in female sexual response.

If sex was important in a woman's life before a cancer diagnosis, it generally remains that way afterwards. Research on couples affected by cancer shows that a majority resume sexual activity in the first few months after treatment ends, while some remain sexually active throughout the cancer experience.[6,7] Surveys show that cancer survivors and their partners have many questions about sex (see Table 20.2): therefore, it is crucial to provide accurate information not only about what to expect and how to respond to changes in function after treatment, but also about what practices are safe during treatment—for example, during chemotherapy and radiation administration, or in the setting of neutropenia and thrombocytopenia. Preparation and prevention are worth a pound of cure: for women especially, there is a use it or lose it aspect to sexual function—that is, regular sexual activity in and of itself tends to maintain vaginal lubrication and elasticity, even in the face of postmenopausal estrogen decline.

TABLE 20.2 COMMON ADVERSE SEXUAL EFFECTS OF SPECIFIC CANCER THERAPIES[1]

Cancer Treatment	Cause of Adverse Effects	Clinical Examples
Surgery	• Cosmetic changes • Removal or damage to critical structures	• Body image issues after mastectomy, radical neck dissection, urostomy, colostomy, surgeries associated with incontinence • Loss of nipple sensation after breast surgery • Reduced genital sensation, blood flow, and muscle contraction after radical pelvic surgery • Discomfort associated with lymphedema, pain syndromes
Radiation therapy	• Damage to critical structures	• Body image issues related to radiation enteritis/fecal incontinence (pelvic irradiation) • Reduced genital sensation, blood flow, and muscle contraction (pelvic irradiation) • Pain on penetration associated with vaginal scarring and stenosis (pelvic irradiation) • Discomfort associated with lymphedema, pain syndromes
Chemotherapy	• Cosmetic changes • Physical inactivity and fatigue • Premature menopause • Peripheral neuropathy	• Body image issues after hair loss, weight gain • Decreased overall stamina and physical fitness • Sexual sequelae associated with atrophic vaginal changes • Decreased genital sensation and discomfort associated with pain syndromes
Hormone therapies	• Anti-estrogen effects	• Atrophic vaginal changes associated with medical menopause induction (GnRH agonists) and anti-estrogens (tamoxifen, aromatase inhibitors) • Discomfort due to vulvar lichen sclerosus (increased incidence in women taking aromatase inhibitors)
Immunotherapies	• Graft-versus-host-disease	• Vulvovaginal scarring and stenosis seen after bone marrow transplantation

[1]Adapted from Potter J, Johnston K. "Sexuality and Intimacy after Cancer" in Davis MP, Feyer P, Ortner P, Zimmermann C. Supportive Oncology. Saunders; Har/Psc edition: 2011.

Some women are at higher risk than others for development of difficulties with intimacy and sexuality. Predisposing factors that have been identified include: poor perceived health, poor body image, vaginal dryness, urinary incontinence, poor dyadic adjustment, a history of pre-existing sexual problems, and having a partner with sexual problems.[8,9,10] For a variety of reasons, younger women seem to be especially vulnerable.[11] Single women frequently articulate the fear that they will be found sexually undesirable or rejected by prospective partners, and express significant anxiety about when to discuss their cancer history during the dating process. Clinicians can help by promptly identifying women who are at risk and instituting appropriate interventions early on.

When women have partners, it is important to include both parties in the evaluation process. When asked directly, a majority of partners—78% in one study—report adverse effects of cancer on their own sexual functioning.[5] This is not surprising, as cancer is known to arouse a multitude of tumultuous reactions in partners, including somatic preoccupations, increased anxiety and/or depression, and fear of cancer recurrence and the eventual death of their spouse. Initially, spouses may keep these fears to themselves, hoping to protect their loved one from additional worry;[12] however, this can lead to loneliness and distance. Since emotional support provided by either partner to the other plays a critical role in each person's adjustment,[13] it is crucial to help couples achieve open communication. Fortunately, coping with cancer tends to strengthen relationships overall.[14]

When women experience difficulties with sexual function, it is the rule rather than the exception that multiple dimensions (biological, psychological, interpersonal, and cultural) are affected and manifestations of difficulty tend to impact several, if not all, sexual function domains (desire/libido, sexual arousal, and orgasm) simultaneously. For interventions to have the greatest success, it is critical to ascertain and address each dimension and domain that is affected. Readers may find it helpful to refer to Figure 20.1, which presents a schematic representation of common bio-psycho-social-cultural factors that impact sexual function in female cancer survivors, and Table 20.2, which depicts domains of sexual function and their neurobiological correlates. When explaining the impact of specific cancer treatments on sexual function to patients, it may also be useful to refer to Table 20.3, which maps various surgical, radiation, chemo-, hormone- and immuno-therapies to their common adverse physiological effects. Questions clinicians can ask to delve into each of these key areas are presented in Table 20.4.

Given the inherent complexity of sexual function, it is not surprising that interventions that address sexual difficulties effectively also tend to be multidimensional and include a variety of techniques including individual and couples counseling, lifestyle and behavioral change, and (when indicated) pharmacological manipulation. In discussing the need to attend to each of these areas, it is helpful to explain the concept of a sexual tipping point (see Figure 20.2). The degree of sexual responsiveness a person experiences at any given point in time is the sum of all of the excitatory psychological, interpersonal, cultural,

TABLE 20.3 QUESTIONS TO ASK WHEN TAKING A HISTORY[1]

Begin with General Opening Questions

Are you satisfied with your sexual life?

Are there things about your (or your partner's) sexual function you wish you could change?

Has cancer treatment affected your sexual function (self image, comfort showing your body to your partner, interest in sex, responsiveness to sexual stimulation) in any way?

Did you experience any problems with sexual intimacy before cancer?

Determine Affected Functional Domains

Desire: Do you notice a change in your interest in sex?

Arousal: Do you become sufficiently lubricated?

Orgasm: Are you able to reach orgasm?

Comfort/Pain: Do you experience any discomfort of pain during sex?

Evaluate Distress and Expectations

How have these changes affected you? Your partner? Your relationship?

Are you interested in trying to change the current situation?

Have you tried any interventions already? If so, what were the results?

Evaluate Relationship Quality

How would you describe the overall quality of your relationship?

Do you feel comfortable talking with your partner about the kinds of stimulation you enjoy?

If you do talk about sex with your partner, have you found her/him to be responsive?

Questions about Orgasm

Have you ever had an orgasm?

If not . . . Are you familiar with female genital structures, such as the clitoris?

Are you aware that most women need clitoral stimulation to become fully aroused?

What kinds of sexual activities do you participate in? Do they involve stimulation of the clitoris?

Is so . . . When did you notice a change? What happens exactly? Are you ever able to achieve orgasm? Does it take longer? Do some kinds of stimulation work better than others?

Can you identify any distracting feelings or thoughts that seem to interfere with orgasm?

Do you expect to have an orgasm every time you have sex? Do you ever feel satisfied without reaching climax?

Questions about Pain / Discomfort

Do you experience any discomfort during sexual activity?

If so, when did it start? Does it occur every time you have sex or just sometimes? Is it related to how turned on you are feeling or how much foreplay you've had?

What does the discomfort feel like? Where do you feel it exactly? At what point during sexual activity does it occur?

Have you experienced pain in the past when using tampons or with speculum insertion during pelvic exam? (symptoms of vaginismus)

TABLE 20.3 QUESTIONS TO ASK WHEN TAKING A HISTORY[1] (*Continued*)

Ask Specific Questions about Each Affected Sexual Domain

Questions about Desire
What was your highest ever level of desire (grade on a 0-10 point scale)? How about now?
Can you identify any inhibiting feelings or thoughts that interfere with your level of desire?
Do you participate in sexual activities even though your level of desire has changed? If so, what motivates you?
Do you experience spontaneous sexual thoughts or fantasies?
Are you turned on by erotic descriptions in books or sex scenes in movies?
Do you find your partner (or other people) attractive?
How often do you masturbate?

Questions about Arousal
Is vaginal dryness a problem? Have you tried using lubricants? Which ones? Are they helpful?
Do you experience pleasurable sensations when you masturbate?
What kinds of sexual activities do you and your partner engage in? Do you experience pleasurable sensations during these activities?
Can you identify any distracting feelings or thoughts that seem to inhibit these sensations?
Have you had any negative experiences that might be interfering with your enjoyment now, such as being sexually abused, raped, or coerced into having sex?

[1]Adapted from Potter J, Johnston K. "Sexuality and Intimacy after Cancer" in Davis MP, Feyer P, Ortner P, Zimmermann C. Supportive Oncology. Saunders; Har/Psc edition: 2011.

and physiological factors that act to turn on the system balanced against all of the inhibitory influences that act to turn it off. An excess of excitatory influences results in more rapid/intense sexual responsiveness (e.g., hot), whereas a preponderance of inhibitory influences results in slower/weaker responsiveness (e.g., not).[15]

Clinicians should take the time to enumerate each opportunity patients and their partners have to tip the scale toward greater intimacy and sexual satisfaction, as this facilitates hope, understanding, and patience, and typically results in both parties becoming actively engaged in working together. It is always important to remind patients/partners that it is not usually possible to accept physical changes or feel open to experimenting with new ways to stimulate sexual interest and arousal until losses have been fully acknowledged and grieved. For example, it may take many months for a woman who used to pride herself on her breasts and achieved exquisite arousal from

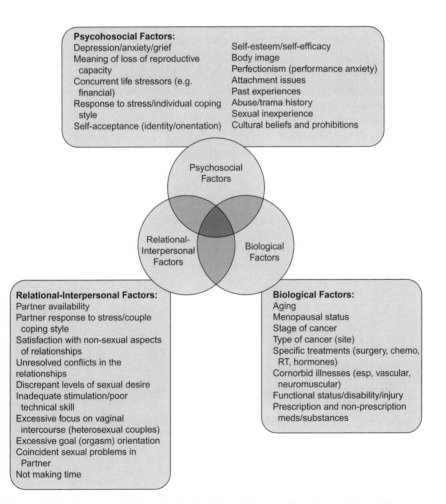

Figure 20.1. Common Bio-Psycho-Socio-Cultural Factors That Impact Sexual Function in Female Cancer Survivors. (Adapted from Potter J, Johnston K. Sexuality and Intimacy after Cancer in Davis MP, Feyer P, Ortner P, Zimmermann C. Supportive Oncology. Saunders; Har/Psc edition: 2011.)

nipple stimulation to be able to bear looking at her post-mastectomy body in the mirror, let alone imagine letting her partner touch her in any intimate fashion.

Table 20.4 lists a wide variety of useful educational, counseling, and lifestyle interventions. As a first step, it is important to identify and address any misconceptions patients and partners have about sex and to help them develop reasonable expectations. In contradistinction to what media hype would have us believe—that good sex requires rapid, multiple and simultaneous orgasms and that magic pharmacological remedies are available whenever problems arise—restoration of emotional and sexual intimacy in the face of the trauma of cancer generally requires substantial dedicated time and effort. A basic review of female sexual anatomy and physiology should also be provided, along with a description of changes that occur naturally with aging and menopause plus discussion of the potential impact of each of the patient's specific cancer therapies. Explaining that cancer treatment frequently causes an acceleration of the physiological changes associated with aging helps put cancer-related changes in context for older individuals and couples who have already learned to accept and adjust to age-related physical changes. It is very reassuring for a spouse to hear that the fact that his partner now requires more intense and prolonged genital stimulation in order to achieve orgasm is an

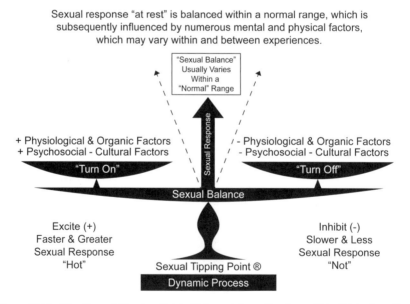

Figure 20.2. The Sexual Tipping Point. (Adapted from Perelman MA. Clinical application of CNS-acting agents in FSD. J Sex Med 2007;4[Suppl 4]:280–290.)

expected consequence of her cancer treatment and not a sign of decreased affection.

One of the most distressing effects of cancer treatment for both women and their partners is decreased libido. While it is important to acknowledge this loss, it is helpful to point out that motivators other than lust (such as the desire to feel close to one's partner) can lead women to initiate contact or respond to their partner's advances, and once engaged in sexual activity, there are many ways to achieve satisfaction (e.g., with appropriate stimulation, arousal may proceed and orgasm may occur, or one may simply take pleasure in one's partner's enjoyment). Women with reduced libido can be taught using cognitive restructuring techniques to identify and celebrate intact motivations to participate in sexual activity, to experiment with positive sexual fantasies and thoughts that spur on arousal, and to deflect negative thoughts that lead to avoidance of sexual activity or anticipation (and therefore a higher likelihood) of experiencing disappointment.

Some women feel betrayed by their bodies after a cancer diagnosis, while others experience their changed bodies as unfamiliar or alien. It can be difficult to engage in intimate sexual activities with a partner under these circumstances, and it is often helpful for patients to spend some time alone first, getting to know their new bodies and learning what locations and types of touch feel good. It is important for clinicians to give women explicit permission to explore masturbation, since some are initially reluctant due to cultural beliefs. For women who are sexually inexperienced it is helpful to provide basic information about erogenous zones and sexual technique. Exploration of previously unappreciated non-genital erogenous areas (e.g., ears, breasts, neck, antecubital and popliteal fossae, etc.) should be encouraged. Once a woman learns how to pleasure her own body, she can show her partner the type of stimulation she enjoys. For a woman who is not comfortable practicing erotic self-touch, massage of non-erogenous areas using a pleasantly scented oil or lotion may be an acceptable alternative.

Referral for counseling is indicated to enhance general coping skills, alleviate depression, anxiety and body image issues, and improve communication between patients and established or prospective partners. Many forms of counseling—individual, couples or groups—can be beneficial; for practical help with sexual communication and technique, dedicated sex therapy is often useful, and for women with significant anxiety, depression, or post-traumatic stress reactions, a combination of psycho- and psychopharmacological therapies may be appropriate. When selecting an anti-anxiety or antidepressant medication, it is always important to consider and discuss potential sexual side effects of treatment (for example, many antidepressants have adverse effects on sexual interest and arousal), and to make sure that there are no untoward interactions with anti-cancer therapies (for example, some selective serotonin reuptake inhibitors reduce the efficacy of tamoxifen in women with breast cancer).

TABLE 20.4 NON-PHARMACOLOGICAL INTERVENTIONS TO IMPROVE SEXUAL FUNCTION[1]

Sexuality Education

1. Identify and address any misconceptions about sex

2. Review sexual anatomy and physiology; expected changes with aging, menopause; and changes associated with specific cancer treatments

3. Distinguish between lust and other motivations for initiating sexual activity or responding to a partner's advances; identify and celebrate these motivations

4. Discuss sexual techniques, including identification of both genital (e.g. the clitoris, in women) and non-genital erogenous zones; encourage exploration and experimentation

Referral for Counseling and/or Psychopharmacology Consultation

1. Individual, couples, or group interventions

2. Sex therapists have expertise providing counseling that focuses on the sexual aspect of relationships, using various behavioral techniques and homework assignments. AASECT provides a national listing of such therapists.

3. For patients with significant anxiety, depression, PTSD, or compulsive sexual behaviors, a combination of psychotherapy and medications may be appropriate.

Lifestyle Changes to Enhance Sexual Satisfaction

1. Create opportunities for intimacy (make "dates", eliminate distractions, create a conducive environment with candles, dimmed lighting, music, etc.)

2. Maximize comfort (encourage use of lubricants, experimentation with position changes, strategic analgesic use, etc.)

3. Give permission to explore (masturbation, new positions, new techniques, sex toys, erotica, etc.)

4. Encourage weight loss and exercise

Use of Mechanical Devices and Pelvic Floor Techniques

1. Vibrator use to enhance the intensity and duration of genital stimulation

2. Clitoral vacuum pump use to increase genital blood flow

3. Vaginal dilators to prevent and treat vaginal stenosis

4. Pelvic floor physical therapy for incontinence

[1] Adapted from Potter J, Johnston K. "Sexuality and Intimacy after Cancer" in Davis MP, Feyer P, Ortner P, Zimmermann C. Supportive Oncology. Saunders; Har/Psc edition: 2011.

Importantly, body image, self-esteem and sexual responsiveness do not occur in a vacuum; instead, a woman's self view is sculpted by the responses of people in her life, and positive regard from others can be profoundly healing.[16] A recent review of couples-based interventions to enhance sexual adjustment and body image after cancer showed that the most effective strategies were couple-focused and included treatment components that educated both partners about the women's diagnosis and treatments; promoted couples' mutual coping and support processes; and included specific sexual therapy techniques to address sexual and body image concerns.[17] Accordingly, dyadic interventions should be considered for women who have partners, while group interventions may have particular power for single women.

Several other strategies may help improve body image. Chemotherapy-induced hair loss is consistently ranked as one of the most distressing effects of cancer treatment, and has a profoundly negative impact on body image.[18] Participation in programs such as the American Cancer Society's Look Good . . . Feel Better program, which provides cosmetic makeovers and hair help, can enhance self-confidence and social comfort for women whose appearance is altered by cancer treatment.[19] For women who have undergone mastectomy without reconstruction and are bothered by the appearance of their surgical scar, strategies such as experimentation with use of temporary chest wall tattoos or consideration of delayed surgical reconstruction can be discussed. Women who are embarrassed by the presence of a urostomy or colostomy bag may feel more comfortable engaging in intimate activities using cleverly-designed lingerie designed for use in this context.

A number of lifestyle and behavioral changes can be implemented to enhance sexual satisfaction. For patients who have partners, it may be helpful to deliberately create opportunities for closeness, such as making dates to spend intimate time together, making sure there will be no distractions, and setting a relaxing and/or romantic mood by choosing a quiet setting, relaxing music, incense, candles, etc. Physical closeness of all kinds should be encouraged: snuggling up to watch a movie and spooning while sleeping create valuable connection too. For survivors who find themselves avoiding sexual activity because of performance anxiety, physical discomfort, or fear of discomfort, sensual touching exercises (sensate focus exercises) that focus on pleasurable sensations associated with non-genital touch are a good place to start. Typically, these exercises begin with non-threatening physical contact, such as a back rub or foot massage, and progress over time to nude, full-body caressing, including the genitals. As discussed earlier, patients who do not have partners often need help planning how and when to discuss their cancer history with prospective partners, and may benefit from practicing these conversations using role play exercises.

Physical comfort during sexual activity may be an issue for many cancer survivors, because of hypersensitivity to touch caused by scarring or neuropathy, lymphedema, or reduced mobility. Helpful suggestions include considering a warm bath prior to sexual activity, optimizing analgesic use, and experimenting with alternative sexual positions. For women who experience discomfort during penetrative sexual activity due to postmenopausal vaginal atrophy, both vaginal moisturizers and sexual lubricants can be recommended. Vaginal moisturizers are used daily to hydrate vulvar and vaginal cells and reduce mucosal fragility, while lubricants are used during sexual activity to reduce friction and facilitate smooth glide. A combination of the

TABLE 20.5 A PROBLEM-ORIENTED APPROACH TO IMPROVING SEXUAL FUNCTION[1]

Affected Functional Domain	Goal of Treatment	Specific Interventions
Desire	• Optimize effect of cognitive motivators • Minimize effect of cognitive inhibitors • Minimize effect of biological inhibitors • Optimize effect of biological motivators	• Encourage sexual fantasies, exploit erotica, maximize opportunities for closeness, etc. • Address body image issues, utilize cognitive behavioral techniques • Address depression/anxiety, avoid medications with sexual side effects, treat hypothyroidism, etc. • Consider referral to an expert to discuss pharmacological management
Arousal	• Optimize effect of cognitive motivator • Minimize effect of cognitive inhibitors • Optimize genital sensation • Optimize genital blood flow • Optimize lubrication • Optimize pelvic floor muscle contraction	• Same as for desire • Same as for desire • Encourage vibrator use • Clitoral vacuum pump • Sexual lubricants (if not contraindicated, consider vaginal estrogen use) • Refer to PT for pelvic floor exercises to enhance pleasurable sensations and restore continence
Orgasm	• Reduce latency to orgasm (frequently caused by SSRI antidepressants)	• Switch to a less sex-negative antidepressant or add an antidote
Comfort / Pain	• Address general comfort • Assess specific issues (e.g. vaginal atrophy and stenosis)	• Strategic analgesic dosing, trying different positions, etc. • Sexual lubricants, vaginal estrogen (if not contraindicated), vaginal dilators

[1]Adapted from Potter J, Johnston K. "Sexuality and Intimacy after Cancer" in Davis MP, Feyer P, Ortner P, Zimmermann C. Supportive Oncology. Saunders; Har/Psc edition: 2011.

two is sometimes more efficacious than either one alone. While this chapter will not review pharmacological interventions in any detail, it should be noted that use of low-dose vaginal estrogen is highly effective in reducing symptoms of vulvar and vaginal atrophy in survivors for whom estrogen administration is an acceptable option.

Use of mechanical devices (e.g., vibrators) may be helpful for women who have experienced vascular or neurological injury to genital structures and therefore need intense and prolonged stimulation to achieve arousal.[20]

Vibrators are available in a wide variety of shapes and sizes and can be bought discreetly from online sex boutiques. Other mechanical devices may be useful in specific circumstances. For example, use of clitoral vacuum pump—the Eros Clitoral Therapy Device—to increase clitoral blood flow during 15–30 minutes of intermittent therapy, four times per week for three months was found to significantly increase desire, arousal, lubrication, orgasm, satisfaction, and to reduce pain in a small (n = 15) group of irradiated cervical cancer patients with sexual dysfunction two years post treatment.[21]

Women who undergo radical pelvic surgery and/or irradiation may benefit from additional interventions. The strongest evidence supports use of topical estrogen and benzydamine in the prevention and treatment of acute radiation-induced vaginal changes.[22] Use of vaginal dilators to prevent vaginal stenosis is frequently recommended, though there is little consensus on when to begin dilatation, how often it should be performed, and for how long.[23] Urinary and fecal incontinence have a profoundly negative on sexual function of affected women and their partners; routinely asking about their presence is crucial as many patients are so mortified they will not initiate discussion spontaneously. The extent to which pelvic floor physical therapy restores continence in post-operative cancer survivors needs to be further evaluated. Referral to an appropriate practitioner is probably reasonable as there is no evidence for harm and one small, non-randomized study demonstrated improved continence in irradiated and non-irradiated postoperative colon cancer survivors who received anal sphincter muscle training.[24]

Last but not least, the importance of restoration and maintenance of a healthy weight and participation in regular physical exercise cannot be overestimated. Weight gain is a frequent complication of cancer treatment and is associated with negative effects on body image and sexual functioning. Obesity after cancer diagnosis is associated with increased recurrence and poorer prognosis,[25,26] higher levels of post-treatment physical activity are associated with better outcomes,[27,28] and moderate weight loss and regular physical activity not only reduce the risk of chronic health conditions other than cancer, but are also associated with improvements in body image and sexual satisfaction specifically.[29] Therefore, all cancer survivors should be encouraged to achieve and maintain a healthy weight and to engage in regular physical activity.

In summary, this chapter outlines a general approach to discussing sexual concerns with female cancer survivors. Key recommendations include (1) initiating the discussion before, during, and after cancer treatment; (2) asking all women, regardless of cancer type, age, or partnership status; (3) considering multiple dimensions (biological, psychological, interpersonal, cultural) and asking about each affected sexual function domain (desire, arousal, orgasm); (4) providing information about the expected impact of cancer treatments on intimacy and sexuality; and (5) discussing simple, non-pharmacological strategies that can be used to facilitate adjustment and adaptation, using a problem-oriented approach (see Table 20.5). These recommendations lie within the purview of the primary care provider or general medical oncologist; however,

TABLE **20.6** RESOURCES[1]

Internet websites

General Sexuality

www.siecus.org. Sexuality Information and Education Council of the United States.

Sexuality after Cancer

www.LAF.org. The Lance Armstrong Foundation.

www.lbbc.org. Living Beyond Breast Cancer.

www.mautnerproject.org. The Mautner Project for Lesbians with Cancer.

www.oncolink.org. Comprehensive, web-based cancer resource.

Books and Other Resources

Body Image

Cash TF. (1997). *The Body Image Workbook: An 8 Step Program for Learning to Like Your Looks.* New York: Harbinger.

"Look Good . . . Feel Good" program offered by the American Cancer Society, 1-800-395-LOOK.

General Sexuality

Heiman JR, LoPiccolo L, LoPiccolo J. (1988). Becoming Orgasmic: A Sexual and Personal Growth Program for Women. New York: Fireside.

Renshaw D. (2004). Seven Weeks to Better Sex. Redondo Beach, CA: Westcom Press.

Sexuality after Cancer

Harpham WS. (1995) After Cancer: A Guide to Your New Life. New York: Harper Perennial.

Hill Schnipper H. (2006). After Breast Cancer: A Common-Sense Guide to Life After Treatment. New York: Bantam Dell.

Kydd S, & Rowett D. (2006). Intimacy after Cancer: A Woman's Guide. Seattle: Big Think Media.

Laken V, & Laken K. (2002). Making Love Again: Hope for Couples Facing Loss of Sexual Intimacy. Ant Hill Press, Sandwich, MA

Mulhall JP. (2008). Saving Your Sex Life: A Guide for Men with Prostate Cancer. Hilton Publishing Company, Chicago.

NCI/PDQ: Sexuality and Reproductive Issues. (2009). National Cancer Institute. Available at http://www.oncolink.org/coping/article.cfm?c=4&s=46&ss=95&id=801.

Schover LR. (1997). Sexuality and Cancer: For the Man Who Has Cancer and His Partner. American Cancer Society.

(Continued)

TABLE 20.6 (*Continued*)

For Referral to a Certified Sex Therapist

Schover LR. (2001). Sexuality and Cancer: For the Woman Who Has Cancer and Her Partner. American Cancer Society, New York.

The American Association of Sex Educators, Counselors and Therapists (AAS-ECT), www.aasect.org; 804-644-3288.

[1]Adapted from reference (2).

lack of familiarity with these topics and competing demands on a provider's time may make it difficult to substantively address these issues. In addition, some women and their partners may wish to pursue pharmacological interventions in addition to the counseling and lifestyle change recommendations outlined here. In either case, clinicians should offer appropriate resources and referrals (please see Table 20.6).

NOTE

This chapter presents a summary and updated version of information published previously in Supportive Oncology (see reference 2). The author would like to acknowledge the contributions Dr. Kate Johnston made to the original manuscript.

REFERENCES

1. Hordern AJ, Street AF. Communicating about patient sexuality and intimacy after cancer: mismatched expectations and unmet needs. *Med J Aust* 2007;186:224–227.

2. Potter J, Johnston K. "Sexuality and Intimacy after Cancer" in Davis MP, Feyer P, Ortner P, Zimmermann C. *Supportive Oncology.* Saunders; Har/Psc edition: 2011.

3. Schover LR. The impact of breast cancer on sexuality, body image and intimate relationships, CA *Cancer J Clin* 1991;41:112–120.

4. Anderson BL & van Der Does J. Surviving gynecologic cancer and coping with sexual morbidity: an international problem. *Int J Gynecol Cancer* 1994;4:225–240.

5. Hawkins Y, Ussher J, Gilbert E, Perz J, Sandoval M, Sundquist K. Changes in sexuality and intimacy after the diagnosis and treatment of cancer: the experience of partners in a sexual relationship with a person with cancer. *Cancer Nurs* 2009;32:271–280.

6. Fobair P, Stewart SL, Chang S, D'Onofrio C, Banks PJ, Bloom JR. Body image and sexual problems in young women with breast cancer. *Psychooncology* (2006 Jul) 15(7):579–594.

7. Wimberly SR, Carver CS, Laurenceau JP, Harris SD, Antoni MH. Perceived partner reactions to diagnosis and treatment of breast cancer: impact on psychosocial and psychosexual adjustment. *J Consult Clin Psychol* (2005 Apr) 73(2):300–311.

8. Greendale GA, Petersen L, Zibecchi L, Ganz PA. Factors related to sexual function in postmenopausal women with a history of breast cancer. *Menopause* 2001; 8:111–119.

9. Carmack Taylor CL, Basen-Engquist K, Shinn EH, Bodurka DC. Predictors of sexual functioning in ovarian cancer patients. *J Clin Oncol* 2004;22:881–889.

10. Ganz PA, Desmond KA, Belin TR, Meyerowitz BE, Rowlnd JH. Predictors of sexual health in women after a breast cancer diagnosis. *J Clin Oncol* 1999;17:2371–2380.

11. Schover LR. Sexuality and body image in younger women with breast cancer. *J Natl Cancer Inst Monogr* 1994;16:177–182.

12. Germino BB, Fife BL, Funk SG. Cancer and the partner relationship: what is its meaning? *Sem Onc Nurs* 1995;11:43–50.

13. Hoskins CN, Baker S, Budin W, Ekstrom D, Maislin G, Sherman D et al. Adjustment among husbands of women with breast cancer. *J Psychsoc Oncol* 1996; 14:41–69.

14. Dorval M, Guay S, Mondor M, Masse B, Falardeau M, Robidoux A, Deschenes L, Maunsell E. Couples who get closer after breast cancer: frequency and predictors in a prospective investigation. *J Clin Oncol* 2005;23:3588–596.

15. Perelman MA. The sexual tipping point: a mind/body model for sexual medicine. *J Sex Med* 2009;6:629–632.

16. Kayser K & Scott J. Helping Couples Cope with Cancer: An Evidence-Based Approach for Practitioners. *Springer Science + Business Media*, New York, 2008.

17. Scott JL & Kayser K. A review of couple-based interventions for enhancing women's sexual adjustment and body image after cancer. *Cancer J* 2009;15:48–56.

18. Lemieux J, Maunsell E, Provencher L. Chemotherapy-induced alopecia and effects on quality of life among women with breast cancer: a literature review. *Psychooncology* 2008;4:317–328.

19. American Cancer Society's Look Good Feel Better program. Information available at: http://www.lookgoodfeelbetter.org/index.htm.

20. Billups KL. The role of mechanical devices in treating female sexual dysfunction and enhancing the female sexual response. *World J Urol* 2002;20:137–141.

21. Schroder MA, Mell LK, Hurteau JA, Collins YC, Rotmensch J, Waggoner SE, Yamada SD, Small W, Mundt AJ. Clitoral therapy device for treatment of sexual dysfunction in irradiated cervical cancer patients. Int *J Radiat Oncol Biol Phys* 2005;61:1078–1086.

22. Denton AS, Maher EJ. Interventions for the physical aspects of sexual dysfunction in women following pelvic radiotherapy. *Cochrane Database Syst Rev.* 2003;(1):CD003750.

23. Lancaster L. Preventing vaginal stenosis after brachytherapy for gynecological cancer: an overview of Australian practices. *Eur J Oncol Nurs* 2004;8:30–39.

24. Allgayer H, Dietrich CF, Rohde W, Koch GF, Tuschhoff T. Prospective comparison of short- and long-term effects of pelvic floor exercise/biofeedback training in patients with fecal incontinence after surgery plus irradiation versus surgery alone for colorectal cancer: clinical, functional and endoscopic/endosonographic findings. *Scand J Gastroenterol.* 2005 Oct;40(10):1168–1175.

25. Carmichael AR. Obesity and prognosis of breast cancer. Obes Rev 2006;4:333–340.

26. Siegel EM, Ulrich CM, Poole EM, Holmes RS, Jacobsen PB, Shibata D. The effects of obesity and obesity-related conditions on colorectal cancer prognosis. *Cancer Control* 2010;17:52–57.

27. Holmes MD, Chen WY, Feskanich D et al. Physical activity and survival after breast cancer diagnosis. JAMA 2005;293:2479–2486.

28. Meyerhardt JA, Giovannucci EL, Holmes MD et al. Physical activity and survival after colorectal cancer diagnosis. *J Clin Oncol* 2006;24:3527–534)

29. Berber JR, Johnson JV, Bunn JY, O'Brien SL. A longitudinal study of the effects of free testosterone and other psychosocial variables on sexual function during the natural traverse of menopause. *Fertil Steril* 2005;83:643–648.

21

THE IMPACT OF ANTI-CANCER TREATMENTS ON FERTILITY AND METHODS FOR FERTILITY PRESERVATION

IRIT BEN-AHARON, MD, PHD,
AND KENNETH MILLER, MD

Novel approaches in early detection and effective management strategies have led to increased rates of cancer survivors throughout the past three decades. In 2005, approximately 1,372,910 people were diagnosed in the United States with cancer and 4% (~55,000 cases) were under the age of 35. The most frequently occurring malignancies in people under 40 are breast cancer, cervical cancer, sarcomas, non-Hodgkin's lymphoma, leukemia, and melanoma.[1] Out of an estimated 2.4 million breast cancer survivors in the United States, 10% are of childbearing age.[3] Seminal advances in anti-cancer therapy as well as supportive care strategies result in improved survival rates, thus yielding an ancillary focus in preservation of an optimum quality of life after cancer treatment. This recognition has paved the way to an increasing research of long-term side effects and an ongoing design of a supportive care system to evaluate and treat long-term adverse effects of cancer treatments, including the impact on fertility and hormone-related disorders.

FERTILITY, MENOPAUSE, AND ANDROPAUSE

In 2006 the American Society of Clinical Oncology (ASCO) developed guidelines for addressing fertility concerns of cancer patients, including fertility preservation. This emphasized the fact that informed decision-making is critical for enhancing the future quality of life of young cancer survivors. Throughout the past decade several studies have addressed the psychological impact of treatment-induced infertility among young cancer patients. Concerns about fertility represent a major issue for young premenopausal cancer patients, regardless of their age and extent of disease. Studies suggest that among young women in particular, cancer-related infertility is associated with a greater risk for emotional distress and poorer quality of life.[5,6] It has been shown that some women are willing to trade some likelihood of survival for the ability to maintain fertility.[7] Female patients were highly concerned of the loss of choice regarding child-bearing.[8] Many young women were also concerned about treatment-related menopause.[9]

In male patients, the term *andropause* is the equivalent to menopause in females and encompasses the spectrum of hormonal-related symptoms. Fewer studies have specifically addressed the impact of infertility and andropause on quality of life in men compared with women. However, these studies have demonstrated that cancer-related infertility in men was associated with long-term distress.[10] Recently, it was demonstrated that young male cancer survivors self-reported a marked impairment in quality of life, energy levels, and quality of sexual functioning. Young male cancer survivors appeared less strong, vital, physically fit, and energetic and had suboptimal sexual function compared with a control population. When hypogonadism was noted, the symptoms became worse.[11]

Although ASCO guidelines have been issued in an attempt to enhance oncologists' attentiveness to fertility concerns of young cancer patients, and to thereby influence clinical practice, several American surveys have shown that oncologists often do not address fertility issues or refer patients to reproductive specialists. In 2009, Quinn et al. reported that only 47% of health care professionals routinely referred their cancer patients of childbearing age to a reproductive endocrinologist.[12] In another survey of academic medical centers, 95% of oncologists reported that they routinely discussed the effect that treatment may have on patients' fertility, but only 39% routinely referred patients to a specialist in reproductive medicine. Regarding sperm conservation, 91% of oncologists agreed it should be offered to eligible men, but only 10% reported actually offering it.[13]

THE IMPACT OF ANTI-CANCER TREATMENTS ON FERTILITY

Several studies have assessed reproductive success after cancer itself, and following anti-cancer treatments. The Childhood Cancer Survivor Study (CCSS) found that female survivors and partners of male survivors were substantially less likely to have live births compared to their siblings. Recently published, the updated CCSS demonstrated that approximately 30% of male childhood cancer survivors had permanent infertility. Men aged 15 to 44 years, who received either testicular radiation at a dose of more than 7.5 Gy, or who were treated with procarbazine or cyclophosphamide, were less likely to achieve a pregnancy. Men diagnosed in early childhood were more likely to father a pregnancy than those diagnosed in adolescence.[14] A study published in 2008 found an increase in the use of assisted reproductive technologies (ART) with both male and female cancer patients, and a significant decrease in first-time parental probability in female patients compared with the general population.[15] Two Scandinavian cohort studies compared approximately 25,000 childhood, adolescent, and young adult survivors with their siblings. These studies found that the relative probability of a cancer survivor having a child was reduced by about 50% for women and about 30–57% for men.[16,17]

There are several obstacles to drawing clear conclusions regarding the gonadotoxic potential (toxic effect to the gonads i.e., the ovaries and testes) of various anti-cancer treatments. The effects of chemotherapy and radiation therapy on fertility depend upon the patient's age, chemotherapeutic regimens, dose and duration, the size and location of the radiation field, type of cancer (mainly in male patients), and pretreatment fertility status of the patient. The major drawback in assessing the rate of infertility is the use of inaccurate parameters such as amenorrhea as gonadal outcomes in most of the studies, as this is only a surrogate marker for infertility; but unfortunately, many women with regular menstrual cycles are not fertile.

Hormonal measurements to evaluate ovarian reserve have been evaluated. Follicle stimulating hormone (FSH) and estradiol measured on day 3 of the menstrual cycle reflects the population of maturing follicles and is indirectly associated with ovarian reserve. Inhibin B, secreted by the granulosa cells lining the follicles is directly associated with loss of oocytes, however the assay is not very reliable. Anti-Mullerian Hormone (AMH), secreted by the granulosa cells of follicles and varies relatively little through the menstrual cycle so can be measured at any time. AMH levels appear to be more sensitive predictors of the loss ovarian reserve, and become abnormal earlier than does early follicular FSH.[18] Ultrasound imaging of the ovaries early in the menstrual cycle (days 2–4) with a count of the antral follicles (measuring 2–10 mm in both ovaries combined) is also a reliable measurement of ovarian reserve.[17] Nevertheless, large, prospective studies are warranted to confirm that these are indeed reliable markers for evaluating chemotherapy-induced ovarian failure.

THE IMPACT OF ANTI-CANCER TREATMENTS ON FEMALE FERTILITY

The impact of anti-cancer treatments on female fertility depends on the women's age at the time of treatment, the chemotherapy protocol, and the duration and total cumulative dose administered.

Age—The high susceptibility of the ovaries to chemotherapy-induced toxicity is related to the physiological decline in the number of oocytes from birth to menopause. Approximately 90% of oocytes within the female ovary will undergo physiologic apoptosis during the fetal or postnatal life.[19,20] The cellular machinery of the follicles has an inherent high susceptibility to apoptosis exerted by many chemotherapeutic agents. Chemotherapy-induced ovarian failure is age dependent, with older age being associated with a greater loss of ovarian reserve. This is due to the lower ovarian reserve in these women prior to treatment due to their older ages.

Type of treatment—Anti-cancer treatments can result in subfertility or infertility due to impacts upon the hypothalamic-pituitary-gonadal axis, causing a hypogonadic state in which the ovary is not adequately stimulated, or due to direct gonadotoxic damage to the germ cells. Cranial irradiation greater than 35 to 40 Gy can impair hypothalamic pituitary function resulting in hypogonadism through gonadotropin-releasing hormone (GnRH) or FSH/ LH deficiency.[21]. Radiation to the pelvis may induce fibrosis which may complicate future pregnancies.

Chemotherapy—Alkylating agents are overall more toxic to the ovary than other chemotherapy classes, although anthracyclines and platinum compounds have also been shown to be toxic to germ cells pre-clinically.[22,23] Several clinical studies have demonstrated that chemotherapy-related amenorrhea (CRA) rates varied between 30% and 76% depending on the average age of the cohort and the chemotherapeutic protocol used.[24–29] Chemotherapy-related amenorrhea occurs in over 90% of patients treated with high-dose chemotherapies, induction therapies prior to bone marrow transplantation, or total body irradiation. Virtually all women undergoing induction chemotherapy and TBI prior to transplantation are irreversibly sterile.[19] There are very limited data regarding infertility risk for patients undergoing newer chemotherapy regimens or targeted biologic agents. The estimated risks of CRA are presented in Table 21.1.

THE IMPACT OF ANTI-CANCER TREATMENTS ON MALE FERTILITY

The impact on male fertility may derive from alteration of the hypothalamic-pituitary-gonadal axis, damage to the germinal epithelium, or functional disruption of ejaculation due to mechanical or emotional factors. Male germ cells are particularly susceptible to injury by chemotherapy and radiation. The seminiferous epithelium of the testes is more sensitive than the testosterone-producing Leydig cells. Therefore, infertility is more likely to be a sequela of anti-cancer treatments than sexual dysfunction.

The most gonadotoxic agents are nitrogen mustard derivates (such as busulphan and melphalan) and alkylating drugs (such as cyclophosphamide and procarbazine).

Temporary impairment of spermatogenesis may remain for up to two years, and an individual's sperm count is at its lowest six months after the completion of therapy.[30] In male patients cancer itself may independently affect fertility. Studies have concluded that the integrity of sperm DNA is compromised before the initiation of treatment in patients with Hodgkin's lymphoma or testicular cancer.[31,32] Testicular cancer is characterized by paracrine secretion of growth factors which can be deleterious to spermatogenesis. The most gonadotoxic agents are nitrogen mustard derivates (such as busulphan and

TABLE 21.1 PRE-TREATMENT OPTIONS

Method	Embryo preservation	Oocyte preservation	Ovarian cryopreservation	Ovarian transposition	Ovarian shielding	Radical Trachelectomy	Ovarian hormonal suppression
Status	Standard	Experimental	Experimental	Standard	Standard	Standard	Experimental
Target population	Pubertal	Pubertal	Pre-pubertal/pubertal	Pre-pubertal/pubertal	Pre-pubertal/pubertal	Pre-pubertal/pubertal	pubertal
Procedure	Oocytes are retrieved following controlled ovulation induction -> fertilized in vitro freezed and stored	Oocytes are retrieved following ovarian stimulation, freezed and stored	Pieces of the ovary are removed, freezed ant stored for future re-implantation	Ovaries are removed to a different body location outside the radiation field	External lead shield protects the reproductive organs if they are in the radiation field	For cervical cancer patients: Removal of the cervix and the uterus remains intact.	GnRH agonists potentially suppress follicular development and hence protect against chemotherapy toxicity
Required time	10–14 days from menses	10–14 days from menses	Variable	Variable	Not applicable	Not applicable	7–10 days before chemotherapy
Setting	Outpatient	Outpatient	Inpatient – surgical procedure	Inpatient – surgical procedure	Throughout radiation	Inpatient – surgical procedure	Outpatient
Success rate	19–31%; depends on age and quality of embryos	900 live births up to now,	Case reports	~50%	Unknown	Unknown. Data shows no higher rates of recurrence.	Unknown – ongoing evaluation in clinical trials
Special consideration	Requires a partner or donor's sperm	Does not require a partner or donor's sperm	Does not require a partner or donor's sperm. May be done in pre-pubertal girls	Does not protect against possible damage from chemotherapy	Does not protect against damage from chemotherapy	Early stage cervical cancer patients; patient selection is critical	Does not protect against possible damage from radiation

TABLE 21.2 Post-Treatment Options

Method	Ovarian hormonal suppression	Donor embryo	Donor oocytes	Gestational surrogate/carrier	Adoption
Status	Experimental	optional	Standard	Standard	Standard
Target population	pubertal	pubertal	pubertal	pubertal	pubertal
Procedure	GnRH agonists potentially suppress follicular development and hence protects against chemotherapy toxicity	Use of embryo donated from other couple and transferred to the uterus	Use of oocyte donated from other women for fertilization and transfer of the embryo to the uterus	A surrogate will carry the pregnancy with the embryo	Parenthood of a born child
Required time	7–10 days before chemotherapy	Variable	Variable	Variable	Variable
Setting	Outpatient	Outpatient	Outpatient	Not applicable	Not applicable
Success rate	Unknown – ongoing evaluation in clinical trials	Unknown	40–50%	~30%	Not applicable
Special consideration	Does not protect against possible damage from radiation	Through fertility clinics or private agency	Ability to choose donor based on individual characteristics	Legal issues vary by country	Medical history may be a factor

melphalan) and alkylating drugs (such as cyclophosphamide and procarbazine).Table 21.2 depicts the classification of drugs according to the risk of testicular toxicity.

High-dose pelvic irradiation in pelvic malignancies may permanently damage testicular function and may also contribute to erectile dysfunction. Cranial irradiation greater than 35 to 40 Gy can impair the hypothalamic pituitary function resulting in hypogonadism through gonadotropin-releasing hormone (GnRH) deficiency.

FERTILITY PRESERVATION IN FEMALE CANCER PATIENTS

Protection of Ovarian Function Prior to Treatment

Postpubertal females can undergo gonadotropin stimulation of the ovaries, followed by embryo cryopreservation prior to cancer treatment. This method has been an established treatment for couples with infertility and is the recommended modality for women as the ability to successfully freeze and thaw embryos is well known. The process involves ovarian stimulation by gonadotropins, oocyte retrieval, fertilization, and freezing and storage of embryos few days later.

For women with hormone-responsive cancers, such as breast cancer, in order to avoid supraphysiologic estradiol levels arising from conventional ovarian stimulation with gonadotropins, several alternative protocols for ovulation induction have evolved. One commonly used protocol employs an aromatase inhibitor combined with a reduced FSH dose resulted in significantly lower estradiol levels. A seven year follow up of women who underwent treatment with this protocol demonstrated that treated women had lower recurrence rates compared with breast cancer survivors who had not been treated for ovulation induction, though this was not a randomized controlled study.[33]

Freezing of mature oocytes after ovarian stimulation is another alternative for women without a male partner or who prefer not to use donor sperm. The process is similar to embryo preservation but without fertilization. Recent technological advances have now improved oocyte cryopreservation mainly due to improvement in the freezing techniques yielding fertilization rates of 60% to 70% with the use of intracytoplasmic sperm injection.[34] More than 900 infants have now been born from cryopreserved oocytes with no apparent increase in congenital anomalies compared with naturally conceived infants.[35]

In women who do not have time to undergo ovarian stimulation and in prepubertal girls, ovarian tissue cryopreservation is an emerging option, yet is still considered experimental due to low yield of recovery of immature oocytes and later lower fertilization rates. This technique involves laparoscopic surgery, removal of an ovary or a portion of the ovarian cortex, and cryopreservation of the ovarian cortex into thin strips containing immature follicles.

Five live births have been reported in women with cancer who underwent autologous transplantation of cryopreserved ovarian tissue.[36,37] Nevertheless, transplantation of ovarian tissue may confer a risk of reintroducing cancer cells from the transplanted tissue and is therefore considered an unfavorable option for fertility preservation, mainly for patients with hematological malignancies such as leukemia or carriers of *BRCA1* and *BRCA2* mutations. Several techniques are being used to screen ovarian tissue for the presence of metastatic disease before transplantation such as histological analysis and real-time PCR.[38] Another technique currently under development is in vitro maturation of follicles obtained from ovarian cortex.

Protection of Ovarian Function during Treatment

During pelvic irradiation, surgical transposition of the ovaries (oophoropexy) outside the radiation field has been shown to decrease ovarian damage and loss of ovarian reserve.

GnRH analogs induce a temporary hypogonadism by decreasing the secretion of pituitary gonadotropins, theoretically resulting in ovarian quiescence, as in a prepubertal state. It has also been postulated that GnRH analogs may cause a reduction of ovarian blood flow, thereby reducing exposure to chemotherapy. However, this option is less well-proven and at best merely increases the probability of resuming menses after therapy, which may not be correlated with fertility potential.[39]

Post-treatment parenthood options for cancer survivors that became infertile include the use of donor oocytes to achieve a pregnancy or donor oocytes with use of gestational surrogacy, or traditional surrogacy in which another woman provides both the ovaries and uterus for the pregnancy.

All methods for fertility preservation in females are summarized in Tables 21.3 and 4.

FERTILITY PRESERVATION IN MALE CANCER PATIENTS

For postpubertal men with cancer, semen cryopreservation prior to chemotherapy is the only established method of fertility preservation. When ejaculation is impaired, some invasive alternatives may be used such as microsurgical epididymal sperm aspiration, where spermatozoa are removed from the epididymal tubules or testicular biopsy. In the small number of patients presenting with azoospermia, testicular biopsy with sperm harvesting may be feasible.[40,41] Intracytoplasmic sperm injection requires only a few viable spermatozoa that can be injected into oocytes as part of in vitro fertilization therapy allows men to father pregnancies when sperm production is minimal.

For prepubertal boys fertility preservation is challenging and is still considered investigational as cryopreservation of testicular tissue is experimental. During radiation, gonad shielding may be used when possible. Ongoing

TABLE 21.3 ESTIMATED RISK FOR CHEMOTHERAPY-RELATED AMENORRHEA

Degree of Risk	Treatment Protocol	Used in
High risk > 80% of women develop amenorrhea after treatment	- Whole abdominal or pelvic radiation doses > 6 Gy in adult women	Multiple cancers
	- Whole abdominal or pelvic radiation doses; >15 Gy in prepubertal girls and > 10 Gy in postpubertal girls - TBI radiation doses BMT/SCT	Wilms tumor, neuroblastoma, sarcoma, Hodgkin's lymphoma
	- CMF, CEF, or CAF X 6 cycles in women age >40	Breast cancer
	- Cyclophosphamide 5 g/m^2 in women age <40	Multiple cancers
	- Cyclophosphamide 7.5 g/m^2 in females age < 20 - Any alkylating agent +TBI or pelvic radiation	NHL, neuroblastoma, ALL, sarcoma conditioning for transplantation BMT/SCT
	- Cranial/brain radiation >40 Gy	Brain tumor
Intermediate risk approximately 30%–70% of women develop amenorrhea after treatment	- |CMF, CEF, or CAF X 6 cycles in women age 30-39 - AC in women age 40	Breast cancer
	- Whole abdominal or pelvic radiation 10 to 15 Gy in prepubertal girls - Whole abdominal or pelvic radiation 5 to 10 Gy in postpubertal girls	Wilms tumor, neuro-blastoma Spinal tumor, brain tumor,
	- Spinal radiation> 25 Gy	neuroblastoma, relapsed ALL or NHL
Low risk <20% of women develop amenorrhea	- AC in women age 30-39	Breast cancer
	- CMF, CEF, or CAF X 6 cycles in women age >30	Breast cancer
	- Nonalkylating chemotherapy	Hodgkin's lymphoma, NHL
	- Anthracycline + cytarabine	AML
	- Multiagent therapies	ALL
Unknown risk	Taxanes Biological agents	Multiple cancers

TABLE 21.4 ESTIMATED RISK FOR IMPAIRED SPERMATOGENESIS

Low Risk	Moderate Risk	High Risk
Vincristine	Cisplatin	Cyclophosphamide
Methotrexate	Carboplatin	Ifosfamide
Dactinomycin	Doxorubicin	Busulfan
Bleomycin		Melphalan
Mercaptopurine		Procarbazine
Vinblastine		Chlorambucil

Male: Adjusted from Wallace et al., 2005 (42).

Female: Adapted from LIVESTRONG, The Lance Armstrong Foundation (http://www.livestrong.org) and from Levine 2010 (41).

Abbreviations: TBI, total-body irradiation; CMF, cyclophosphamide, methotrexate, and fluorouracil; CEF, cyclophosphamide, epirubicin, and fluorouracil; CAF, cyclophosphamide, doxorubicin, and fluorouracil; BMT, bone marrow transplantation; SCT, stem-cell transplantation; NHL, non-Hodgkin's lymphoma; AML, acute myeloid leukemia; ALL, acute lymphoblastic leukemia; AC, doxorubicin and cyclophosphamide.

research includes in vitro maturation of spermatogonia into spermatocytes or germ-cell transplantation into native testicular tissue.[42]

CONCLUSIONS

Cancer therapy may lead to impaired fertility and hormone production in women and men with cancer. The overwhelming comprehension of cancer diagnosis is complicated by the potential loss of fertility in reproductive-age patients. Complex psychosocial and ethical decisions must be made regarding the possibilities of future parenthood. Health care professionals play key roles in informing patients about the potential impact of treatment on fertility. Timely referral to a reproductive endocrinologist is essential due to the period of time required for fertility preservation procedures and to avoid lengthy delays prior to the start of cancer treatments. Fertility preservation counseling should address several important issues: potential gonadotoxic effects, options available to patients prior to treatment as well as discussion of parenthood post treatment. Education resources should be offered to patients to improve their understanding.

While strategies for fertility preservation in post pubertal patients are becoming standard of care, there is a paucity of valid options for younger patients. As the rate of young cancer survivors has grown, fertility issues have become more relevant. Providing cancer patients with timely information related to fertility preservation and referring them to a reproductive specialist may partially alleviate the emotional burden that accompanies the commencement of anti-cancer treatment and later on facilitate the transition from a cancer patient to a cancer survivor.

REFERENCES

1. Jemal A, Murray T, Ward E, et al. Cancer statistics. CA Cancer J Clin 2005;55: 10–30.

2. Ries LAG, Melbert D, Krapcho M, et al: SEER Cancer Statistics Review, 1975-2004. Bethesda, MD, National Cancer Institute. http://seer.cancer.gov/csr/1975_2004.

3. American Cancer Society: Breast Cancer Facts and Figures 2007–2008. Atlanta, GA, American Cancer Society Inc, 2007.

4. Lee SJ, Schover LR, Partridge AH, et al. American society of clinical oncology recommendations on fertility preservation in cancer patients. *J Clin Oncol* 2006;24:2917–2931.

5. Ganz PA, Rowland JH, Desmond K, Meyerowitz BE, Wyatt GE. Life after breast cancer: understanding women's health-related quality of life and sexual functioning. J Clin Oncol. 1998;16:501–514.

6. Ganz PA, Greendale GA, Petersen L, Kahn B, Bower JE. Breast cancer in younger women: reproductive and late health effects of treatment. J Clin Oncol. 2003;21:4184–4193.

7. Tesauro GM, Rowland JH, Lustig C. Survivorship resources for post-treatment cancer survivors. Cancer Pract. 2002;10:277–283.

8. Jeffrey Dunn SKS. Young women's experience of breast cancer: defining young and identifying concerns. Psycho-Oncology 2000;9:137–146.

9. Partridge AH, Gelber S, Peppercorn J, Ginsburg E, Sampson E, Rosenberg R, Przypyszny M, Winer EP. Fertility and menopausal outcomes in young breast cancer survivors. Clin Breast Cancer. 2008;8:65–69.

10. Green D, Galvin H, Horne B. The psycho-social impact of infertility on young male cancer survivors: a qualitative investigation. Psycho-Oncology 2003;12:141–152.

11. Greenfield DM, Walters SJ, Coleman RE, Hancock BW, Snowden JA, Shalet SM, DeRogatis LR, Ross RJ. Quality of life, self-esteem, fatigue, and sexual function in young men after cancer: a controlled cross-sectional study. Cancer. 2010;15:1592–601.

12. Quinn GP, Vadaparampil ST, Lee JH, et al Physician referral for fertility preservation in oncology patients: a national study of practice behaviors. J Clin Oncol. 2009;27:5952–5957.

13. Forman EJ, Anders CK, Behera MA. A nationwide survey of oncologists regarding treatment-related infertility and fertility preservation in female cancer patients. Fertil Steril. 2010;94:1652–1656.

14. Green DM, Kawashima T, Stovall M, et al. Fertility of male survivors of childhood cancer: a report from the Childhood Cancer Survivor Study. J Clin Oncol 2010; 28:332–339.

15. Magelssen H, Melve KK, Skjaerven R, Fosså SD. Parenthood probability and pregnancy outcome in patients with a cancer diagnosis during adolescence and young adulthood. Hum Reprod. 2008;23:178–186.

16. Madanat LM, Malila N, Dyba T, Hakulinen T, Sankila R, Boice JD Jr, Lähteenmäki PM. Probability of parenthood after early onset cancer: a population-based study. Int J Cancer. 2008;123:2891–2898.

17. Schover LR. Premature Ovarian Failure and Its consequences: Vasomotor Symptoms, Sexuality, and Fertility JCO 2008; 26:753–758.

18. Seifer DB, Maclaughlin DT. Mullerian Inhibiting Substance is an ovarian growth factor of emerging clinical significance. Fertil Steril. 2007;88:539–546.

19. Lobo RA. Potential options for preservation of fertility in women. N Engl J Med. 2005;353:64–73.

20. Johnson J, Canning J, Kaneko T, et al: Germline stem cells and follicular renewal in the postnatal mammalian ovary. Nature 2004;28:145–150.

21. Littley MD, Shalet SM, Beardwell CG, et al.: Hypopituitarism following external radiotherapy for pituitary tumours in adults. Q J Med 1989;70:145–160.

22. Gonfloni S, Di Tella L, Caldarola S, Cannata SM, Klinger FG, Di Bartolomeo C, Mattei M, Candi E, De Felici M, Melino G, Cesareni G. Inhibition of the c-Abl-TAp63 pathway protects mouse oocytes from chemotherapy-induced death. Nat Med. 2009;15:1179–1185.

23. Ben-Aharon I, Bar-Joseph H, Tzarfaty G, Kuchinsky L, Rizel S, Stemmer SM, Shalgi R. Doxorubicin-induced ovarian toxicity. Reprod Biol Endocrinol. 2010;4:8–20.

24. Bines J, Oleske DM, Cobleigh MA. Ovarian function in premenopausal women treated with adjuvant chemotherapy for breast cancer. J Clin Oncol. 1996;14:1718–1729.

25. Goodwin PJ, Ennis M, Pritchard KI, Trudeau M, Hood N. Risk of menopause during the first year after breast cancer diagnosis. J Clin Oncol. 1999;17:2365–2370.

26. Burstein HJ, Winer EP. Primary care for survivors of breast cancer. N Engl J Med. 2000;343:1086–1094.

27. Stone ER, Slack RS, Novielli A, et al. Rate of chemotherapy related amenorrhea (CRA) associated with adjuvant Adriamycin and Cytoxan (AC) and Adriamycin and Cytoxan followed by Taxol (ACT) in early stage breast cancer [abstract]. Breast Cancer Res Treat. 2000;64:61. Abstract 224.

28. Parulekar WR, Day AG, Ottaway JA, Shepherd LE, Trudeau ME, Bramwell V, Levine M, Pritchard KI; National Cancer Institute of Canada Clinical Trials Group. Incidence and prognostic impact of amenorrhea during adjuvant therapy in high-risk premenopausal breast cancer: analysis of a National Cancer Institute of Canada Clinical Trials Group Study—NCIC CTG MA.5.J Clin Oncol. 2005;23:6002–6008.

29. Abusief ME, Missmer SA, Ginsburg ES, Weeks JC, Partridge AH. The effects of paclitaxel, dose density, and trastuzumab on treatment-related amenorrhea in pre-menopausal women with breast cancer. Cancer 2010;116:791–798.

30. Hart R: Preservation of fertility in adults and children diagnosed with cancer. BMJ 2008; 337:a2045.

31. O'Flaherty C, Vaisheva F, Hales BF, Chan P, Robaire B. Characterization of sperm chromatin quality in testicular cancer and Hodgkin's lymphoma patients prior to chemotherapy. Hum Reprod 2008; 23:1044–1052.

32. Tempest HG, Ko E, Chan P, Robaire B, Rademaker A, Martin RH. Sperm aneuploidy frequencies analysed before and after chemotherapy in testicular cancer and Hodgkin's lymphoma patients. Hum Reprod 2008;23:251–258.

33. Oktay K, Lee SH, Moy F. A Prospective Controlled Analysis of Fertility Preservation by Oocyte and Embryo Cryopreservation Using an Aromatase Inhibitor-Gonadotropin Protocol: Treatment Outcomes and Safety in Young Women with Breast Cancer. [P2-14-01], San-Antonio Breast Cancer Symposium 2010.

34. Fabbri R, Porcu E, Marsella T, Rocchetta G, Venturoli S, Flamigni C. Human oocyte cryopreservation: new perspectives regarding oocyte survival. *Hum Reprod.* 2001;16:411–416.

35. Noyes N, Porcu E, Borini A. Over 900 oocyte cryopreservation babies born with no apparent increase in congenital anomalies. *Reprod Biomed Online.* 2009; 18:769–776.

36. Donnez J, Dolmans MM, Demylle D, et al. Livebirth after orthotopic transplantation of cryopreserved ovarian tissue. Lancet 2004;364:1405–1410.

37. Meirow D, Levron J, Eldar-Geva T, et al. Pregnancy after transplantation of cryopreserved ovarian tissue in a patient with ovarian failure after chemotherapy. N Engl J Med 2005;353:318–321.

38. Meirow D, Hardan I, Dor J, et al. Searching for evidence of disease and malignant cell contamination in ovarian tissue stored from hematologic cancer patients. Hum Reprod 2008;23:1007–1013.

39. Ben-Aharon I, Gafter-Gvili A, Leibovici L, Stemmer SM. Pharmacological interventions for fertility preservation during chemotherapy: a systematic review and meta-analysis. Breast Cancer Res Treat. 2010;122:803–811.

40. Schrader M, Muller M, Sofikitis N, Straub B, Krause H, Miller K. "Onco-tese": testicular sperm extraction in azoospermic cancer patients before chemotherapy—new guidelines? Urology 2003;61:421–425.

41. Jensen JR, Morbeck DE, Coddington CC. Fertility Preservation. Mayo Clin Proc. 2011;86:45–49.

42. Levine J, Canada A, Stern CJ. Fertility preservation in adolescents and young adults with cancer. J Clin Oncol. 2010;28:4831–4841.

43. Wallace WH, Anderson RA, Irvine DS. Fertility preservation for young patients with cancer: who is at risk and what can be offered? *Lancet Oncol.* 2005; 6: 209–218.

22

Breast Cancer Survivorship

Kathryn Ruddy, MD

Introduction

Breast cancer is second only to lung cancer in incidence in American women, affecting one in eight over the course of a lifetime. Though comparatively rare in men, there are still nearly 2,000 male breast cancers diagnosed per year in the United States. Owing to improvements in early detection and treatment there are now more than 2.3 million breast cancer survivors in the United States.[1] The longitudinal care for this population is complex and includes management of the long-term physical side effects of treatments, psychological distress, issues of sexuality and fertility, and the need for surveillance for recurrent disease.

Currently, early stage breast cancer is treated with breast surgery. Most women also receive one or more of the following treatments: radiation, chemotherapy, and hormonal therapy. The long-term consequences of local therapies may include chest wall pain, lymphedema, and sexual dysfunction. Many other long-term issues for survivors result from systemic treatments (chemotherapy and hormonal therapy) including neuropathy, menopausal symptoms, and rarely, permanent cardiac compromise. By one year after diagnosis, any prescribed surgery, radiation, or chemotherapy is usually finished, but hormonal therapy for hormone-receptor positive cancers typically continues for at least five years.

Progress in Disease Treatments Affects Survivorship Care

The number of breast cancer survivors is rising as therapies for breast cancer become more targeted, optimizing the benefits and minimizing the risks of treatment. For early stage disease, tumor gene signature tests such as Oncotype Dx and Mammaprint have been shown to help identify which women do not benefit from chemotherapy and therefore should be spared the toxicities that result from those drugs. From a surgical standpoint, the advent of sentinel lymph node biopsy has allowed many women to avoid the greater potential for lymphedema and pain associated with full axillary dissection. Furthermore, for metastatic disease, there has been a move toward less aggressive systemic treatments that allow women to preserve quality of life over a long period. For women who do need chemotherapy either in the early or late stage setting, there are new targeted antineoplastic agents that have changed practice over the past decade. For example, the introduction of trastuzumab, a monoclonal antibody, has dramatically improved outcomes for the 20% of breast cancers that overexpress Her2/neu. More incrementally, the recent use of aromatase inhibitors in postmenopausal women has reduced rates of recurrence of hormone receptor positive cancers in postmenopausal women.

Breast cancer survivors have specific needs that are associated with the physical and psychological sequelae of this disease and its treatment. Because new breast cancer therapies are continually being developed, and each therapy causes unique toxicities, optimal survivorship care evolves over time as well. For example, as more women are taking hormonal therapy for periods greater than five years (based on data suggesting superior efficacy when tamoxifen and an aromatase inhibitor are given sequentially), it is becoming more important to address the consequences of longer estrogen deprivation. Likewise, recommended cardiac monitoring for patients on trastuzumab is more intense than for previous breast cancer therapies, and more research is needed to evaluate long term cardiovascular symptoms that may be associated with trastuzumab and bevacizumab.

Toxicities of Local Therapies

Surgery

The standard surgeries used to treat early stage breast cancer are lumpectomy (removal of part of the breast, also termed partial mastectomy) or mastectomy (removal of the entire breast). Mastectomy is more likely to cause motor restriction and chest wall pain, though this is not permanent in most people. Frozen shoulder can result from prolonged shoulder immobility, and nerve damage at the time of the surgery can cause long-term post-operative pain.[2] Although reconstructive surgery can be very valuable to a woman's body image and psychological health, reconstructive procedures can add physical discomfort in the survivorship period. Pectoralis muscle spasms are common while expanders are in place for reconstruction after a mastectomy, and procedures that use autologous tissue to form the breast mound (e.g. TRAM, DIEP) may cause persistent numbness, weakness, and pain at the site from which tissue was removed. Even after lumpectomy, the least invasive breast cancer surgery, women can have persistent discomfort from tissue injury. This is often compounded by radiation (see Table 22.1).

Radiation

The acute toxicities of radiation include skin and soft tissue damage and fatigue. Fatigue may become severe, but it usually resolves within six weeks after the last dose of radiation. Pectoralis muscles may become tight due to radiation, temporarily impeding patients from turning the steering wheel while driving, pushing open doors, and participating in many sports. Stretching and massage may help improve range of motion.[2] Radiation to the chest wall can also cause costochondritis. This inflammation of cartilage can present as tenderness to palpation or pain exacerbated by deep breathing or lifting.

Both surgery and radiation can cause lymphedema of the arm, hand, and chest, which can significantly interfere with quality of life for some breast cancer survivors. The ALMANAC trial found that risks of severe lymphedema were 1% after sentinel lymph node biopsy and 2–3% after full axillary dissection. In that study, risks of mild lymphedema were 3–4% after sentinel node biopsy and 10–14% after full axillary dissection.[3] Lymphedema may begin soon after treatment or many years later (often triggered by an infection, heavy exertion, or trauma to the tissue causing flow of lymph to that area). Efforts to minimize lymphedema focus on avoiding these possible triggers (often including venipuncture and blood pressure monitoring on that arm), though the utility of such measures is not well proven.[4] Exercise is particularly controversial, as some patients may experience worsening lymphedema with exercise, but exercise that helps maintain a healthy weight or induce weight loss may prevent and treat lymphedema. Lymphedema is commonly managed using a compression sleeve and gauntlet, massage, and physical therapy. However, prior to treating a new-onset lymphedema in a breast cancer survivor, it is important to evaluate for alternate causes of swelling including tumor recurrence, infection, and thrombosis.

Other long-term risks of radiation include secondary malignancies, hypothyroidism, pneumonitis and pulmonary fibrosis, cataracts and xerophthalmia, and cardiac damage. Modern radiation techniques shield most non-breast tissues, minimizing the likelihood of these toxicities. However, most masses that appear near a radiation field should be imaged or biopsied due to the possibility of a radiation-induced cancer. These can include sarcomas, cancers of the lung and esophagus, second breast cancers, and myeloid leukemia. Secondary solid tumors tend to occur at least ten years after radiation, but leukemia tends to occur within five years of the exposure to radiation.[5]

According to a SEER database query, only 1/300 breast cancer patients who received radiation for breast cancer between 1973 and 1997 subsequently developed sarcomas over the following 15 years (compared with 1 in 500 breast cancer patients who did not receive radiation).[6] In this study, it appeared that outcomes were similar between radiation-induced sarcomas and non-radiation induced sarcomas. In another study, performed within a Norwegian cancer registry, the median time between radiation and development of sarcoma was found to be 13.6 years,[7] suggesting that the lifetime risk of sarcoma after radiation may be higher than that found with relatively short follow-up in the SEER study.

Toxicities of Systemic Therapies

Chemotherapy

Standard chemotherapies for early stage breast cancer include doxorubicin-cyclophosphamide (AC), docetaxel-cyclophosphamide (TC), and doxorubicin-cyclophosphamide-paclitaxel (AC-T), among others. Trastuzumab is used for breast cancers that overexpress the Her2neu proto-oncogene. The acute side effects of standard breast cancer chemotherapy regimens are commonly hematologic, gastrointestinal, and dermatologic. Fatigue and alopecia are nearly universal. More rarely, cardiac and pulmonary toxicities occur (see Table 22.1).

TABLE 22.1 Common Long-Term and Late Effects of Breast Cancer Treatment

Effect	Management Options
Surgical	
• Cosmetic effects	• Plastic surgery
• Functional disability of arm or chest wall, pain	• Physical therapy
	• Plastic surgery
• Scarring/adhesions	• Physical therapy, avoid trauma to
• Lymphedema	involved arm
Radiation	
• Second malignancies	• Image masses arising near radiation field
• Xerophalmia, cataracts	• Regular visits to ophthalmologist
• Hypothyroidism	• Check TSH if symptoms of hypothyroidism
• Pneumonitis, pulmonary fibrosis	
• Cardiac damage	• Symptomatic management
• Lymphedema	• Lifestyle risk-reduction (diet, exercise)
	• As above
Systemic Therapy	
• Second malignancies (myelodysplasia and leukemia)	• Check CBC if symptoms of leukemia arise
• Ototoxicity (e.g., cisplatin)	• Symptomatic management
• Cardiomyopathy (e.g., anthracyclines)	• Symptomatic management
• Renal toxicity (e.g., cisplatin)	• Symptomatic management
• Premature menopause & infertility (e.g., alkylating agents)	• Referral to infertility specialist
	• SSRI, SSNRI, gabapentin, counseling

(Continued)

TABLE 22.1 (*Continued*)

Effect	Management Options
• Menopausal symptoms & sexual dysfunction • Osteoporosis (e.g., hormonal therapy, chemotherapy) • Neuropathy (e.g., taxanes and platinums) • Cognitive dysfunction, weight gain, fatigue	• Calcium, vitamin D, exercise, bisphosphonate • Symptomatic management • Exercise, rule out depression and anemia

From Hayes DF: Clinical practice. Follow-up of patients with early breast cancer. N Engl J Med 356:2505–13, 2007.8

Cardiac

Regimens that contain anthracyclines such as doxorubicin or epirubicin and/or that contain trastuzumab carry a risk of cardiac damage and congestive heart failure. On one adjuvant chemotherapy trial (N9831), 5% of women who received AC experienced decreases in ejection fraction that precluded trastuzumab therapy. Of the 95% whose post-AC ejection fractions allowed subsequent paclitaxel-trastuzumab (TH), 8–10% experienced an asymptomatic reduction in ejection fraction that required temporary or permanent cessation of trastuzumab (50% temporary).[9] The risk of congestive heart failure or cardiac death after this AC-TH regimen was 3.3% at three years.[9] Older women who have hypertension and/or other cardiac risk factors are at greater risk of congestive heart failure due to these regimens.[10] For some women who have significant cardiac comorbidity, non-anthracycline containing regimens such as TC and docetaxel-carboplatin-trastuzumab (TCH) for Her2+ cancers may therefore be preferable. It does not appear that dose dense regimens (giving AC every two weeks rather than every three) increases the risk of cardiotoxicity.[11,12] Cardiac ejection fraction should be monitored intermittently during trastuzumab therapy so that cardioprotective medications can be introduced and/or doses can be delayed if need be. The same principles apply for neoadjuvant (before surgery) as adjuvant (after surgery) chemotherapy for early stage disease. After a cardiotoxic chemotherapy regimen is finished, there are no recommendations to perform routine cardiac monitoring, but any cardiac symptoms should be evaluated.

Case Example: P.R. is a 66 year old overweight woman who presents with a stage 2B ER+Her2+ breast cancer. She receives AC-TH chemotherapy after her lumpectomy and full axillary dissection. Her ejection fraction is initially 66%, and after AC it is 62%. After 12 weekly doses of TH, her repeat MUGA shows an EF of 49%. She reports no shortness of breath, chest pain, or palpitations, but she does report new bilateral ankle edema. Systolic blood pressures are approximately 130–140/70–80. She is started on lisinopril 2.5 mg orally daily, and her trastuzumab is held for one month. Before resuming trastuzumab, an echocardiogram is performed, revealing a stable ejection fraction of 49%. Blood pressure is still 130/70. Her ankle edema has resolved and no new symptoms have developed, so her lisinopril dose is increased to 5 mg daily and she resumes trastuzumab, eventually completing a year of therapy with echocardiograms every three months showing stable ejection fractions of 49–50%. No further cardiac testing is performed after trastuzumab is finished, and she remains without cardiac symptoms five years later.

Hematologic

The most common hematologic consequences of chemotherapy for breast cancer are temporary anemia and leucopenia due to bone marrow suppression. Thrombocytopenia is less common. Blood cell counts usually normalize within a few months of the final dose of chemotherapy. More troublesome is the fact that alkylating agents such as cyclophosphamide and topoisomerase II inhibitors such as doxorubicin can cause myelodysplastic syndrome and leukemia. AC causes leukemia in approximately 0.2–1% of women (with possibly higher rates in older women and in those who also receive radiation).[13,14] Leukemia that is related to exposure to an alkylating agent usually occurs three to seven years after the exposure in the context of myelodysplastic syndrome. These are often M1 or M2 acute myeloid leukemias that have chromosome 5 or 7 abnormalities and poor prognoses. Leukemias that are related to exposure to a topoisomerase II inhibitor (e.g. doxorubicin) generally occur within the first three years after exposure, exhibit M4 or M5 phenotypes, are not associated with myelodysplastic syndrome, and carry an 11q23 chromosomal translocation.[15,16] Although this remains controversial, a recent large meta-analysis suggests that G-CSF does not appear to increase the risk of secondary leukemias.[14]

Case example: A 55-year-old woman has been on tamoxifen for 3 years since she completed AC for a high grade stage 1 breast cancer. She reports severe fatigue for two weeks at a routine follow-up visit. A CBC is sent, and she is found to have a peripheral blood monocytosis and a cytogenetic study revealed t(9;11) (p22;q23). Bone marrow biopsy confirms the diagnosis of 11q23 AML, so she is given standard 7 + 3 induction and HiDAC consolidation chemotherapy and achieves a remission. She resumes tamoxifen to complete her 5-year course, and she remains cancer-free 10 years later.

Musculoskeletal

Neuropathy is a common side effect of taxane chemotherapies and platinum agents. Cisplatin can cause permanent hearing loss, and taxanes cause peripheral neuropathy that is usually reversible, but sometimes permanent. Glutamine and amitriptyline have demonstrated some efficacy in treating taxane-related neuropathy.[17]

Case example: 40-year-old woman with a stage 3A ER-Her2+ breast cancer receives neoadjuvant AC-TH, but she complains of significant numbness and painful tingling after her first dose of TH, and by her fifth dose, she reports that she feels unsteady on her feet and she cannot button her shirts anymore. Her breast mass size has decreased from 8 cm to 4 cm by that time. Due to her neuropathy, her paclitaxel dose is held that week, and the following week she reports substantial improvement. Her paclitaxel is resumed at 75% of the standard dose, and her neuropathy does not worsen. She undergoes mastectomy and radiation and then starts to see her medical oncologist every three to six months for history and physical exam. Six months later, she still reports that she has uncomfortable paresthesias in her palms, so her oncologist starts her on amitriptyline 25 mg orally daily. This is titrated up to 50 mg, which provides substantial relief. One year later, she no longer reports any paresthesias, so she is able to titrate off amitriptyline.

Cognitive

Many breast cancer patients complain of cognitive dysfunction (i.e., chemo brain) during and after chemotherapy. Breast cancer patients who received chemotherapy have been shown to score lower on neurocognitive tests than those who did not, but interestingly, in at least one study, patient self-report did not correlate with scores on neurocognitive testing.[18] In another study of long-term survivors of breast and lymphoma, results suggested that verbal memory and psychomotor functioning were inferior in those who had received chemotherapy even five years later.[19] However, most patients were still functioning in the normal range, and deficits were subtle. Preliminary data suggest that women who complain of chemo brain may benefit from Memory and Attention Adaptation Training (MAAT)[20] and/or medications that enhance alertness (e.g., modafinil).[21]

Hormonal therapy

Antiestrogenic medications such as tamoxifen and aromatase inhibitors commonly cause menopausal symptoms such as hot flashes and night sweats. These can interfere with sleep and cause significant discomfort. Selective serotonin reuptake inhibitors (SSRIs) and venlafaxine, a serotonin and norepinephrine reuptake inhibitor (SNRI), have been shown to reduce hot flashes,[22,23] as has gabapentin.[24,25] However, some of the antidepressants (including fluoxetine, paroxetine, sertraline, and bupropion) are contraindicated in patients receiving tamoxifen due to a concern that they interfere with the metabolism of tamoxifen into its active metabolite, endoxifen.

Other common toxicities of aromatase inhibitors include vaginal dryness, arthralgias/myalgias, and bone thinning. The musculoskeletal symptoms that occur on aromatase inhibitor therapy can be significant impediments to quality of life in many patients. In a recent survey of 200 women taking aromatase inhibitors, nearly half complained of joint pain and joint stiffness.[26] Exercise and non-steroidal anti-inflammatory drugs (NSAIDs) such as ibuprofen 600 mg two to three times daily can be helpful to ameliorate joint stiffness and pain due to aromatase inhibitors. Pain usually resolves within weeks of stopping the offending medication (for some women, symptoms are severe enough to prompt a switch to tamoxifen or a cessation of therapy).[27]

Vaginal discharge is a common side effect of tamoxifen, and rarer side effects of this drug include venous blood clots and uterine cancer. Patients over age 50 are most susceptible to these serious toxicities. It is controversial whether tamoxifen increases stroke risk. In women receiving tamoxifen for prevention, the risk of pulmonary embolus was increased 3-fold and the risk of endometrial cancer 2.5 fold, but still the absolute risk of both is low (< 1% risk of pulmonary embolus, deep venous thrombosis, stroke, or endometrial cancer over five years of treatment with tamoxifen).[28,29]

PSYCHOSOCIAL ISSUES

Many breast cancer patients face major psychological hurdles as they transition out of active treatment. Relationships may change during and after a breast cancer diagnosis, roles at work and home may be altered, and finances may be strained, all of which may contribute to distress in this population. It is natural that patients and their loved ones worry about their risk of recurrence, and sometimes this anxiety can make it difficult for all to move forward mentally and emotionally.

In a study of 202 early stage breast cancer patients no older than 60, 48% were found to report depression or anxiety during the first year after the diagnosis.[30] Over time, distress tends to wane. Out of 116 Dutch patients who were two to four years after their primary surgical treatment, only 7% met frank DSM-IV criteria for anxiety or depression. Still, some psychological sequelae of breast cancer, particularly post-traumatic stress disorder symptoms, may persist for 20 years or more.[31] Support from friends and family, counseling, and psychiatric medications can all help breast cancer survivors cope with their psychosocial challenges.

IMPACT OF TREATMENTS ON SEXUALITY

Women may experience sexual dysfunction during and after treatment for breast cancer due to side effects of systemic treatments, psychological results of treatment, strains on relationships with sexual partners, and changes in appearance. Breast surgery can be disfiguring and can impair body image, perhaps most substantially when a woman has mastectomy without immediate reconstruction.[32] Hormonal therapies and loss of ovarian function due to chemotherapy often cause vaginal dryness and atrophy, necessitating use of vaginal moisturizers (such as Replens®) and water-based lubricants (such as

Astroglide®). Arousal, orgasm, lubrication, sexual satisfaction, and absence of dyspareunia have been found to correlate strongly with relationship satisfaction, though it is unclear which is the cause and which is the effect.[33] Depression and older age have been shown to be associated with sexual dysfunction.[33]

FERTILITY

Concern about infertility is common among young breast cancer survivors.[34] Women who are interested in having biologic children after they are treated for breast cancer may face several obstacles. The first is that data are limited regarding the safety of post-breast cancer pregnancies, though most studies suggest that there is no increased risk of cancer recurrence if a woman does go on to become pregnant. In fact, most studies show lower rates of recurrence among these women, though all are probably confounded by a healthy mother effect (i.e., women who are healthier and have tumors that are less likely to recur are the ones who choose to pursue a future pregnancy).[35] Some experts recommend that patients wait two years before attempting conception in order to avoid pregnancy during the time of highest relapse risk, but there are actually data that suggest that earlier pregnancies are not detrimental.[36] There are also data demonstrating that prior breast cancer treatments do not cause congenital malformations in future offspring.[37]

The second obstacle to fertility is that those who are on hormonal therapy should not attempt conception until they have stopped it. Tamoxifen can cause birth defects, particularly when a fetus is exposed in the first trimester.[38] Some women opt to stop tamoxifen early, before the recommended five years, because they know that their fertility naturally wanes over time, and they prioritize child-bearing over optimal cancer recurrence risk reduction.

The third obstacle to fertility after breast cancer is that chemotherapy, unlike hormonal therapy, directly damages the ovaries, causing temporary or permanent amenorrhea in most premenopausal patients, and reducing fertility in all.[39] Thus, even patients with estrogen receptor and progesterone receptor negative cancers, who are not delayed by ongoing hormonal therapy, may face difficulty conceiving if they have received chemotherapy (as most do). Reproductive specialists with expertise treating breast cancer patients may be very helpful in this setting, though patients will have the most fertility preservation options if they see a fertility expert before chemotherapy is begun.

SURVIVORSHIP CARE FOR MEN WITH BREAST CANCER

Men only comprise approximately 1% of all breast cancer patients, so there is little data on how best to treat them, particularly during the survivorship period. In general, in the absence of data, breast cancer therapy in men mimics that in women. As breast cancer survivors, men are therefore also at risk for the long-term toxicities of local treatments (e.g. lymphedema and pain) and of systemic treatments (e.g. cardiac compromise, leukemia, and neuropathy). However, the relative rates and severities of these toxicities in men compared to women have not been well-studied. Men are more likely than women to undergo mastectomy (due to less concern about the cosmetic consequences of the surgery), but little is known about the impact of this surgery upon men's lives. Side effects of hormonal therapies may be especially different between the sexes due to different baseline hormone levels and physiology. Based on prostate cancer literature, we know that ovarian suppression can reduce bone mineral density in men as it does in women,[40] but we do not know how much an aromatase inhibitor might contribute to this. If men have better baseline bone mineral densities than women the same age, ovarian suppression and aromatase inhibitors may not increase their risk of fracture as much as they do in women. However, sexual dysfunction may be equally or more problematic in men on these therapies. One small study of 24 men on tamoxifen found that 2 (8%) stopped tamoxifen within a year due to loss of libido, 2 (8%) stopped due to hot flashes, and 1 (4%) stopped due to deep venous thrombosis.[41] Additional research is needed to evaluate the survivorship needs of male breast cancer patients.

One factor that should be considered in all men with breast cancer is genetic risk, as BRCA mutations (particularly BRCA2 mutations) predispose to male breast cancer and likely account for approximately 10% of cases.[42] Therefore, all men should be counseled about genetic testing in the survivorship period if they were not tested at the time of diagnosis. BRCA testing is appropriate for many female survivors as well (particularly those diagnosed under the age of 40, with Ashkenazi heritage, or with strong family history of breast and/or ovarian cancer). Men with BRCA mutations may want to consider contralateral mastectomy, though there are few data to guide this decision. There is debate regarding whether male breast cancer patients as a whole face increased risks of other subsequent cancers.[43]

LIFESTYLE MODIFICATIONS

Recent studies suggest that alcohol intake may be associated with an increased risk of breast cancer recurrence. An abstract presented at the 2009 San Antonio Breast Cancer Symposium reported that breast cancer survivors in the Life After Cancer Epidemiology (LACE) study who drank more than 6 grams of alcohol daily had higher rates of recurrence and death than those who drank less than 0.5 grams of alcohol per day. Overweight and postmenopausal women seemed to experience the greatest harm from alcohol intake as measured by breast cancer recurrence risk.[44] Thus, breast cancer survivors should be counseled that minimizing alcohol intake (to less than three to four drinks weekly) may improve their prognoses.

All breast cancer survivors should also be counseled to assure that they are exercising enough (working up a sweat for at least 30 minutes three times a week). There is some evidence that exercise and prevention of weight gain may reduce the risk of breast cancer recurrence.[45–47] Exercise has also been proven to enhance quality of life, cardiopulmonary function, and bone mineral density in breast cancer patients.[48–51] One study showed that an oncologist's recommendation to a breast cancer survivor to exercise did increase self-reported exercise over the next five weeks, though referral to an exercise specialist did not further raise levels of self-reported exercise.[52] Calcium and vitamin D supplementation and avoidance of tobacco may also help reduce bone loss after breast cancer.[53]

SURVEILLANCE RECOMMENDATIONS

After treatment for an early stage breast cancer, patients are advised to undergo annual screening of residual breast tissue with mammography. Breast MRIs are not routinely recommended, nor are scans of the rest of the body or bloodwork to evaluate for metastatic disease. Several large studies have shown no improvements in outcomes when women are screened for distant recurrence with labs and imaging.[54–56] As imaging techniques and therapies for metastatic breast cancer improve, it is possible that more intensive imaging will become useful in the follow-up period, but currently, we recommend against imaging and labs in the absence of symptoms for breast cancer survivors. Please see Table 22.2 for surveillance recommendations.

- Criteria for annual screening with breast MRI:
  - Confirmed presence of BRCA1 or BRCA2 mutation; *or*
  - First degree blood relative with BRCA1 or BRCA2 mutation and are untested; *or*
  - Have a lifetime risk of breast cancer of 20–25 percent or more using standard risk assessment models (BRCAPRO, Claus model, Gail model, or Tyrer-Cuzick); *or*
  - Carry or have a first-degree relative who carries a genetic mutation in the TP53 or PTEN genes (Li-Fraumeni syndrome and Cowden and Bannayan-Riley-Ruvalcaba syndromes); or

TABLE 22.2 FOLLOW-UP CARE RECOMMENDATIONS AFTER EARLY STAGE BREAST CANCER

Recommended	Not Recommended
History and PE every 3–6 months for 3 years, every 6–12 months for years 4–5, then annually	Routine blood tests (e.g. complete blood counts, liver function tests)
Mammograms every 6–12 months starting 1 year after initial image that diagnosed cancer, but not earlier than 6 months after radiation	Breast MRI except in rare cases*
Monthly self-breast examination	Other imaging studies (e.g. CT, FDG-PET)
Patient education regarding symptoms of recurrence	Tumor markers

Adapted from Khatcheressian JL, Wolff AC, Smith TJ, et al.: American Society of Clinical Oncology 2006 update of the breast cancer follow-up and management guidelines in the adjuvant setting. J Clin Oncol 24:5091–97, 2006.57

• Received radiation treatment to the chest between ages 10 and 30 years, such as for Hodgkin disease.

The majority of recurrences of breast cancer occur within five years, but a steady recurrence rate persists for estrogen receptor positive tumors for many years. Triple negative (not expressing the estrogen receptor, progesterone receptor, or Her2/neu protein) cancers have a high risk of recurrence for the first three to four years, but they are very unlikely to recur after more than five to six years.

COORDINATED CARE

Breast cancer patients should be encouraged to maintain relationships with their primary care providers throughout their treatment. During the survivorship period, primary care providers take on more of the surveillance responsibilities as patients see their oncologists less frequently. It is important that oncologists communicate well with primary care providers and with other members of their patients' health care teams. Communication may be facilitated by the creation of a survivorship care plan that delineates the breast cancer treatments the patient has received and also the care she or he should receive in the future from various providers.[58] After five years of follow-up, some oncologists will transition the care of breast cancer survivors entirely to their primary care providers, though others continue to see these patients annually indefinitely. Please see Table 22.3 for an age-based approach to primary care for breast cancer

TABLE 22.3 AGE-BASED PRIMARY CARE RECOMMENDATIONS FOR CARE OF BREAST CANCER SURVIVORS

Recommendation	Age <30	Age 30–40	Age 41–50	Age 51–65	Age >65
Counseling	Recommendation for exercise (≥ 30 minutes 3 times a week), calcium 1200-1500mg QD, vitamin D 800IU QD; achievement or maintenance of healthy body weight with behavioral interventions offered if BMI > 30; cessation of tobacco use; reduce alcohol use to <4 drinks per week; dietary counseling if patient has cardiovascular disease or diet-related disease				
Gyn	Pap smear and pelvic manual exam yearly	Pap smear every 3 years if 3 prior were nl			May stop Pap if had 3 normal and none abnormal in prior 10 yrs
Bone density	For women who are menopausal or functionally post-menopausal (i.e. on ovarian suppression, s/p oophorectomy, or experiencing chemo-induced				DEXA Q1-2 yrs

TABLE 22.3 (*Continued*)

	amenorrhea), DEXA every 2 years; If high risk for osteoporosis as described below under * and age 60–64, consider yearly scans	
Genetic testing	Based on young age at diagnosis alone, women should be offered genetic counseling for BRCA testing	Family history should be updated at each visit and genetic counseling for BRCA testing should be offered if patient may meet criteria for >10% risk of a mutation.
Blood pressure	Blood pressure should be checked every 2 years if BP < 120/80 and yearly if 120-139/80-90; treat if >140/90 on 2 separate occasions at least 1 week apart.	
Other Cardiovascular	If menopause or functional meno-pause occurs, yearly assessment for modifiable heart disease risk factors (smoking, obesity, lack of exercise). Fasting glucose and lipid profile at least every 5 yrs starting at age 45.	Yearly assessment for modifiable heart disease risk factors. Fasting glucose and lipid profile at least Q5 yrs
Infectious Disease	Chlamydial/gonorrheal screen for sexually active women and those under 25; HIV/syphilis test if at increased risk	Chlamydial, gonorrhea, HIV, and syphilis screen-ing for any women at in-creased risk of infection.
Vaccines	Td booster every 10 years or one dose Tdap; MMR once or twice before age 50; varicella vaccine if no evidence of prior infection or vaccination; consider influenza Qyr; pneumococcal vaccine once before age 65; consider hepA, hepB, and menigococcal vaccines	Td booster Q10yrs or one dose Tdap; MMR x1 after 50; varicella vaccine if no prior infec-tion or vacc; influenza Qyr; pneumococ vx x1 before and x1 after 65; zoster vaccine x1 after 60; consider hepA/B & menigococ vx

survivors. Research suggests that primary care doctors are equally capable of performing appropriate testing and counseling to survivors, with no difference found in quality of life or breast cancer outcome between patients who see primary care providers and those who see oncologists for long-term follow-up.[59]

- Criteria for high risk of osteoporosis:
  - Body weight less than 70 kg, history of nontraumatic fracture or sedentary lifestyle

- Tobacco use, more than 2 alcoholic drinks per day, on chronic steroid medication, or on AI
- Hyperthyroidism, liver disease, eating disorder, or family history of osteoporosis

REFERENCES

1. Institute NC: Estimated U.S. Cancer Prevalence.

2. Kaelin C: The Breast Cancer Survivor's Fitness Plan, President and Fellows of Harvard College, 2007.

3. Goyal A, Newcombe RG, Chhabra A, et al.: Morbidity in breast cancer patients with sentinel node metastases undergoing delayed axillary lymph node dissection (ALND) compared with immediate ALND. *Ann Surg Oncol* 15:262–67, 2008.

4. Burstein HJ, Winer EP: Primary care for survivors of breast cancer. *N Engl J Med* 343:1086–94, 2000.

5. Roychoudhuri R, Evans H, Robinson D, et al: Radiation-induced malignancies following radiotherapy for breast cancer. *Br J Cancer* 91:868–72, 2004.

6. Yap J, Chuba PJ, Thomas R, et al: Sarcoma as a second malignancy after treatment for breast cancer. *Int J Radiat Oncol Biol Phys* 52:1231–37, 2002.

7. Bjerkehagen B, Smeland S, Walberg L, et al: Radiation-induced sarcoma: 25-year experience from the Norwegian Radium Hospital. *Acta Oncol* 47:1475–82, 2008.

8. Hayes DF: Clinical practice. Follow-up of patients with early breast cancer. *N Engl J Med* 356:2505–13, 2007.

9. Perez EA, Suman VJ, Davidson NE, et al: Cardiac safety analysis of doxorubicin and cyclophosphamide followed by paclitaxel with or without trastuzumab in the North Central Cancer Treatment Group N9831 adjuvant breast cancer trial. *J Clin Oncol* 26:1231–38, 2008.

10. Tan-Chiu E, Yothers G, Romond E, et al: Assessment of cardiac dysfunction in a randomized trial comparing doxorubicin and cyclophosphamide followed by paclitaxel, with or without trastuzumab as adjuvant therapy in node-positive, human epidermal growth factor receptor 2-overexpressing breast cancer: NSABP B-31. *J Clin Oncol* 23:7811–19, 2005.

11. Morris PG, Dickler M, McArthur HL, et al.: Dose-dense adjuvant Doxorubicin and cyclophosphamide is not associated with frequent short-term changes in left ventricular ejection fraction. *J Clin Oncol* 27:6117–23, 2009.

12. Dang C, Fornier M, Sugarman S, et al.: The safety of dose-dense doxorubicin and cyclophosphamide followed by paclitaxel with trastuzumab in HER-2/neu overexpressed/amplified breast cancer. *J Clin Oncol* 26:1216–22, 2008.

13. Smith RE, Bryant J, DeCillis A, et al: Acute myeloid leukemia and myelodysplastic syndrome after doxorubicin-cyclophosphamide adjuvant therapy for operable breast cancer: the National Surgical Adjuvant Breast and Bowel Project Experience. *J Clin Oncol* 21:1195–1204, 2003.

14. Lyman GH, Dale DC, Wolff DA, et al.: Acute Myeloid Leukemia or Myelodysplastic Syndrome in Randomized Controlled Clinical Trials of Cancer Chemotherapy With Granulocyte Colony-Stimulating Factor: A Systematic Review. *J Clin Oncol.* Lyman GH, Dale DC, Wolff DA, Culakova E, Poniewierski MS, Kuderer NM, Crawford J: *J Clin Oncol.* 2010 Jun 10;28(17):2914–24. Epub 2010 Apr 12. Review.PMID: 20385991

15. Patt DA, Duan Z, Fang S, et al: Acute myeloid leukemia after adjuvant breast cancer therapy in older women: understanding risk. *J Clin Oncol* 25:3871–76, 2007.

16. Akerley W: Secondary leukemia: twice is a coincidence? *Cancer* 88:497–99, 2000.

17. Makino H: Treatment and care of neurotoxicity from taxane anticancer agents. *Breast Cancer* 11:100–104, 2004.

18. van Dam FS, Schagen SB, Muller MJ, et al: Impairment of cognitive function in women receiving adjuvant treatment for high-risk breast cancer: high-dose versus standard-dose chemotherapy. *J Natl Cancer Inst* 90:210–18, 1998.

19. Ahles TA, Saykin AJ, Furstenberg CT, et al: Neuropsychologic impact of standard-dose systemic chemotherapy in long-term survivors of breast cancer and lymphoma. *J Clin Oncol* 20:485–93, 2002.

20. Ferguson RJ, Ahles TA, Saykin AJ, et al: Cognitive-behavioral management of chemotherapy-related cognitive change. *Psychooncology* 16:772–77, 2007.

21. Kohli S, Fisher SG, Tra Y, et al: The cognitive effects of modafinil in breast cancer survivors: A randomized clinical trial. ASCO Annual Meeting Proceedings Part I 25:9004, 2007.

22. Loprinzi CL, Pisansky TM, Fonseca R, et al: Pilot evaluation of venlafaxine hydrochloride for the therapy of hot flashes in cancer survivors. *J Clin Oncol* 16:2377–81, 1998.

23. Loprinzi CL, Sloan JA, Perez EA, et al: Phase III evaluation of fluoxetine for treatment of hot flashes. *J Clin Oncol* 20:1578–83, 2002.

24. Loprinzi CL, Kugler JW, Barton DL, et al: Phase III trial of gabapentin alone or in conjunction with an antidepressant in the management of hot flashes in women who have inadequate control with an antidepressant alone: NCCTG N03C5. *J Clin Oncol* 25:308–12, 2007.

25. Loprinzi CL, Sloan J, Stearns V, et al.: Newer antidepressants and gabapentin for hot flashes: an individual patient pooled analysis. *J Clin Oncol* 27:2831–37, 2009.

26. Crew KD, Greenlee H, Capodice J, et al: Prevalence of joint symptoms in postmenopausal women taking aromatase inhibitors for early-stage breast cancer. *J Clin Oncol* 25:3877–83, 2007.

27. Burstein HJ, Winer EP: Aromatase inhibitors and arthralgias: a new frontier in symptom management for breast cancer survivors. *J Clin Oncol* 25:3797–99, 2007.

28. Gail MH, Costantino JP, Bryant J, et al: Weighing the risks and benefits of tamoxifen treatment for preventing breast cancer. *J Natl Cancer Inst* 91:1829–46, 1999.

29. Fisher B, Costantino J, Redmond C, et al: A randomized clinical trial evaluating tamoxifen in the treatment of patients with node-negative breast cancer who have estrogen-receptor- positive tumors. *N Engl J Med* 320:479–84, 1989.

30. Burgess C, Cornelius V, Love S, et al: Depression and anxiety in women with early breast cancer: five year observational cohort study. Bmj 330:702, 2005.

31. Kornblith AB, Herndon JE, 2nd, Weiss RB, et al: Long-term adjustment of survivors of early-stage breast carcinoma, 20 years after adjuvant chemotherapy. *Cancer* 98:679–89, 2003.

32. Al-Ghazal SK, Sully L, Fallowfield L, et al: The psychological impact of immediate rather than delayed breast reconstruction. *Eur J Surg Oncol* 26:17–19, 2000.

33. Speer JJ, Hillenberg B, Sugrue DP, et al: Study of sexual functioning determinants in breast cancer survivors. *Breast J* 11:440–47, 2005.

34. Ruddy K, Ginsburg E, Gelber S, et al.: Infertility concerns in premenopausal breast cancer survivors, Fourth Biennial Survivorship Research Conference. Atlanta, GA, 2008.

35. Sankila R, Heinavaara S, Hakulinen T: Survival of breast cancer patients after subsequent term pregnancy: "healthy mother effect". *Am J Obstet Gynecol* 170:818–23, 1994.

36. Ives A, Saunders C, Bulsara M, et al: Pregnancy after breast cancer: population based study. Bmj 334:194, 2007.

37. Sutton R, Buzdar AU, Hortobagyi GN: Pregnancy and offspring after adjuvant chemotherapy in breast cancer patients. *Cancer* 65:847–50, 1990.

38. Cunha GR, Taguchi O, Namikawa R, et al: Teratogenic effects of clomiphene, tamoxifen, and diethylstilbestrol on the developing human female genital tract. *Hum Pathol* 18:1132–43, 1987.

39. Partridge AH, Ruddy KJ: Fertility and adjuvant treatment in young women with breast cancer. *Breast* 16 Suppl 2:S175–81, 2007.

40. Smith MR, McGovern FJ, Zietman AL, et al: Pamidronate to prevent bone loss during androgen-deprivation therapy for prostate cancer. *N Engl J Med* 345:948–55, 2001.

41. Anelli TF, Anelli A, Tran KN, et al: Tamoxifen administration is associated with a high rate of treatment-limiting symptoms in male breast cancer patients. *Cancer* 74:74–77, 1994.

42. Ottini L, Rizzolo P, Zanna I, et al: BRCA1/BRCA2 mutation status and clinical-pathologic features of 108 male breast cancer cases from Tuscany: a population-based study in central Italy. *Breast Cancer Res Treat* 116:577–86, 2009.

43. Grenader T, Goldberg A, Shavit L: Second cancers in patients with male breast cancer: a literature review. *J Cancer Surviv* 2:73–78, 2008.

44. Kwan ML: Alcohol consumption and breast cancer recurrence and survival among women with early-stage breast cancer, San Antonio Breast Cancer Symposium, 2009.

45. Friedenreich CM, Gregory J, Kopciuk KA, et al: Prospective cohort study of lifetime physical activity and breast cancer survival. *Int J Cancer* 124:1954–62, 2009.

46. Holick CN, Newcomb PA, Trentham-Dietz A, et al: Physical activity and survival after diagnosis of invasive breast cancer. *Cancer Epidemiol Biomarkers Prev* 17:379–86, 2008.

47. Chlebowski RT, Aiello E, McTiernan A: Weight loss in breast cancer patient management. *J Clin Oncol* 20:1128–43, 2002.

48. Courneya KS, Mackey JR, Bell GJ, et al: Randomized controlled trial of exercise training in postmenopausal breast cancer survivors: cardiopulmonary and quality of life outcomes. *J Clin Oncol* 21:1660–68, 2003.

49. Schwartz AL, Winters-Stone K, Gallucci B: Exercise effects on bone mineral density in women with breast cancer receiving adjuvant chemotherapy. *Oncol Nurs Forum* 34:627–33, 2007.

50. Milne HM, Wallman KE, Gordon S, et al: Effects of a combined aerobic and resistance exercise program in breast cancer survivors: a randomized controlled trial. *Breast Cancer Res Treat* 108:279–88, 2008.

51. Courneya KS, Segal RJ, Mackey JR, et al: Effects of aerobic and resistance exercise in breast cancer patients receiving adjuvant chemotherapy: a multicenter randomized controlled trial. *J Clin Oncol* 25:4396–4404, 2007.

52. Jones LW, Courneya KS, Fairey AS, et al: Effects of an oncologist's recommendation to exercise on self-reported exercise behavior in newly diagnosed breast cancer survivors: a single-blind, randomized controlled trial. *Ann Behav Med* 28:105–13, 2004.

53. Vondracek SF, Hansen LB, McDermott MT: Osteoporosis risk in premenopausal women. *Pharmacotherapy* 29:305–17, 2009.

54. Rosselli Del Turco M, Palli D, Cariddi A, et al: Intensive diagnostic follow-up after treatment of primary breast cancer. A randomized trial. *National Research Council Project on Breast Cancer follow-up.* Jama 271:1593–97, 1994.

55. Rojas MP, Telaro E, Russo A, et al: Follow-up strategies for women treated for early breast cancer. Cochrane Database Syst Rev:CD001768, 2005.

56. Impact of follow-up testing on survival and health-related quality of life in breast cancer patients. A multicenter randomized controlled trial. The GIVIO Investigators. Jama 271:1587–92, 1994.

57. Khatcheressian JL, Wolff AC, Smith TJ, et al: American Society of Clinical Oncology 2006 update of the breast cancer follow-up and management guidelines in the adjuvant setting. *J Clin Oncol* 24:5091–97, 2006.

58. Ganz PA, Hahn EE: Implementing a survivorship care plan for patients with breast cancer. *J Clin Oncol* 26:759–67, 2008.

59. Grunfeld E, Levine MN, Julian JA, et al: Randomized trial of long-term follow-up for early-stage breast cancer: a comparison of family physician versus specialist care. *J Clin Oncol* 24:848–55, 2006.

23

Colon Cancer Survivorship

Nadine Jackson McCleary, MD

Overview

Defining Survivorship in GI Cancer

For the purposes of this chapter, a gastrointestinal (GI) cancer survivor is defined as individual diagnosed with GI cancer that completed active treatment, surgery, chemotherapy, and radiation. This is consistent with the Institute of Medicine 2005 report, From Cancer Patient to Cancer Survivor; Lost in Transition, and in keeping with the more broadly applied definition of a cancer survivor established by the National Coalition for Cancer Survivorship.[1] Those with colorectal cancer account for 10% of the 11.4 million cancer survivors as of 2006 in the United States.[2] Of that overall group, the majority (60%) are age 60 or older.[2] Given the increasing incidence and prevalence of GI malignancies in the older population, it is anticipated that the majority of the GI cancer survivors will also be comprised of older individuals (Figures 23.1 and 2).[3]

With improvements in access to care, diagnostic techniques and treatment options, all gastrointestinal malignancies have increased rates of survival over the last 30 years (Table 23.1). Among the GI cancers, colorectal cancer has the highest survival rate at five years, followed by stomach, esophagus, liver, biliary tract, and pancreatic cancers successively in rates of survival at five years.

While the majority of cancer survivors continue to be evaluated by their oncologist during the survivorship period, those with more complicated medical histories, e.g., more than three concurrent medical conditions, tend to be cared for predominantly by their primary care provider, possible due to need for frequent medical attention.[4] Given this shared responsibility for cancer survivors,[5] it is imperative that key surveillance issues are discussed and monitored collaboratively.

This chapter will review the key features of GI cancer survivorship for individuals who have completed active treatment and have no evidence of residual disease, including the impact of treatment over time and recommendations for surveillance following comparison of primary treatment.

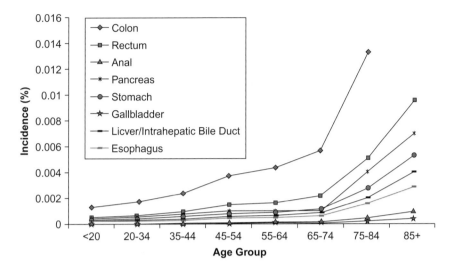

Figure 23.1. Percentage of Incident Cases by Age Group for GI Malignancies (2000–2003). Adjusted for 2003 U.S. Census. (*Source:* Jackson N, Enzinger P: Chapter 98: Gastrointestinal Malignancies, in Halter J, Ouslander J, Tinetti M, et al. (Eds.): Hazzard's Geriatric Medicine and Gerontology (Ed. 6). New York, McGraw Hill, 2009, pp. 1167–1176.)

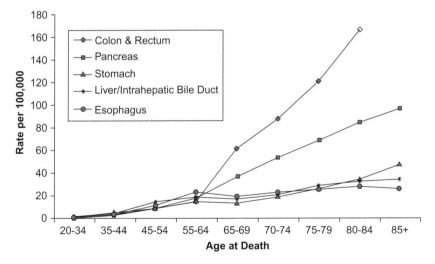

Figure 23.2. Mortality Rates for Gastrointestinal Malignancies (2000–2003) by Age at Death. (*Source:* Jackson N, Enzinger P: Chapter 98: Gastrointestinal Malignancies, in Halter J, Ouslander J, Tinetti M, et al. (Eds.): Hazzard's Geriatric Medicine and Gerontology (ed 6). New York, McGraw Hill, 2009, pp. 1167–1176.)

TABLE 23.1 TREND IN FIVE-YEAR SURVIVAL RATE, BY CANCER SITE, FROM PERIOD
OF 1975–1977 TO 1999–2006 FOR GASTROINTESTINAL MALIGNANCIES

Cancer site	5-year survival rate %		% Increase
	1975–1977	1999–2006	
Esophagus	5.1	18.9	13.8
Stomach	15.9	26.7	10.8
Liver, biliary tract	3.7	14.4	10.7
Pancreas	2.5	5.7	3.2
Colon	51.7	65.8	4.1
Rectum	49.4	68.5	19.1
Anus	NR	NR	---

Focus on Colorectal Cancer

Given the prevalence of colorectal cancer, the majority of research in gastrointestinal cancer survivorship focuses on this diagnosis. As such, this chapter will highlight findings relevant to colorectal cancer which may also apply to other GI cancer sites. As diagnostic and treatment options improve for esophageal, gastric, hepatic, biliary tract, and hepatic cancers, further research is warranted for the expected increase in survivors of these cancers.

Colorectal cancer is the third leading cause of cancer-related diagnosis and death for men and women within the United States.[6] Given that half of colorectal cancers are diagnosed in individuals 70 years of age, and that rates of death from this disease have decreased over time,[6] there will continue to be an increasing number of survivors, particularly, older individuals living with a history of colorectal cancer. The trend of increased survival can partially be attributed to improvements in access to colorectal cancer screening, funding for screening, as well as improved screening methodology.[7–9]

Further improvements are also noted for surgical resection of primary tumors as well as metastatic lesions in addition to initiation of appropriate chemotherapy (and radiation therapy where applicable).[10,11] Individuals diagnosed with colorectal cancer undergoing surgical resection of their tumor without lymph node involvement are expected to have five-year survival rates exceeding 60–90%.[3,12] Those noted to have lymph node involvement have five-year survival rates of 30–70%, depending on the depth of tumor invasion.[3,12] Less than 10% of individuals noted to have metastatic spread of colorectal

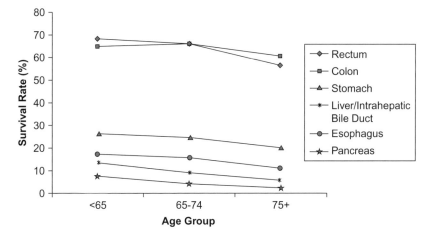

Figure 23.3. Five-Year Survival Rates for Gastrointestinal Malignancies by Age Group. (*Source:* Jackson N, Enzinger P: Chapter 98: Gastrointestinal Malignancies, in Halter J, Ouslander J, Tinetti M, et al. (Eds.): Hazzard's Geriatric Medicine and Gerontology (ed 6). New York, McGraw Hill, 2009, pp. 1167–1176.)

cancer are expected to survive beyond 5 years.[3] Improved survival rates are linked to adequacy of surgical staging (≥12 lymph nodes resected, negative tumor margins, and higher volume of surgeries performed by the operating surgeon).[13–17] Lastly, improvements in chemotherapy regimens, particularly in the adjuvant setting, further extend duration of survival. For colorectal cancer, treatment with 5-fluorouracil based chemotherapy following surgical resection of the primary tumor results in 30% risk reduction in mortality.[18,19] Addition of oxaliplatin further improves survival for patients,[20] although conflicting data exist regarding benefit in those age 70 and older.[20–23] What is not clear from available survival data is the quality of that survival period—specifically the impact of diagnosis and treatment on physical function, emotional outlook, and social interaction.[24]

MEDICAL CONCERNS

Several studies report that survivors of gastrointestinal malignancies, comprised mainly of colorectal cancer, report fewer long-term effects of treatment compared to other cancer survivor groups.[25–29] In fact, one study demonstrated that the majority of colorectal cancer survivors have resolution of treatment effects within four years of diagnosis.[30] Prevalent persistent symptoms include fatigue, diarrhea following radiation therapy, and abdominal discomfort following chemotherapy. Those with lower baseline levels of physical function (due to older age or increased concurrent medical conditions) were more likely than others to report persistent physical and psychologic effects of treatment.[30,31] As Denlinger et al.[32] notes, it is important to keep in mind the specific diagnosis and treatment rendered when discussing potential effects of treatment with patients or other clinicians as they differ by cancer site and treatment modality.

Toxicities Due to Disease, Treatment

Acute Toxicities

Acute toxicities may be defined as those occurring during active treatment or within six months of completion. For gastrointestinal malignancies, toxicities often include alterations in bowel habits, nutritional intake, wound healing, and energy level as well as less tangible impact on the individual's emotional outlook.[33] Rates of acute toxicities correspond to treatment regimen used as well as the dose and duration (also known as dose intensity, or the proportion of total planned dose actually administered) of that treatment. Despite similar dose intensity among older and younger patients demonstrated in some[34,35,] but not all clinical trials,[36] fewer older patients receive indicated therapy outside of clinical trials. Those who do receive lower doses and shorter durations than their younger counterparts,[37,38] which may correspond with reduced benefit or decrease in rates of late toxicities in those older than 75, as noted in one study.[38]

Chronic Toxicities

Chronic toxicities may be defined as those effects occurring six months or more following completion of active treatment. Chronic toxicities may also refer to those acute toxicities that persist throughout the survivorship period. The various systems affected by surgical, radiation, and chemotherapy treatment will be reviewed here.

Neurologic

Neuropathy is a common adverse effect of chemotherapy agents used to treat gastrointestinal malignancies leading to symptoms of pain, paresthesia, and alterations in sensation as well as affecting gross and fine motor skills. More pronounced manifestations, including urinary retention or transient visual loss, have been observed with oxaliplatin use.[39-41] Specifically, use of either oxaliplatin or gemcitabine can result in peripheral neuropathy, dependent on the dose and duration of therapy. As yet, there is no recommended screening test to detect patients at risk for neuropathy prior to treating with these agents. Typically, cessation of the offending agent can stop further progression of the neuropathy symptoms, but the noted time to regression of those symptoms is less predictable.

Oxaliplatin-induced neuropathy typically occurs once the cumulative dose exceeds 780 mg/m^2 due to dysfunction of calcium-dependent voltage-gated sodium channels and direct toxicity to the dorsal root ganglia.[39,40] Of the 2,246 patients enrolled in the MOSAIC study, 138 (12.5%) receiving

FOLFOX4 (fluorouracil, leucovorin, oxaliplatin) in the postoperative setting experienced grade 3 or higher peripheral sensory neuropathy compared to 0.2% of the FU/LV arm (fluorouracil, leucovorin).[20] At 18 and 48 months follow-up, 0.7% of patients continued to report grade 3 or higher peripheral sensory neuropathy. Patient self-report rating scales of neuropathy symptoms can be helpful to track the onset and progression of this symptom.[42] Interventions using calcium and magnesium infusions showed promise in retrospective studies,[43,44] although clear recommendations based on prospective studies cannot be made presently.

Cardiac

Long-term cardiac complications of colorectal cancer treatment appear to be uncommon, but may be understudied. Bevacizumab is an anti-angiogenic inhibitor approved for use in advanced[45] but not resected colon cancer.[36] It is the most common cause of cardiac complications related to colorectal cancer treatment. Potential cardiovascular complications of bevacizumab use include hypertension with possible progression to reversible posterior leukoencephalopathy syndrome, and arterial and venous thromboembolism (myocardial infarction, cerebrovascular events, deep venous thrombosis, intra-abdominal thrombosis).[46] Frequency of long-term sequelae from these cardiovascular manifestations is not known. Fluoropyrimidines, fluorouracil (FU) and capecitabine (an oral prodrug of FU), can cause reversible coronary vasospasm.[47,48] Depending on dose and schedule, fluoropyrimidine-induced vasospasm can persist, inducing cardiac arrhythmias, ischemia, or cardiogenic shock requiring more long-term cardiac management.

Pulmonary

Frequency of pulmonary complications due to gastrointestinal cancer treatment is low. One meta-analysis noted a 1% increased incidence of dyspnea among patients receiving cetuximab, a chimeric monoclonal antibody to the epidermal growth factor receptor, for colorectal cancer.[49] For patients undergoing resection of metastatic pulmonary lesions, complications directly relate to decreased pulmonary reserve, although surgery quantification of this effect over time remains unknown.[50]

Secondary Cancer

Data regarding rates of secondary malignancies for adult survivors of childhood cancers are well established,[51] yet data is limited for adult survivors of gastrointestinal malignancies. Based on data from adult survivors of childhood cancers, rates of subsequent malignant neoplasms increase to 15% at 20 years following diagnosis and are the leading cause of death unrelated to primary cancer recurrence.[52] Secondary (hematologic) cancer due to treatment with alkylating agents (e.g. platinum agents) or topoisomerase II inhibitors occur within three years[52] and are less likely to occur given regimens used in treatment of gastrointestinal malignancies. However, radiation-induced secondary (solid) cancers can occur after 10 years of treatment[52] and are more likely given the frequency of radiation therapy use for gastrointestinal malignancies. Extrapolating from recommendations for adult survivors of childhood cancers, adult cancer survivors should be screened for possible treatment related secondary cancers up to 10 years following diagnosis, dependent on their particular treatment exposure.[52]

Dermatologic

Use of epidermal growth factor receptor inhibitors, cetuximab and panitumumab, are associated with increased rates of acneiform rash. At present, these drugs are approved for use in the advanced colorectal cancer setting, but studies are ongoing evaluating their use in the postoperative setting as well as in other cancer sites.[53] The resulting cutaneous toxicity is related to the dose and duration of drug used. Left untreated, the rash can be severe and debilitating, negatively impacting body image and increasing risk of infection and hospitalization. Appropriate treatment includes use of gentle skin cleansers, topical and systemic antibiotic therapy, skin emollients, and limited sun exposure to avoid further skin irritation. Following completion of treatment, patients are expected to have full recovery of intact skin.[53]

Gastrointestinal

Radiation therapy increases the risk of chronic diarrhea and stool incontinence for survivors of anal and rectal cancer, reported in up to 50% of survivors up to 10 years following treatment.[31] Cancer survivors should be aware of this potential chronic effect as well as strategies to cope, including changes in diet, antidiarrheal and stool bulking agents, and use of protective undergarments.[32] Symptoms of bowel dysfunction are associated with poor body image and can interfere with social functioning, leading to decreased quality of life. Colorectal cancer survivors of at least 10 years report having long-term complications following an ostomy or colorectal anastomosis of hernia, urinary retention, bleeding, intestinal obstruction, and fistula.[54] Although ostomy survivors appear to have more early complications, complications rates in both groups converge over time.[54]

Fertility

While chemotherapy can transiently impact desire for sexual intimacy as well as fertility, the majority of cancer survivors remain interested in restoring these abilities once treatment is completed. Limited data is available specifically regarding male fertility following treatment of GI cancer or the impact of drugs used to treat GI cancer on sperm count, oocyte maturation, or induction of menopause. In general, factors leading to increased rates of ovarian failure following chemotherapy include increased age and increased dose of gonadotoxic agents.[55,56] An increased dose of gonadotoxic agents also deleteriously impacts male fertility. In contrast to ovarian failure due to treatment effect on mature oocytes, younger males are more at risk of decreased spermatogenesis as chemotherapy adversely impacts maturing sperm.[55] Radiation to the pelvis can also lead to ovarian failure, uterine function, and decreased spermatogenesis.[55] For both males and females, cisplatin and carboplatin are associated with moderate risk of ovarian/testicular failure, while fluorouracil is associated with low risk.[55] Less than 10% of new colorectal cancer cases occur in women of child-bearing age (<40 years).[57] For these women, pregnancy remains an option, although potentially with higher rates of complications.[57–59] A wide variety of fertility methods for both males and females exist for those wanting to conceive as well as contraceptive methods for those wishing to defer or avoid pregnancy, including surgical procedures, hormonal contraception, barrier methods, or behavioral techniques.[57,58,60] Fortunately, several studies show no increase in rates of congenital abnormalities or malignancies in offspring of cancer survivors.[55]

PSYCHOLOGIC CONCERNS

Psychologic Distress

High levels of psychologic distress may persist among cancer survivors, particularly those reporting decreased perception of control and uncertainty regarding their diagnosis, including anxiety related to risk of cancer recurrence.[61–64] Manifestations of psychologic distress range from mild levels of anxiety and demoralization to major depression and symptoms of post-traumatic stress, which may not be recognized by patients or providers. Issues of psychologic distress may be further increased among older individuals who report higher rates of psychologic distress and comprise the majority of patients diagnosed with gastrointestinal malignancy.[32] However, all patients should be screened for symptoms of psychologic distress specific to their disease and provided with a mechanism to address those needs, which may include counseling via a social worker or psychologist or medication treatment via a psychiatrist.[65–67]

Body Image, Sexuality, and Intimacy

Body image concerns are particularly prevalent among individuals with a permanent ostomy for colorectal cancer or feeding tube for esophageal or gastric cancer.[54,68–71] Although ostomies and feeding tubes have not been shown to impact physical or social functioning, cancer survivors do report persistent negative impact on body image as for as four years from diagnosis.[30] The presence of an ostomy can further impact desire for sexual intimacy.[72] Further, cancer survivors report two-times higher rates of sexual dysfunction (including erectile dysfunction, vaginal dryness, and dyspareunia) following abdomino-perineal resection compared to low anterior resection for rectal cancer,[73,74] symptoms that may also follow radiation treatment to the pelvis.[75] Targeted intervention trials for sexual and urinary dysfunction among rectal cancer survivors are warranted.[76]

FINANCIAL CONCERNS

Colon cancer survivors are less likely to return to the workforce, particularly those of older age or with increased risk of disease recurrence (higher stage).[77,78] Cancer survivors have reported pessimism regarding ability to obtain another job should they lose employment.[79] This loss of income may be attributed to lingering effects of treatment given that cancer survivors are more likely than age-matched controls to have poor health and more concurrent medical conditions.[80,81] This further compounds the individual's ability to maintain health care insurance coverage needed for health surveillance during the survivorship period.

PROVIDER, CAREGIVER CONCERNS

Components of Active Disease Surveillance

While concise disease surveillance guidelines for each type of gastrointestinal malignancy do not exist, oncologists do agree on regularly scheduled visits and restaging studies to monitor patients for disease recurrence. The American Society of Clinical Oncology published specific surveillance guidelines for colorectal cancer in 2005.[82] The surveillance guidelines endorse use of a Colon Cancer Survivorship Care Plan.[83] The practice guideline recommends medical oncologist evaluation with history and physical examination every three to six months following treatment for three years, then semi-annually until five years following treatment, after which time medical oncology follow-up is optional. An annual CT scan of the chest and abdomen is advised for three years following treatment for colon cancer and annual CT scan of the pelvis for three years following treatment for rectal cancer. Colonoscopy is recommended within three years of operative treatment, then every five years if there is no evidence of recurrence for colon cancer. Flexible proctosigmoid-oscopy is advised semi-annually for five years for rectal cancer. A blood test for carcinoembryonic antigen is recommended every three months for three years following treatment for colon or rectal cancer.

In addition to a survivorship care plan, reviewing a treatment summary (a summary of the treatment provided and relevant indications for that treatment) may further improve cancer care during the survivorship period, allowing coordination of surveillance care with primary care providers and patients with their treating oncologist.[83–85] Data regarding the utility of this approach to survivorship care is forthcoming in gastrointestinal malignancies but may be limited by the challenge of recruiting cancer survivors to participate in such research.[1]

Lifestyle Modification

Smoking

Ample evidence exists linking tobacco exposure to the incidence and prevalence of both pre-malignant states, such as colon adenomas, and malignant states, such as colorectal, pancreatic, biliary, gastric, esophageal, and hepatic cancers.[86-90] Similar to lung cancer, the impact of tobacco exposure on the development of a gastrointestinal malignancy appears to be dose-dependent— that is, higher incidence of cancer among those with longer duration or higher dose of tobacco exposure. One retrospective study suggested that tobacco exposure earlier in life may be particularly prognostic among colorectal cancer survivors.[23] Health care providers play a pivotal role in encouraging cancer survivors to discontinue smoking, but often miss the opportunity to provide resources for patients to do so.[91] Smoking cessation among cancer survivors may impact future risk of disease recurrence and should be strongly recommended.[92,93]

Diet and Exercise

The effect of diet and dietary supplements is difficult to study in the cancer survivor population given potential bias introduced by observational or retrospective studies. However, a well-conducted prospective observational study showed that patient who had a higher intake of a Western-patterned diet (comprised of high red meat intake, refined grains, sugary desserts, and high fat content) had increased likelihood of recurrence and increased mortality compared to those with relatively lower intake of such a diet. Other studies have demonstrated that patients who had higher vitamin D blood levels or were consistent aspirin users may further reduce colon cancer recurrence and increase survival.[94,95] Prospective studies are underway to confirm these findings. Physical activity is also beneficial for cancer survivors. Meyerhardt et al. demonstrated a nearly 50% increase in disease-free survival for survivors of stage III colon cancer who engaged in at least 18 metabolic equivalent task hours of physical activity per week compared to those who were inactive with less than three metabolic equivalent task hours per week.[96] This finding was further supported by another study of colon cancer survivors, demonstrating improved overall survival for individuals who increased their level of physical activity following diagnosis.[97] Further, a body mass index exceeding 35 kg/m^2 is associated with lower overall survival in colon cancer increased cancer recurrence in colon and rectal cancer.[98,99] Hence, exercise and avoidance of obesity should be encouraged to potentially decreasing the risk of colorectal cancer recurrence among survivors.

CONCLUSION

Further study of the course of survivorship among individuals diagnosed with GI malignancies is warranted. As diagnostic techniques and treatment modalities continue to improve, documentation of the ways in which individuals are affected over time is imperative. Oncologists are advised to coordinate surveillance care with primary care providers to comprehensively address the needs of their patients. This may best be achieved through treatment summary plans and survivorship care plans, as is recommended for colorectal cancer by the American Society of Clinical Oncology. In so doing, cancer survivors are supported in maximizing the quality of improved survival derived from treatment.

SUGGESTED READING

See References 1, 12, 17, 76, 82, 84, and 85.

REFERENCES

1. Biganzoli L, Aapro M, Balducci L, et al.: Adjuvant therapy in elderly patients with breast cancer. *Clin Breast Cancer* 5:188–95; discussion 196–7, 2004.

2. National Cancer Institute. Cancer Survivorship Research.

3. Surveillance Epidemiology and End Results (SEER).

4. Haggstrom DA, Arora NK, Helft P, et al.: Follow-up care delivery among colorectal cancer survivors most often seen by primary and subspecialty care physicians. *J Gen Intern Med* 24 Suppl 2:S472–9, 2009.

5. Hong S, Nekhlyudov L, Didwania A, et al.: Cancer survivorship care: exploring the role of the general internist. *J Gen Intern Med* 24 Suppl 2:S495–500, 2009.

6. Jemal A, Siegel R, Ward E, et al.: Cancer statistics, 2009. *CA Cancer J Clin* 59:225–49, 2009.

7. Guessous I, Dash C, Lapin P, et al.: Colorectal cancer screening barriers and facilitators in older persons. *Prev Med* 50:3–10.

8. Cronin-Fenton DP, Norgaard M, Jacobsen J, et al.: Comorbidity and survival of Danish breast cancer patients from 1995 to 2005. *Br J Cancer* 96:1462–8, 2007.

9. Chen X, White MC, Peipins LA, et al.: Increase in screening for colorectal cancer in older Americans: results from a national survey. *J Am Geriatr Soc* 56:1511–6, 2008.

10. Jackson GL, Melton LD, Abbott DH, et al.: Quality of Nonmetastatic Colorectal Cancer Care in the Department of Veterans Affairs. *J Clin Oncol* 2010 Jul 1;28(19):3176–81. Epub 2010 Jun 1.

11. Neeff H, Horth W, Makowiec F, et al.: Outcome after resection of hepatic and pulmonary metastases of colorectal cancer. *J Gastrointest Surg* 13:1813–20, 2009.

12. Ogino S, Meyerhardt JA, Kawasaki T, et al.: CpG island methylation, response to combination chemotherapy, and patient survival in advanced microsatellite stable colorectal carcinoma. Virchows Arch 450:529–37, 2007.

13. Hodgson DC, Zhang W, Zaslavsky AM, et al.: Relation of hospital volume to colostomy rates and survival for patients with rectal cancer. *J Natl Cancer Inst* 95:708–16, 2003.

14. Kapiteijn E, Marijnen CA, Nagtegaal ID, et al.: Preoperative radiotherapy combined with total mesorectal excision for resectable rectal cancer. *N Engl J Med* 345:638–46, 2001.

15. Meyerhardt JA, Tepper JE, Niedzwiecki D, et al.: Impact of hospital procedure volume on surgical operation and long-term outcomes in high-risk curatively resected rectal cancer: findings from the Intergroup 0114 Study. *J Clin Oncol* 22:166–74, 2004.

16. Swanson RS, Compton CC, Stewart AK, et al.: The prognosis of T3N0 colon cancer is dependent on the number of lymph nodes examined. *Ann Surg Oncol* 10:65–71, 2003.

17. Meyerhardt JA, Mayer RJ: Systemic therapy for colorectal cancer. *N Engl J Med* 352:476–87, 2005.

18. Laurie JA, Moertel CG, Fleming TR, et al.: Surgical adjuvant therapy of large-bowel carcinoma: an evaluation of levamisole and the combination of levamisole and fluorouracil. The North Central Cancer Treatment Group and the Mayo Clinic. *J Clin Oncol* 7:1447–56, 1989.

19. Moertel CG, Fleming TR, Macdonald JS, et al.: Levamisole and fluorouracil for adjuvant therapy of resected colon carcinoma. *N Engl J Med* 322:352–8, 1990.

20. Andre T, Boni C, Navarro M, et al.: Improved overall survival with oxaliplatin, fluorouracil, and leucovorin as adjuvant treatment in stage II or III colon cancer in the MOSAIC trial. *J Clin Oncol* 27:3109–16, 2009.

21. Yothers G: 5-FU and leucovorin with or without oxaliplatin for adjuvant treatment of stage II and III colon cancer: Long-term follow-up of NSABP C-07 with survival analysis (abstract # 401). ASCO Gastrointestinal Oncology Symposium 2010, 2010.

22. Haller DG CJ, Tabernreo J, Marou J, de Braud D, Proce T, van Cutsem E, Hill M, Gilberg F, Schmoll H-J: Phase III trial of capecitabine + oxaliplatin vs. bolus 5-FU/LV in stage III colon cancer (NO16968): impact of age on disease-free survival (abstract #284). 2010.

23. Jackson McCleary NA MJ, Green E, Yothers G, de Gramont A, Van Cutsem E, O'Connell M, Twelves C, Saltz L, Sargent L and The ACCENT Collaborative Group Impact of older age on the efficacy of newer adjuvant therapies in >12,500 patients (pts) with stage II/III colon cancer: Findings from the ACCENT Database. *J Clin Oncol* 27:4010, 2009.

24. Extermann M, Hurria A: Comprehensive geriatric assessment for older patients with cancer. *J Clin Oncol* 25:1824–31, 2007.

25. Stommel M, Kurtz ME, Kurtz JC, et al.: A longitudinal analysis of the course of depressive symptomatology in geriatric patients with cancer of the breast, colon, lung, or prostate. *Health Psychol* 23:564–73, 2004.

26. Wingard JR, Curbow B, Baker F, et al.: Health, functional status, and employment of adult survivors of bone marrow transplantation. *Ann Intern Med* 114:113–8, 1991.

27. Arndt V, Merx H, Stegmaier C, et al.: Quality of life in patients with colorectal cancer 1 year after diagnosis compared with the general population: a population-based study. *J Clin Oncol* 22:4829–36, 2004.

28. Arndt V, Merx H, Stegmaier C, et al.: Restrictions in quality of life in colorectal cancer patients over three years after diagnosis: a population based study. *Eur J Cancer* 42:1848–57, 2006.

29. Rauch P, Miny J, Conroy T, et al: Quality of life among disease-free survivors of rectal cancer. *J Clin Oncol* 22:354–60, 2004.

30. Schneider EC, Malin JL, Kahn KL, et al.: Surviving colorectal cancer: patient-reported symptoms 4 years after diagnosis. *Cancer* 110:2075–82, 2007.

31. Ramsey SD, Andersen MR, Etzioni R, et al.: Quality of life in survivors of colorectal carcinoma. *Cancer* 88:1294–303, 2000.

32. Denlinger CS, Barsevick AM: The challenges of colorectal cancer survivorship. *J Natl Compr Canc Netw* 7:883–93; quiz 894, 2009.

33. Gusani NJ, Schubart JR, Wise J, et al.: Cancer survivorship: a new challenge for surgical and medical oncologists. *J Gen Intern Med 24 Suppl* 2:S456–8, 2009.

34. Goldberg RM, Tabah-Fisch I, Bleiberg H, et al.: Pooled analysis of safety and efficacy of oxaliplatin plus fluorouracil/leucovorin administered bimonthly in elderly patients with colorectal cancer. *J Clin Oncol* 24:4085–91, 2006.

35. Haller D: Phase III trial of capecitabine + oxaliplatin vs. bolus 5-FU/LV in stage III colon cancer (NO16968): Impact of age on disease-free survival (abstract # 284). ASCO *Gastrointestinal Oncology Symposium* 2010, 2010.

36. Wolmark N YG, O'Connell MJ, Sharif S, Atkins JN, Seay TE, Feherenbacher L, O'Reilly S, Allegra CJ for the National Surgical Adjuvant Breast and Bowel Project: A phase III trial comparing mFOLFOX6 to mFOLFOX6 plus bevacizumab in stage II or III carcinoma of the colon: Results of NSABP Protocol C-08. *J Clin Oncol* 27:18s, 2009.

37. Schrag D, Cramer LD, Bach PB, et al.: Age and adjuvant chemotherapy use after surgery for stage III colon cancer. *J Natl Cancer Inst* 93:850–7, 2001.

38. O'Connell MJ, Mailliard JA, Kahn MJ, et al: Controlled trial of fluorouracil and low-dose leucovorin given for 6 months as postoperative adjuvant therapy for colon cancer. *J Clin Oncol* 15:246–50, 1997.

39. Cersosimo RJ: Oxaliplatin-associated neuropathy: a review. *Ann Pharmacother* 39:128–35, 2005.

40. Grothey A: Oxaliplatin-safety profile: neurotoxicity. *Semin Oncol* 30:5–13, 2003.

41. O'Dea D, Handy CM, Wexler A: Ocular changes with oxaliplatin. *Clin J Oncol Nurs* 10:227–9, 2006.

42. Kiernan MC, Krishnan AV: The pathophysiology of oxaliplatin-induced neuro-toxicity. *Curr Med Chem* 13:2901–7, 2006.

43. Gamelin L, Boisdron-Celle M, Delva R, et al.: Prevention of oxaliplatin-related neurotoxicity by calcium and magnesium infusions: a retrospective study of 161 patients receiving oxaliplatin combined with 5-Fluorouracil and leucovorin for advanced colorectal cancer. *Clin Cancer Res* 10:4055–61, 2004.

44. Marshall JL, Haller DG, de Gramont A, et al.: Adjuvant Therapy for Stage II and III Colon Cancer: Consensus Report of the International Society of Gastrointestinal Oncology. *Gastrointest Cancer Res* 1:146–54, 2007.

45. Saltz LB, Clarke S, Diaz-Rubio E, et al.: Bevacizumab in combination with oxaliplatin-based chemotherapy as first-line therapy in metastatic colorectal cancer: a randomized phase III study. *J Clin Oncol* 26:2013–9, 2008.

46. Saif MW: Managing bevacizumab-related toxicities in patients with colorectal cancer. *J Support Oncol* 7:245–51, 2009.

47. Ang C, Kornbluth M, Thirlwell MP, et al: Capecitabine-induced cardiotoxicity: case report and review of the literature. *Curr Oncol* 17:59–63.

48. Bathina JD, Yusuf SW: 5-Fluorouracil-induced coronary vasospasm. *J Cardio-vasc Med* (Hagerstown) 11:281–4.

49. Hoag JB, Azizi A, Doherty TJ, et al: Association of cetuximab with adverse pulmonary events in cancer patients: a comprehensive review. *J Exp Clin Cancer* Res 28:113, 2009.

50. Fiorentino F, Hunt I, Teoh K, et al: Pulmonary metastasectomy in colorectal cancer: a systematic review and quantitative synthesis. *J R Soc Med* 103:60–6.

51. Seehusen DA, Baird D, Bode D: Primary care of adult survivors of childhood cancer. *Am Fam Physician* 81:1250–5.

52. Bhatia S: Secondary Malignancies: What, when, why, in whom?, NCCN Clinical Practice Oncology Forum, 2008.

53. Jean GW, Shah SR: Epidermal growth factor receptor monoclonal antibodies for the treatment of metastatic colorectal cancer. *Pharmacotherapy* 28:742–54, 2008.

54. Liu L, Herrinton LJ, Hornbrook MC, et al.: Early and late complications among long-term colorectal cancer survivors with ostomy or anastomosis. *Dis Colon Rectum* 53:200–12, 2010.

55. Knopman JM, Papadopoulos EB, Grifo JA, et al: Surviving childhood and re-productive-age malignancy: effects on fertility and future parenthood. *Lancet Oncol* 11:490–8.

56. Wo JY, Viswanathan AN: Impact of radiotherapy on fertility, pregnancy, and neonatal outcomes in female cancer patients. *Int J Radiat Oncol Biol Phys* 73:1304–12, 2009.

57. Spanos CP, Mamopoulos A, Tsapas A, et al: Female fertility and colorectal cancer. *Int J Colorectal Dis* 23:735–43, 2008.

58. Schwarz EB, Hess R, Trussell J: Contraception for cancer survivors. *J Gen Intern Med* 24 Suppl 2:S401–6, 2009.

59. Madanat LM, Malila N, Dyba T, et al: Probability of parenthood after early onset cancer: a population-based study. *Int J Cancer* 123:2891–8, 2008.

60. Lee SJ, Schover LR, Partridge AH, et al.: American Society of Clinical Oncology recommendations on fertility preservation in cancer patients. *J Clin Oncol* 24:2917–31, 2006.

61. Goldzweig G, Hubert A, Walach N, et al: Gender and psychological distress among middle- and older-aged colorectal cancer patients and their spouses: an unexpected outcome. *Crit Rev Oncol Hematol* 70:71–82, 2009.

62. Clark KL, Loscalzo M, Trask PC, et al: Psychological distress in patients with pancreatic cancer-an understudied group. *Psychooncology.*2010 Dec;19(12):1313–20. doi: 10.1002/pon.1697.

63. Tavoli A, Mohagheghi MA, Montazeri A, et al: Anxiety and depression in patients with gastrointestinal cancer: does knowledge of cancer diagnosis matter? *BMC Gastroenterol* 7:28, 2007.

64. Kurtz ME, Kurtz JC, Stommel M, et al: Predictors of depressive symptomatology of geriatric patients with colorectal cancer: a longitudinal view. *Support Care Cancer* 10:494–501, 2002.

65. Hurria A, Gupta S, Zauderer M, et al: Developing a cancer-specific geriatric assessment: a feasibility study. *Cancer* 104:1998–2005, 2005.

66. Dunn J, Lynch B, Rinaldis M, et al: Dimensions of quality of life and psycho-social variables most salient to colorectal cancer patients. *Psychooncology* 15:20–30, 2006.

67. Lynch BM, Steginga SK, Hawkes AL, et al: Describing and predicting psychological distress after colorectal cancer. *Cancer* 112:1363–70, 2008.

68. Sideris L, Zenasni F, Vernerey D, et al: Quality of life of patients operated on for low rectal cancer: impact of the type of surgery and patients' characteristics. *Dis Colon Rectum* 48:2180–91, 2005.

69. Guren MG, Eriksen MT, Wiig JN, et al: Quality of life and functional outcome following anterior or abdominoperineal resection for rectal cancer. *Eur J Surg Oncol* 31:735–42, 2005.

70. Padilla GV, Grant MM: Psychosocial aspects of artificial feeding. *Cancer* 55:301–4, 1985.

71. Roberge C, Tran M, Massoud C, et al: Quality of life and home enteral tube feeding: a French prospective study in patients with head and neck or oesophageal cancer. *Br J Cancer* 82:263–9, 2000.

72. Ramirez M, McMullen C, Grant M, et al.: Figuring out sex in a reconfigured body: experiences of female colorectal cancer survivors with ostomies. *Women's Health* 49:608–24, 2009.

73. Mannaerts GH, Schijven MP, Hendrikx A, et al.: Urologic and sexual morbidity following multimodality treatment for locally advanced primary and locally recurrent rectal cancer. *Eur J Surg Oncol* 27:265–72, 2001.

74. Hendren SK, O'Connor BI, Liu M, et al: Prevalence of male and female sexual dysfunction is high following surgery for rectal cancer. *Ann Surg* 242:212–23, 2005.

75. Bruheim K, Guren MG, Dahl AA, et al: Sexual function in males after radiotherapy for rectal cancer. *Int J Radiat Oncol Biol Phys* 76:1012–17.

76. Donovan KA, Thompson LM, Hoffe SE: Sexual function in colorectal cancer survivors. *Cancer Control* 17:44–51.

77. Earle CC, Chretien Y, Morris C, et al.: Employment among survivors of lung cancer and colorectal cancer. *J Clin Oncol* 28:1700–5.

78. Morris M, Platell C, de Boer B, et al.: Population-based study of prognostic factors in stage II colonic cancer. *Br J Surg* 93:866–71, 2006.

79. Norredam M, Meara E, Landrum MB, et al.: Financial status, employment, and insurance among older cancer survivors. *J Gen Intern Med 24 Suppl* 2:S438–45, 2009.

80. Ramsey SD, Berry K, Moinpour C, et al.: Quality of life in long term survivors of colorectal cancer. *Am J Gastroenterol* 97:1228–34, 2002.

81. Given CW, Given B, Azzouz F, et al.: Comparison of changes in physical functioning of elderly patients with new diagnoses of cancer. *Med Care* 38:482–93, 2000.

82. Desch CE, Benson AB, 3rd, Somerfield MR, et al: Colorectal cancer surveillance: 2005 update of an American Society of Clinical Oncology practice guideline. *J Clin Oncol* 23:8512–9, 2005.

83. American Society of Clinical Oncology. Colorectal Cancer Treatment Plan and Summary Resources.

84. Faul LA, Shibata D, Townsend I, et al: Improving survivorship care for patients with colorectal cancer. *Cancer Control* 17:35–43.

85. Earle CC: Failing to plan is planning to fail: improving the quality of care with survivorship care plans. *J Clin Oncol* 24:5112–6, 2006.

86. Liang PS, Chen TY, Giovannucci E: Cigarette smoking and colorectal cancer incidence and mortality: systematic review and meta-analysis. *Int J Cancer* 124:2406–15, 2009.

87. Iodice S, Gandini S, Maisonneuve P, et al.: Tobacco and the risk of pancreatic cancer: a review and meta-analysis. *Langenbecks Arch Surg* 393:535–45, 2008.

88. Ladeiras-Lopes R, Pereira AK, Nogueira A, et al.: Smoking and gastric cancer: systematic review and meta-analysis of cohort studies. *Cancer Causes Control* 19:689–701, 2008.

89. Bosetti C, Gallus S, Peto R, et al.: Tobacco smoking, smoking cessation, and cumulative risk of upper aerodigestive tract cancers. *Am J Epidemiol* 167:468–73, 2008.

90. Kerr D GR, Quirke P, Watson D, Yothers G, Lavery IC, Lee M, O'Connell MJ, Shak S, Wolmark N, Quasar Colon Teams: A quantitative multigene RT-PCR assay for prediction of recurrence in stage II colon cancer: Selection of the genes in four large studies and results of the independent, prospectively designed QUASAR validation study. *J Clin Oncol* 27 2009.

91. Coups EJ, Dhingra LK, Heckman CJ, et al.: Receipt of provider advice for smoking cessation and use of smoking cessation treatments among cancer survivors. *J Gen Intern Med* 24 Suppl 2:S480–6, 2009.

92. Tseng TS, Lin HY, Martin MY, et al.: Disparities in smoking and cessation status among cancer survivors and non-cancer individuals: a population-based study from National Health and Nutrition Examination Survey. *J Cancer Surviv* 2010 Dec;4(4):313–21. Epub 2010 May 13.

93. Mamounas E, Wieand S, Wolmark N, et al.: Comparative efficacy of adjuvant chemotherapy in patients with Dukes' B versus Dukes' C colon cancer: results from four National Surgical Adjuvant Breast and Bowel Project adjuvant studies (C-01, C-02, C-03, and C-04). *J Clin Oncol* 17:1349–55, 1999.

94. Ogino S NK, Irahara N, Shima K, Baba Y, Kirkner G, Meyerhardt J, and Fuchs C: Prognostic Significance and Molecular Associations of 18q Loss of Heterozygosity: A Cohort Study of Microsatellite Stable Colorectal Cancers. *J Clin Oncol* 22:8858, 2009.

95. Ng K, Meyerhardt JA, Wu K, et al.: Circulating 25-hydroxyvitamin d levels and survival in patients with colorectal cancer. *J Clin Oncol* 26:2984–91, 2008.

96. Meyerhardt JA, Heseltine D, Niedzwiecki D, et al.: Impact of physical activity on cancer recurrence and survival in patients with stage III colon cancer: findings from CALGB 89803. *J Clin Oncol* 24:3535–41, 2006.

97. Meyerhardt JA, Giovannucci EL, Holmes MD, et al.: Physical activity and survival after colorectal cancer diagnosis. *J Clin Oncol* 24:3527–34, 2006.

98. Meyerhardt JA, Catalano PJ, Haller DG, et al.: Impact of diabetes mellitus on outcomes in patients with colon cancer. *J Clin Oncol* 21:433–40, 2003.

99. Jackson N BJ, Soufi-Mahjoubi R, Marshall J, Mitchell E, Zhang X, Meyerhardt J.: Safety and Efficacy of First-Line Irinotecan/Fluoropyrimidine Combinations in Elderly versus Nonelderly Patients with Metastatic Colorectal Cancer: Findings from the BICC-C Study. *Cancer*, 2008, In Press.

100. SEER: 5-year survival.

24

Prostate Cancer Survivorship

Lindsay Haines, BS and Aymen Elfiky, MD

Prostate Cancer and Survivor Demographics

It is estimated that in the United States, one in six men will be diagnosed with prostate cancer at some point in their lifetime.[1] Prostate cancer patients represent approximately 20% of cancer survivors by site of disease in the United States, second only to breast cancer patients.[2] In 2010, 217,730 men were diagnosed with prostate cancer and 86,220 men died of this disease, making it both the second most common and the second deadliest form of cancer among men.[1,3]

Age is considered to be the most significant risk factor for prostate cancer, which occurs primarily in older men. Between 2003 and 2007, the median age of men diagnosed with prostate cancer was 67.[4] Table 24.1 shows the percentage of prostate cancer patients diagnosed by the disease in each age group.[4] The table illustrates that a majority of prostate cancer patients (65.2%) are between the ages of 55 and 74.[4] The probability that a man will develop prostate cancer increases with age as does the probability that a prostate cancer patient will die from the disease.[3] The median age at death for a prostate cancer survivor, however, is 80 years old, indicating that many patients live for many years either with the disease or in remission.[3]

Besides age, race also plays a role in prostate cancer incidence and survival. Black men have a higher incidence of and mortality rate due to prostate cancer compared to men of other races in every age group.[3,4,5] All other racial and ethnic groups—Asian/Pacific Islander, Hispanic, and Native American/Alaska Native—however, have lower prostate cancer incidence and mortality rates as compared to black and white men.[3,5] Figure 24.1 illustrates the incidence of prostate cancer for black and white patients.[6] This figure shows the age-adjusted rates of prostate cancer per 100,000 people from 1999 to 2007.[6] Both prostate cancer incidence and mortality rate are higher for black men. Figure 24.2 illustrates age-adjusted prostate cancer mortality rates per 100,000 people from 1975 to 2007.[6] The figure illustrates that although mortality rates for all races have declined since the 1990s, blacks are much more likely to die of prostate cancer than patients of other races.[6]

Several studies have examined racial disparities in prostate cancer mortality and have found that black patients were diagnosed at later stages for prostate cancer, likely contributing to the increased mortality rate.[7,8,9] Figure 24.3 shows relative survival rates for prostate cancer survivors.[6] Blacks and whites

TABLE 24.1 INCIDENCE OF PROSTATE CANCER
BASED ON AGE[4]

Age (years)	% of prostate patients
Under 20	0.0%
20–34	0.0%
35–44	0.6%
45–54	8.9%
55–64	29.9%
65–74	35.3%
75–84	20.7%
Over 85	4.6%

Table Data Courtesy of SeerStat http://seer.cancer.
gov/statfacts/html/prost.html[4]

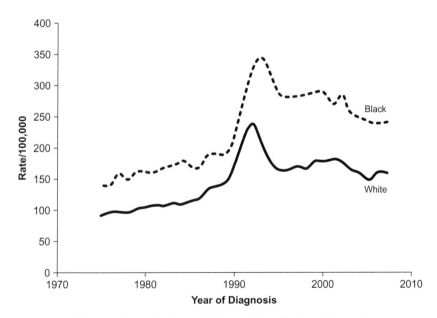

Figure 24.1. Prostate Cancer Incidence by Race. (Data Retrieved from the SEER239*Stat Database, http://seer.cancer.gov/.)

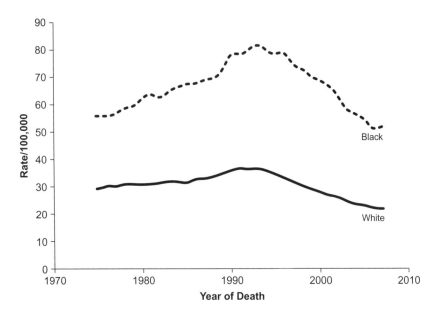

Figure 24.2. Prostate Cancer Mortality by Race. (Data Retrieved from the SEER*Stat Database, http://seer.cancer.gov/.)

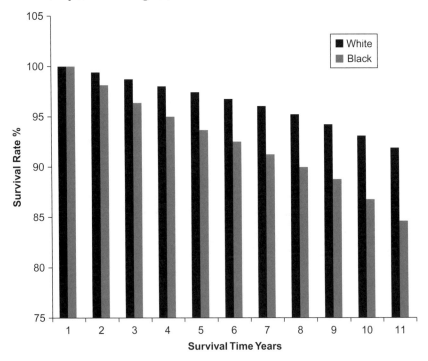

Figure 24.3. Relative Survival Rates by Clinical State and Race for Prostate Cancer Survivors (All Ages), 1988–2006. (Data Retrieved from the SEER*Stat Database, http://seer.cancer.gov/.)

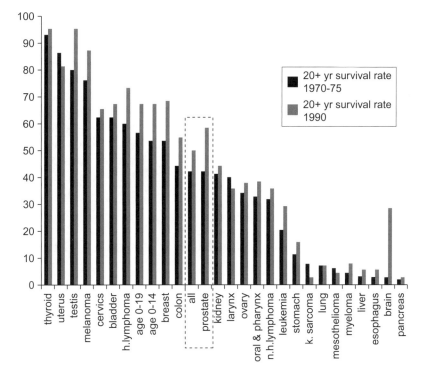

Figure 24.4. Twenty or More Year Survival Rate for Prostate Cancer Patients Diagnosed in 1970–1975 and 1990. (Data Retrieved from the SEER*Stat Database, http://seer.cancer.gov/.)

have a 98.3% and 99.6% survival rate, respectively within the first year of diagnosis, but over time survival rates drop more drastically for black patients.[6] According to this data, survival rates for black patients were lower than for white patients for each time frame.

Despite significant disparities, when black and white patients received uniform equal-access health care—as seen in a 1995 study of military personnel treated through the VA system—they had similar survival rates.[7] During the same time frame, however, national data suggests that black patients had a 7–17% lower prostate cancer survival rate.[9,10] This study indicates that cancer survival may be in large part due to access to care. Other studies indicate that prostate cancer mortality is dependent to some extent on socioeconomic status helping to explain the results of the VA study.[3] Another study found that prostate cancer mortality rates in black men with less than 12 years of education were two times higher than mortality rates in black men with more than 12 years of education.[11] A similar, though not as drastic, difference was seen when comparing white men with less than 12 years of education to white men with more than 12 years of education.[11] Additionally, there was a substantial decrease in prostate cancer mortality rates between 1993 and 2001, but the decrease was greater among men who had completed high school and went on to complete one or more years of college or vocational school.[3,12]

The number of prostate cancer survivors in the United States has grown over time as illustrated in Figure 24.4, and the prostate cancer survivor population now makes up 20% of the entire cancer survivor population. As shown, long term survival rates (>20 years since diagnosis) for those patients diagnosed between 1970 and 1975 is 42% while the survival rate for those patients diagnosed in 1990 is 58%, growing faster than the overall increase in the cancer survivor population as seen in the figure.[6] Although there is still clearly a need for further research and support for prostate cancer patients to lower the mortality rate, there is also a clear need for a greater emphasis on prostate cancer survivorship to help the growing number of men that are now a part of this demographic.

EMERGENCE OF SURVIVORSHIP CARE IN PROSTATE CANCER

While many men remain asymptomatic, others face a spectrum of physical and psychosocial challenges as a result of their diagnosis and/or treatment. Improvements in diagnostic and treatment options for this disease has allowed practitioners to diagnose prostate cancer in more patients at early stages and to treat the disease more effectively. In the same vein, this has highlighted the fact that prostate cancer care is a multidisciplinary effort requiring the concerted input of clinicians, nurses, social workers, nutritionists, and others. Notably, gains in survival reflect a systematic evidence-based approach to the patient involving the above stakeholders. Unfortunately, established approaches to definitive therapy have not been balanced by the development of formal protocols for the follow-up care of survivors.

In 2006, the Institute of Medicine (IOM) published a report on adult cancer survivors in which survivorship was defined as a distinct phase in the cancer care trajectory when acute treatment is completed, and the patient transitions into a period of less intensive medical follow-up.[2] The recommendations of the IOM with regard to cancer survivorship required raising awareness of survivor needs, establishing survivorship as a distinct phase of care, and acting to ensure appropriate care as a coordinated effort. In the specific case of prostate cancer survivors, this underscores the need for coordinated advocacy such as which, for example, should exist between a patient's oncologist and primary care provider to manage short-term and late effects of treatment, prevention of late sequelae, surveillance for new cancers, and enforcement of routine preventive health measures such as weight control. Additionally, the IOM recommended that patients be outfitted with a survivorship care plan that is developed and implemented on the using evidence-based guidelines for that care.[2] At present, post-therapy care of the prostate cancer patient is characterized by clinic and office-based practices directed at problem solving, with no standards for follow-up testing or visit frequency, with an increasing number of patients not being seen more than ten years following treatment.

The paucity of research on long-term care and few evidence-based criteria for testing and intervention further contributes to the fragmented care shared between the general practitioner, oncologist, urologist, and other specialists.

ISSUES FACING PROSTATE CANCER SURVIVORS

According to the IOM Report, prostate cancer survivors face a variety of challenges including cancer recurrence, second primary cancer, psychosocial problems, sexual dysfunction, bladder dysfunction, bowel dysfunction, osteoporosis, and cognitive dysfunction.[13] These issues pose potentially major complications for a prostate cancer patient and may have a significant impact on quality of life (QOL). One study found that some survivors (16%) regretted their treatment decision and had lower quality of life scores.[13,14] Indeed, prostate cancer survivors may need more follow-up care to improve QOL as seen in an early study on prostate cancer survivorship, which found that QOL predictors for prostate cancer survivors decreased over time compared to lung cancer survivors who maintained consistent quality of life scores over time and colon cancer survivors who had increased quality of life scores over time.[15] It is important to appreciate how medical and survivorship issues impact the survivor's QOL, which studies have shown do impact QOL for these patients.[13,16] In the same vein, the psychosocial aspects of QOL are impacted by the intimate nature of the physical manifestations.

Although many of the issues that prostate cancer survivors face are similar, because of the wide variety of treatment options available to prostate cancer survivors and the fact that this disease affects patients of all ethnicities and socioeconomic backgrounds, QOL may differ significantly amongst this population. This is illustrated in a recent study that shows that the health issues prostate cancer survivors faced differed based on the type of treatment received.[16] The study found that patients with adjuvant hormone therapy had worse overall outcomes, and depending on the treatment type, patients experienced differing severity of bladder, bowel, and sexual dysfunction.[16] These symptoms were worse in patients who were obese, had enlarged prostates, had a high prostate specific antigen (PSA) score, or were older in age.[16] Another study found that prostate cancer survivors of a racial minority had lower quality of life scores as compared to white survivors and that these quality of life scores were closely linked to health behaviors, including post-treatment follow-up care.[17] Taken as a whole, QOL issues bear upon the success of a patient's treatment, their well-being, and their long-term outcomes as encompassed by survivorship care.

CANCER RECURRENCE

Research is currently being conducted to study prostate cancer recurrence in the effort to establish clear evidence based clinical guidelines for prostate cancer follow-up screening.[13] One study found that 35% of radical prostatectomy patients developed a biochemical recurrence—as seen by an elevated PSA score—within ten years of their first treatment indicating the need for consistent screening guidelines to monitor prostate cancer survivors for recurrences.[18] Unfortunately, there is currently no one consensus on follow-up screenings. As noted in the IOM publication, the 1995 Prostate Cancer Clinical Guidelines Panel Summary Report on the Management of Clinically Localized Prostate Cancer reported that making recommendations on the outcomes of localized prostate cancer was too difficult due to the differences in treatment.[19] This was considered too difficult to do because the variety of treatment options that differ based on age, tumor, grade, and several other factors.

In 2007, the guidelines were once again reviewed. Although more consistent treatment guidelines were established, the review concluded that specific screening recommendations for prostate cancer recurrences were varied.[20] Although PSA recurrence is utilized to monitor long-term disease control, the review found that it does not correlate well with long term outcomes and is inconsistently defined.[18] The heterogeneity associated with prostate cancer treatment makes the creation of standardized guidelines difficult, but it also highlights the importance of more in-depth research in this field.

Despite a lack of consistent screening options, some organizations have published their own guidelines for follow-up screening. The National Comprehensive Cancer Network, for example, recommends that prostate cancer survivors be screened with a PSA every six months for the first five years after treatment and annually after this period in addition to annual rectal exam.[13,21] The American Urological Association (AUA) recommends that prostate cancer survivors obtain PSAs periodically to screen for a recurrence.[22] For patients who were treated surgically, the AUA recommends that survivors obtain serum PSAs and proper imaging when necessary; patients treated with radiotherapy are encouraged to get PSAs periodically and those who have serum PSAs over 2.0 ng/mL or have three PSAs that each show an increase in serum PSA are considered to indicate a biochemical recurrence.[22] For those patients who are undergoing active surveillance, a serum PSA, DRE, prostate biopsy, and imaging are all encouraged to monitor the progression of the disease.[22] The AUA however, does not give specific time intervals for these procedures.

In addition to medical concerns associated with prostate cancer recurrence, many survivors have a significant fear of recurrence, which has been seen to persist two years after treatment has been completed.[13,23] In some cases, fear of recurrence increases over time, as seen in one study that found that 41% of the prostate cancer patient population reported an increased fear of recurrence over time.[24] This fear of recurrence may be due to secondary health issues that result from the treatment. For instance, one study found that those patients who had low confidence about cancer control were more likely to have adverse medical issues such as increased PSAs.[25] Although prostate cancer is a slow growing disease, anxiety over recurrence may significantly affect quality of life.[26]

SECOND PRIMARY CANCER

Like all cancer survivors, prostate cancer survivors are also at risk of developing second primary cancers. Studies show that prostate cancer survivors have a higher rate of bladder cancer when compared to the rest of the population.[13,27] One study found that 5.5% of prostate cancer survivors were diagnosed with urinary bladder cancer at some point within a 20-year period after the completion of their prostate cancer treatment.[27] Those prostate cancer survivors who do develop second primary bladder cancer tend to be older, white, have a low income, and have a low education level.[28] Additionally, bladder cancer has been found to be more prominent in those prostate cancer patients treated with radiation therapy, and one study found that those treated with radiation therapy were twice as likely as those treated with radical prostatectomies to develop bladder cancer.[28] This study also found that although smokers have an independent increased risk of bladder cancer, prostate cancer patients who both smoked and were treated with radiation therapy were four times as likely to develop bladder cancer.[28]

Other studies have shown an increase in endocrine-related cancers, such as male breast cancer. Additionally, patients who have undergone prostate irradiation are at increased risk for rectal cancer.[29,30] Providers should be aware of these risks and screening prostate cancer survivors accordingly.

PSYCHOSOCIAL ISSUES

Most cancer survivorship studies about psychosocial issues are performed on breast cancer survivors due in part to the fact that they make up the majority of the survivor population. While these studies may help to some extent to describe the psychosocial issues of prostate cancer survivors, it is unclear whether the survivorship experience differs amongst men and women, and studies focusing on men and specifically prostate cancer survivors will be important when creating care plans for this group. As mentioned previously, the psychosocial issues may differ significantly from patient to patient due to differences in demographics and treatment.

One study found that patients diagnosed with more advanced stages of prostate cancer are at higher risk of distress because of lower physical quality of life and that patients who have had recurrences had greater distress and lower QOL scores.[31] Of the studies that have been done regarding psychosocial issues in prostate cancer survivors, it has been found that younger men have a harder time adjusting to life after treatment.[13,32] Although the reasons for this are unknown, it is speculated that older survivors tend to have pre-existing health issues, such as urinary and sexual problems, that younger men only develop after treatment, making the adjustment period more difficult.[13] Another study, however, found that a year after treatment, younger men (under the age of 55) were more likely to have improved urinary and sexual function when compared to older men.[13,33]

Although the prostate cancer survivor plan is focused primarily on the survivor, there is evidence that partners of prostate cancer survivors also face significant psychosocial distress and can contribute to the psychological health of the survivor as well.[13] One study found that wives of prostate cancer survivors had high levels of anxiety and depression, and another found that spouses were not confident that the disease was being effectively managed and that as a spouse they lacked proper support.[13,31,34] A partner, however, can also have a positive impact on a patient's survivorship journey as seen in other studies that found that those survivors with partners had a higher QOL.[35] Additional studies on both partners and the effect of partners on psychosocial health may be important in helping to maximize the quality of life for prostate cancer survivors.

SEXUAL DYSFUNCTION

Psychosocial distress is also significantly impacted by sexual dysfunction, which affects nearly all prostate cancer survivors at some point in their survivor journey.[13,3] As the IOM report indicates, sexual dysfunction is a consequence of nearly all commonly used prostate cancer therapies, and it is reported that nearly two-thirds of prostate cancer survivors treated with a nerve sparing prostatectomy, three-fourths of prostate cancer survivors treated with a non-nerve sparing prostatectomy, nearly a quarter of prostate cancer survivors treated with brachytherapy, 40% of prostate cancer survivors treated with brachytherapy and external beam radiation, and 40% of prostate cancer survivors treated with external beam radiation struggle with erectile dysfunction a year after treatment.[13] Over the long term, however, sexual dysfunction tends to decrease. When a cohort of prostate cancer survivors treated with radical prostatectomies were followed over a five year time period, it was found that 9% of the patients had erections firm enough to have intercourse six months after diagnosis, and this percentage increased to 22% and 28% after two years and five years, respectively.[36] Although there is increase in sexual function between two and five years, it was not considered statistically significant, indicating that after longer time periods, sexual function remains the same.[36] The same study found that after two years since diagnosis 54% of patients reported that sexual functioning was a moderate to great problem while only 46% reported moderate to great issues with sexual functioning after five years.[36] The study also found that younger men (under 60) were more likely to find erection aids useful.[36]

Issues with sexual dysfunction vary significantly amongst prostate cancer survivors and many psychosocial factors contribute to the level of concern patients have with sexual dysfunction.[37] Most prostate cancer survivors, however, do express dissatisfaction about their sexual function after treatment.[13] Although sexual issues have improved due to new less invasive and nerve sparing therapies as well as medical advances in sexual dysfunction, it is still a significant issues for prostate cancer survivors and certainly needs to be addressed by providers.[36]

BLADDER DYSFUNCTION

Bladder dysfunction is also an issue seen in nearly all prostate cancer survivors immediately after treatment, but for most patients improves to a manageable degree over time. Bladder dysfunction can also play a significant role in quality of life, but the effect of the issue on individual patients is highly variable. Urinary leakage is primarily seen in patients who have undergone radical prostatectomies.[13] Patients with brachytherapy were reported to have long lasting urinary irritation.[16] Patients with prostatectomies also experience urinary incontinence but saw improvement over time.[16] Another study found that the percent of prostate cancer survivors experiencing urinary issues increased over time from 10% after two years and 14% after five years.[36] Although bladder dysfunction may not be a significant issue to many prostate cancer survivors, it does significantly affect others and should be addressed and treated as necessary.

OTHER ISSUES

Other less common issues also exist for prostate cancer survivors, depending on the type of treatment they received. For those patients treated with radiotherapy, bowel dysfunction may occur.[38] The study found that dysfunction increased with increased radiation volume but not with increased dosage.[38] Prostate cancer patients treated with androgen deprivation therapy also face additional post-treatment complications such as osteoporosis and cognitive dysfunction.[13] This therapy decreases bone mineral density in turn increasing risk of osteoporosis and bone fractures.[13] The therapy can also result in cognitive dysfunction, including impaired memory, shortened attention span, and reduced ability to perform executive functions.[13] Most of these side effects, however, were reversed within a year after treatment, but in some rare cases cognitive dysfunction remained for more than two years.[13]

CONCLUSIONS AND FUTURE DIRECTIONS

Prostate cancer survivors face a myriad of medical and psychosocial issues that can significantly impact their quality of life at various stages of therapy. The approach to actualizing comprehensive survivorship care requires collaborative and complementary efforts by the spectrum of stakeholders. Specifically, there must be a strategic emphasis on overall wellness, respecting and building from individual's strengths and limitations, active rehabilitation when necessary, support and coaching as a complement to patient education, and relationship building.

Dedicated research is required in parallel with the above efforts. Within the medical realm, there are ongoing endeavors directed at development of tools for use in informed decision making and risk stratification. At the same time, clinical trials should be designed to better include QOL analyses that make use of demographic, biologic, and genetic markers. With regard to psychosocial considerations, avenues of research include group think investigations, outcomes analyses, and risk stratification determinations. Lastly, the scope of cancer disparities research must be expanded to include specific survivorship determinants.

REFERENCES

1. "What are the Key Statistics about Prostate Cancer?" *American Cancer Society: Information and Resources for Cancer: Breast, Colon, Prostate, Lung, and Other Forms.* Nov 22, 2010. Accessed Jan 27, 2011. http://www.cancer.org/cancer/prostatecancer/de tailedguide/prostate-cancer-key-statistics.

2. Hewitt M, Greenfield S, and Stovall E. *From Cancer Patient to Cancer Survivor: Lost in Transition.* National Academies. Washington, D.C. (2006).

3. *Cancer Facts and Figures 2010.* American Cancer Society. Atlanta (2010).

4. Data retrieved by Haines L from Altekruse SF, Kosary CL, Krapcho M, Neyman N, Aminou R, Waldron W, Ruhl J, Howlader N, Tatalovich Z, Cho H, Mariotto A, Eisner MP, Lewis DR, Cronin K, Chen HS, Feuer EJ, Stinchcomb DG, Edwards BK. *SEER Cancer Statistics Review, 1975–2007,* National Cancer Institute. Bethesda, MD (2010) Accessed on Jan 27, 2011. http://seer.cancer.gov/statfacts/html/prost.html.

5. "CDC—Prostate Cancer Rates by Race and Ethnicity." Centers for Disease Control and Prevention. Accessed Jan 27, 2011. http://www.cdc.gov/cancer/ prostate/ statistics/race.htm.

6. Haines L. Data Retrieved from the SEER*Stat Database (http://seer.cancer. gov/). Rates are per 100,000 and are age-adjusted to the 2000 U.S. Standard Population (19 age groups-Census P25–1130). Regression lines are calculated using the Joinpoint Regression Program Version 3.4.3, April 2010, National Cancer Institute.

7. Virnig BA, Baxter NN, Habermann EB, Feldman RD, Bradley CJ. A Matter of Race: Early-Versus-Late-Stage Cancer Diagnosis. *Cancer. January/February* (2009):160–168.

8. Ramsey SD, Zeliadt SB, Hall IJ, Ekwueme DU, Penson DF, On the Importance of Race, Socioeconomic Status and Comorbidity When Evaluating Quality of Life in Men with Prostate Cancer. *The Journal of Urology, Vol. 177,* June (2007): 1992–1999.

9. Campbell LC, Keefe FJ, Scipio C, McKee DC, Edwards CL, Herman SH, Johson LE, Colvin OM, McBride CM, Donatucci C. Facilitating Research Participation and Improving Quality of Life for African American Prostate Cancer Survivors and Their Intimate Partners. *Cancer 109, 2* Suppl. (2007): 414–424.

10. Optenberg SA, Thompson IM, Friedrichs P, Wojcik B, Stein C, Kramer B. Race, Treatment, and Long-term Survival from Prostate Cancer in an Equal-Access Medical Care Delivery System. *JAMA, November 22/29* (1995): 1599–1605.

11. Albano JD, Ward E, Jemal A, et al. Cancer mortality in the U.S. by education level and race. *J Natl Cancer Inst.* Sept 19, 2007; 99(18): 1384–1394.

12. Kinsey T, Jemal A, Liff J, Ward D, Thun M. Secular trends in mortality from common cancers in the U.S. by educational attainment, 1993–2001. *J Natl Cancer Inst.* Jul 16, 2008; 100(14): 1003–1012.

13. Hewitt M, Greenfield S, and Stovall E. "Medical and Psychological Concerns of Cancer Survivors: Prostate Cancer." *From Cancer Patient to Cancer Survivor: Lost in Transition.* Washington, D.C.: National Academies, 2006.

14. Wright JL, Cowan JE, Carroll PR, Litwin M. Quality of life in young men after radical prostatectomy. *Prostate Cancer and Prostatic Diseases 11(1)*. Mar 2008: 67–73.

15. Schag, C.A.C., P.A. Ganz, D.S. Wing, M. -S. Sim, and J.J. Lee. "Quality of Life in Adult Survivors of Lung, Colon and Prostate Cancer." *Quality of Life Research* 3.2 (1994): 127–41. Print.

16. Sanda MG, Dunn RL, Michalski J, Sandler HM, Northouse L et al. Quality of life and satisfaction with outcome among prostate-cancer survivors. *New England Journal of Medicine* 358 (2008): 1250–1261.

17. Penedo FJ, Dahn JR, Shen BJ, Schneiderman N, Antoni MH. Ethnicity and Determinants of Quality of Life After Prostate Cancer Treatment. *Urology 67* (2006): 1022–1027.

18. Freedland SJ, Humphreys EB, Mangold LA, Eisenberger M, Dorey FJ, Walsh PC, Partin AW. Risk of prostate cancer-specific mortality following biochemical recurrence after radical prostatectomy. The Journal of the American Medical Association 294(4). 2005: 433–439.

19. Middleton RG, Thompson IM, Austenfeld MS, Cooner WH, Correa RJ, Gibbons RP, Miller HC, Oesterlin JE, Resnick MI, Smalley SR, Wasson JH. Prostate cancer clinical guidelines panel summary report on the management of clinically localized prostate caner. *Clinical Urology 154(6)*, Dec. 1995: 2144–2148.

20. Thompson I, Thrasher JB et al. Prostate cancer: guideline for the management of clinically localized prostate cancer: 2007 update. American Urological Association (2007) 1–81.

21. NCCN. 2004. Clinical Practice Guidelines in Oncology V1. 2004. Prostate Cancer [online] available: http://www.nccn.org/professionals/ physician_gls/PDF/prostate.pdf.

22. Prostate-Specific Antigen Best Practice Statement: 2009 Update. Rep. *American Urological Association Education and Research,* 2009. Print.

23. Mehta SS, Lubeck, DP, Pasta DJ, Litwin MS. 2003. Fear of cancer recurrence in patients undergoing definitive treatment for prostate cancer: results from CaPSURE. *J Urol 170(5):* 1931–1933.

24. Fradet V, Paciorek A, Knight SJ, Carroll PR. Change over time of fear of cancer recurrence in prostate cancer survivors: are there clinical predictors? *2008 Genitourinary Cancer Symposium. Abstract 272.* 2008.

25. Clark JA, Talcott JA. Confidence and uncertainty long after initial treatment for early prostate cancer: survivors' view of cancer control and the treatment decisions they made. *Journal of Clinical Oncology* 24(27) 2006: 4457–4463.

26. Hart SL, Latini DM, Cowan JE, Carroll PR et al. Fear of recurrence, treatment satisfaction, and quality of life after radical prostatectomy for prostate cancer. Supportive Care in Cancer 16(2) 2007: 161–169.

27. Pawlish KS, Schottenfeld D, Severson R, Montie JE. Risk of multiple primary cancers in prostate cancer patients in the Detroit metropolitan area: a retrospective cohort study. *The Prostate 33(2)* October 1997: 75–86.

28. Boorjian S, Cowan JE, Konety BR, DuChane J et al. Bladder cancer incidence and risk factors in men with prostate cancer: results from cancer of the prostate strategic urologic research endeavor. *The Journal of Urology* 177(3) 2007: 883–888.

29. Thellenberg C, Malmer B, Tavelin B, Gronberg H. 2003. Second primary cancers in men with prostate cancer: an increased risk of male breast cancer. *J Urol 169 (4):* 1345–1348.

30. Grady WM, Russell K. 2005. Ionizing radiation and rectal cancer: victims of our own success. *Gastroenterology 128(4):* 1114–1117.

31. Northouse LL, Mood DW, Montie JE, Sandler HM, Forman JD, Hussain M et al. Living with prostate cancer: patients' and spouses' psychosocial status and quality of life. *Journal of Clinical Oncology* 25(27) 2007: 4171–4177.

32. Eton DT, Lepore SJ, Helgeson VS. 2001. Early quality of life in patients with localized prostate carcinoma: an examination of treatment-related, demographic, and psychosocial factors. *Cancer 92(6):* 1451–1459.

33. Hu JC, Kwan L, Saigal CS, Litwin MS. 2003. Regret in men treated for localized prostate cancer. *J Urol 196(6):* 2279–2283.

34. Manne SL. 2002. Prostate cancer support and advocacy groups: their role for patients and family members. *Semin Urol Oncol 20(1):* 45–54.

35. Gore JL, Krupski T, Kwan L, Maliski S, Litwin MS. 2005. Partnership status influences quality of life in low-income, uninsured men with prostate cancer. *Cancer 104(1):* 191–198.

36. Penson DF, McLerran D, Feng Z, Li L et al. Five-year urinary and sexual outcomes after radical prostatectomy: results from the prostate cancer outcomes study. *The Journal of Urology* 179(5): S40–S44. 2008.

37. Robinson JW, Mortiz S, Fung T. 2002. Meta-analysis of rates of erectile function after treatment of localized prostate carcinoma. *Int J Radiat Oncol Biol Phys 54(4):* 1063–1068.

38. Nguyen PL, Chen RC, Hoffman KE, Trofimov A et al. Gastrointestinal quality of life after conventional and high-does radiation for prostate cancer: a subgroup analysis of a randomized trial. *International Journal of Radiation Oncology Biology Physics* 78(4). 2010: 1081–1085.

25

Sarcoma Survivorship

Andrea Marrari, MD, and Suzanne George, MD

Background: Sarcomas as a Heterogeneous Disease

Sarcomas are a heterogeneous group of malignant neoplasms, representing less than 1% of all human tumors.[1,2,3] Depending of which classification system one employs, there can be more than 50 different sarcoma subtypes. In addition, with the use of molecular diagnostics, further heterogeneity among specific subtypes is increasingly apparent, accounting for the diverse natural history and sensitivity to therapy seen within this group of diseases.[4]

In addition to pathologic heterogeneity, there is also significant heterogeneity in the anatomic site of primary sarcomas which leads to challenges in treatment and in the post-treatment phase.[1] The anatomic distribution of sarcomas in adults is as follows: extremities 50% of cases, retroperitoneum 15%, trunk 15%, and head and neck 5%. Visceral sarcomas account for approximately 15% of the cases (see Figure 25.1).

General Treatment Principles

The treatment of choice for the vast majority of localized sarcoma is surgery with wide, negative margins.[1,2] Thoracic, retroperitoneal, and head and neck sarcomas may pose unique surgical challenges due to anatomic constraints.

Radiotherapy is often employed to reduce the risk of local recurrence. The decision to use radiation as part of the treatment plan is based on tumor size, tumor grade, and depth of the primary tumor.[1,2] The specific details of each case will define the optimal treatment plan. Generally, surgery alone is typically used to treat tumors which are low grade, < 5 cm and/or superficial. Radiotherapy is often given in addition to surgery in the case of high grade tumors, deep tumors, and/or tumors which are greater than 5 cm. Radiotherapy may also be required for a resected sarcoma with microscopically positive or close margins if a wider surgical excision is not feasible, for example in the head and

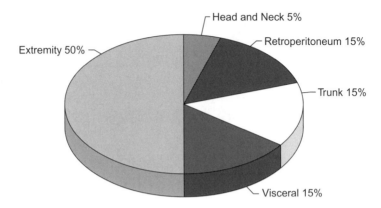

Figure: 25.1. Distribution of Sarcomas.

neck. Although these general principles hold for most soft tissue sarcomas, each case is unique and the ultimate treatment plan should be defined by a multi-disciplinary team following an expert pathology review of diagnostic material.

With the exception of rhabdomyosarcoma, Ewing's sarcoma and osteosar-coma[5-8] in which the introduction of multi-agent chemotherapy resulted in a significant increase in overall survival, the benefits of chemotherapy are still uncertain in patients with localized soft tissue sarcoma.[9] Systemic therapies, including standard cytotoxic chemotherapy as well as novel targeted therapies, such as tyrosine kinase inhibitors, remain the mainstay of therapy for patients with advanced/metastatic sarcomas.

Survivorship in Sarcoma

The NCI definition of a cancer survivor is any person diagnosed with cancer from the time of diagnosis, through the end of life. This definition of cancer survivor is most appropriate for patients diagnosed with a sarcoma. Patients may be treated and cured with surgery alone, required multiagent intensive chemotherapy along with radical surgery and radiotherapy, or live with metastatic disease, on chronic anti-cancer directed therapy for years.

The issues each survivor faces are unique to each patient, based in part on the age of diagnosis, the specific surgery and chemotherapy required as well as the patients prognosis. In addition, consideration of each patient's personal priorities is critical to ensuring their needs are best met and addressed following the diagnosis.

Specific Treatment Related Considerations: Effect of Local Control Limb-Sparing Surgery versus Amputation

In the last decades, the close collaboration between medical oncologists, surgeons, pathologists, and radiation oncologists has led to an improvement in treatment options for localized sarcoma, which has translated into a major improvement in quality of life. Over the last 30 years, the rate of amputation for a sarcoma of the extremities has dramatically fallen.[10,11] In 1982, Rosenberg published the results of a randomized study comparing amputation to limb sparing surgery and postoperative radiation therapy in patients with localized soft tissue sarcomas.[12] Both arms also received postoperative chemotherapy with doxorubicin, methotrexate, and cyclophosphamide. With a median follow-up over nine years, no differences in local recurrence, disease free, and overall survival rate were detected. Currently, less than 10% of the patients undergo amputation for localized soft tissue sarcoma.

Despite the development of limb sparing procedures,[10] musculoskeletal morbidity due to locoregional treatments remains an important issue, and includes premature osteoporosis, early joint aging in case of joint replacements, asymmetric stress and altered function, short stature, osteonecrosis, loss of muscle tissue, and strength and amputation in patients not amenable of conservative surgery.

Radiation therapy may worsen local function. Based on the primary site, the volume of the disease and the administered dose, an increased rate of pathologic bone fractures, decreased limb strength and range of motion is commonly seen.[13]

Neural sacrifice due to either surgery and high dose radiation therapy and neurosensory deficits caused by cisplatin and vinka-alkaloids may also have an impact on motility.

Physical disabilities are therefore amongst the most common long term consequences in sarcoma survivors.[14] In the International Classification of Function, Disability and Health, the World Health Organization (WHO) defines disability in a broad way, in relation to body structure and function, the ability to perform activities and participate in community, social and civil life and to develop interpersonal interaction and relationship, and considers also external environmental that may impact disability. The majority of sarcoma survivors reported some degree of physical disability.[14–16] When compared to age and sex matched controls, the physical performance and endurance of sarcoma survivors are reduced. However these limitations go beyond the local sequelae of treatment, demonstrating a more generalized impairment of functions.

This has huge repercussions, especially on the adolescent young adult population. These physical impairments and disabilities put in perspective their autonomy, their personal vocations, and their self-worth and sexual development, among others.[17]

Individuals with physical disabilities do benefit from early interventions aimed at restoring lost functions. These measures will not only prevent further loss of function due to inactivity and disuse but, in turn, will positively affect self esteem and promote interpersonal relations.

Despite these advances, certain patients may present specific sarcoma subtypes which, due to the location of the disease, and unique biologic characteristics, may require radical surgery.

Case 1

A 23-year old man presented with a slow growing superficial mass in his left thigh. He presented to his primary care physician and imaging studies were performed. However, imaging studies demonstrated the presence of multiple soft tissue nodules, involving the musculature of the thigh, extending from the knee to the groin. Additional imaging revealed no evidence of disease beyond the leg. Biopsy revealed an epithelioid sarcoma. Although his disease was extensive in the limb, there was no evidence of distance disease.

The patient was seen by a multidisciplinary sacoma team. Expert pathology review confirmed a unique subtype of epitheliod sarcoma, which is unlikely to spread beyond the limb. Chemotherapy has no known role in this disease, and therefore surgery was recommended to provide the best attempt at disease control. Due to the distribution of the disease, the patient underwent hip disarticulation followed by radiation therapy to reduce the risk of local recurrence at the proximal margin.

Due to the significant functional challenges with his surgery, the patient started intensive physical therapy soon after surgery. In addition, the patient clearly articulated that his priorities were to remain as active as possible. He became very active in support programs directed toward young adults and began his recovery through increased activity through adaptive sports. In addition, he opted for semen preservation prior to his radiation. Today, after seven years from surgery, he is an avid cyclist, skier, school teacher, and a proud father and husband.

Effect of Systemic Cytoxic Therapies

As stated above, some subtypes of sarcoma, such as Ewings sarcoma, osteosarcoma, and rhabdomyosarcoma, require intensive multiagent chemotherapy, in addition to local control, in order to optimize the likelihood of long term disease control. These intensive treatment programs come along with significant short and long term toxicities that may impact survivorship.

Case 2

A 30-year old female presented with back pain, and acute and severe shortness of breath. Her work-up revealed a large calcified mass arising from her sixth thoracic rib posteriorly, and involving the associated spinous process.

Her initial treatment plan included preoperative chemotherapy, with doxorubicin and cisplatin, radical surgery with reconstruction of the chest wall and spine, and postoperative chemotherapy with ifosfamide and etoposide. Moreover, given the extent of the disease and its location, the risk of local recurrence was considered extremely high. Therefore, radiation therapy was administered to region near the spine. Her course was complicated by an empyema requiring long term antibiotics.

Postoperative, she has faced challenges with decreased mobility, chronic pain, neurologic toxicity related to her chemotherapy, and antibiotics.

> *Her post-treatment course has been focused on physical therapy with slow, but steady improvements in pain, function, and mobility. In addition, reproductive endocrinology has been extensively involved.*
>
> *Seven years after her surgery, thanks to the early and intensive strategies to improve her residual limb function, which are still ongoing, she carries out a fully rewarding life.*

EFFECT OF SYSTEMIC TREATMENTS

Cardiotoxicity

Anthracyclines are one of the most effective classes of agents in sarcoma. Anthracyclines may be associated with cardiac dysfunction in a dose dependent manner. Chest radiation therapy, young age, female sex, and preexisting conditions may further decrease cardiac function.[18-20]

In retrospective studies on unselected cancer patients receiving anthracyclines, the incidence of cardiac dysfunction in adults, ranged between 7 and 15% after a cumulative dose > 450 mg/mq with no cardioprotection,[18] while pediatric patients showed a relative risk of developing symptomatic CHF of about 10% at 15 years from treatment. However, subclinical cardiac dysfunctions affect as many as 50% of these patients.

A prospective longitudinal evaluation of cardiotoxicity in pediatic osteosarcoma and Ewing's sarcoma patients showed a 7.5% incidence of cardiac dysfunction, both clinical and subclinical, after a mean cumulative doxorubicin dose of $300 + 103$ mg/m^2 and mean follow-up time of $34+12$ months.[21] Two patients out of 265 developed cardiac dysfunction after a cumulative dose of 80 mg/m^2 underlying that a subgroup of patient might be particularly prone to develop anthracyclines-induced cardiac toxicity.

Some of these patients were started on anticongestive therapy with some degree of improvement.

Determination of LVEF is generally performed before and throughout treatment. The guidelines developed by the Children's Oncology Group (http://www.childrensoncologygroup.org/disc/le/) advise us to the most appropriate cardiologic follow-up after treatment, according to age at first treatment, total anthracyclines dose and a history of prior radiation therapy to the chest. However, any symptom of CHF should be promptly evaluated. If CHF develops, it must be treated regardless the etiology.

Fertility

Fertility is probably one of the major concerns among adolescent and young adult cancer survivors.[22] Factors such as sex, age, type of cancer, and treatment options need to be considered to predict the probability of infertility.

Fertility issues should be addressed as soon as possible, prior to the initiation of any therapy. Unfortunately, recent surveys among cancer survivors have pointed out that only a minority of them actually recalls a discussion about this issue with their oncologists.[22]

Since parenthood has been recognized as one of the most important predictors of emotional well being and satisfaction in cancer survivors, the risks of infertility linked to cancer treatments should be fully addressed together with the available fertility sparing options and reproductive technologies. Collaboration with reproductive endocrinologists to explore fertility preservation options is often very helpful in this situation.

In addition, it is important to reassure patients that no study has demonstrated a higher rate of chromosomal aberrations among children born to cancer survivors compared to the general population.[23]

The risk of gonadal damage varies greatly among anticancer compounds. Adriamycin and methotrexate, frequently used in some sarcomas, have a low risk of gonadal failure. Cisplatin, often used in osteosarcoma is gonadotoxic. However, its effect is generally transient, with most of the patients recovering within two and five years from treatment.

The gonadotoxic effect of alkylating agents is well known. Cyclophosphamide and ifosfamide are two active and widely employed drugs in sarcoma. The largest series addressing fertility issues in sarcoma are focused on pediatric and AYA patients with osteosarcoma and Ewing's sarcoma. Male sex and cumulative dose of alkylating agents correlates with the risk of long term gonadotoxicity and infertility.[24–28]

Nephrotoxicity

Methotrexate, cisplatin, and ifosfamide are three well known nephrotoxic drugs commonly used in sarcoma. Vigorous hydration and urine alkalinization remain two essential strategies to reduce the risk of renal failure during therapy. However, despite these supportive measures, some the risk for kidney damage remains.

Widemann reported on the development of methotrexate induced nephrotoxicity in patients receiving high dose of the drug for the treatment of osteosarcoma.[29] Despite hydration, urine alkalinization, and leucovirin rescue, 1.8% of the patients developed grade ≥ 2 nephrotoxicity, with a mortality rate among these patients of 4.4%. Since methotrexate is eliminated primarily by the kidneys, its high plasma levels following renal damage favor the development of other methotrexate associated toxicities, such as myelosuppression, toxic hepatitis, dermatitis, and mucositis.

Cisplatin nephrotoxicity may lead to a reduction of glomerular filtration rate and/or electrolyte alterations.[30] Of note, most of the patients have normal serum creatinine.

Up to 90% of the patients receiving cisplatin develop asymptomatic hypomagnesaemia during treatment. Cisplatin nephrotoxicity generally improves after the completion of treatment, although 10–20% of the patients has long term magnesium disturbances.

The toxic effect of ifosfamide is on the proximal tubules, leading to sub-clinical tubular dysfunction in up to 90% of the patients as loss of phosphate, bicarbonate, glucose, amino acids, and low weight proteins. However, Fanconi syndrome develops in about 10% of the cases.[31] Glomerular dysfunction may also develop. The prognosis of ifosfamide induced nephrotoxicity is unclear: after the completion of treatment, complete resolutions, improvements but also deteriorations of kidney function can be seen.

Neurotoxicity

Many chemotherapeutic agents are neurotoxic. Some of them exhibit an acute toxicity, such as high dose methotrexate and ifosfamide, which is generally reversible and easily prevented with supportive measures. Neu-rotoxicity related to cisplatin and vinca may be irreversible. This may pres-ent as peripheral neurotoxicity, affecting sensory fibers, and is partially reversible over time. However, one of the biggest concerns using cisplatin is its bilateral sensoneural hearing loss. This impacts mainly high frequen-cies but, also low frequencies in the most severe cases. Although cisplatin-induced ototoxicity depends on its cumulative dose, treatment, and admin-istration schedule, and on some patients' characteristics, such as young age, around 40% of the patients with osteosarcoma who received methotrexate, adryamicin, and cisplatin developed some degree of hearing loss.[32] Ototox-icity is unlikely to improve over time. Rather, in the 15–20% of the cases, it worsens.

Hearing loss has the greatest impact on the pediatric patients, causing de-layed and reduced language development. Moreover, it has been estimated that children with minimal sensoneural hearing loss are more likely to fail in school, when compared to their peers.

It is therefore mandatory that patients who received cisplatin undergo careful and audiologic evaluations to avoid further deterioration of their audiometry and, at the same time, improve their social and educational status.

Second Malignancies

The development of therapy induced secondary cancer (SC) is probably one of the most devastating complications of primary cancer therapy. Both radiation therapy and chemotherapy have been implicated in the onset of SC. The risk of SC depends on many factors, such as high dose alkylating agents and topoisomerase II inhibitors and, for radiation therapy, on the volume and the total administered dose. In the majority of cases, myelodysplastic syn-dromes, acute myeloid leukemia and sarcoma, most commonly osteosarcoma, are seen. Acute leukemia may develop after a few years from the completion of therapy, while sarcoma generally have a longer latency.

Ginsberg and colleagues recently reported on the long term follow up of a group of long term Ewing's sarcoma survivors, treated between 1970 and 1986 and diagnosed before the age of 21.[26] The cumulative incidence of treatment induced neoplasms at 25 years from diagnosis was 9.0%. Therefore, patients who died of acute leukemia within five years have not been included in the study.

Although the advances in radiation therapy delivery and the introduction of multi-agent chemotherapy protocols, which comprise high dose cyclofosfamide, ifosfamide, adriamycin, and etoposide, led to significant improvements in survival, we should all be constantly aware of the late effects of such treatments. Moreover a recent report estimates that the incidence of radiation therapy is destined to increase with the new radiation therapy delivery techniques, making it even more important that patients are followed for this late effect.[33]

EFFECTS OF LONG-TERM KINASE INHIBITION: GIST AND THE ROLE OF IMATINIB AND SUNITINIB

Before 2000, the median survival time of a patient with metastatic gastrointestinal stromal tumor (GIST) was less than two years.[34] Chemotherapy was not active, although adriamycin and dacarbazine based regimens were frequently administered in the attempt to slow down the progression of the disease. The response rate was extremely disappointing, less than 10%, despite the well known toxicity of these agents. The clinical history of these patients was characterized by reiterated debulking surgeries. The morbidity associated with these procedures over time was considerable.

Imatinib gained an accelerated FDA approval for metastatic GIST patients in 2001, after having showed an impressive clinical response rate.[35]

Case 3

In early 2000, a 32-year old man presented with fatigue and profound anemia. His work-up included a CT scan of abdomen and pelvis, which showed an 8-cm mass of the small bowel with extensive soft tissue thickening throughout the omentum. Liver metastatsis were also identified. Five years prior, a small bowel tumor had been resected. The patient was told this was benign and no follow-up occurred. Biopsy of the new liver metastasis in 2001was compared to the original tumor and reviewed by a pathologist with expertise is sarcoma pathology. The pathology was consistent with GIST. Since the role of adjuvant imatinib was yet to be established, the patient did not receive further treatment.

The patient was started on imatinib, and remains on therapy with excellent disease control today.

Although this patient does not have a curable sarcoma, he remains living well with cancer, now for more than a decade. It is critically important that patients such as this be considered among cancer survivors.

Although the median time to progression on imatinib is two years, it is not uncommon to see patients with a longer disease response. We have recently celebrated a group of metastatic GIST patients still responding to imatinib after 10 years of treatment.

Since patients may be on imatinib indefinitely, every physician involved in their care must be aware of both short and long term imatinib side effects. Imatinib is a relatively well tolerated drug. One of its earliest and commonest side effects is fluid retention, mainly as morning peri-orbital and lower extremities edema. If mild, it requires no treatment, otherwise diuretics might be employed. Daily monitoring of body weight is recommended.

Other common side effects include skin rash and itching, muscle cramps and joint pain, nausea, diarrhea, fatigue and anemia, and an increase in serum transaminases.

The onset of kinase inhibitor-associated depression has been recently described.[36] Of note, although the causal relation might be hard to define in this patient population, response to standard antidepressant drugs has been inconsistent while dose reduction or discontinuation of treatment proved to be helpful.

Endocrine side effects of imatinib have been described. Imatinib may cause secondary hyperparathyroidism and altered bone turnover over time.[37] Its effects on glucose metabolism are contrasting, and the underlying molecular mechanisms are still unclear.

Sunitinib is a broad spectrum kinase inhibitor which is approved for patients with metastatic GIST who are intolerant or resistant to imatinib. As with imatinib, sunitinib use may be indefinite. Sunitinib has many unique toxicities, including the development of hypertension, rare incidence of heart failure, hypothyroidism, and hand-foot skin reaction. These toxicities should be screened for and treated when they occur.

Although most of this management will fall within the realm of the treating oncologist, as patients continue to live well with GIST, the primary care team may be involved in seeing these patients to evaluate these findings.

In addition, within the realm of sarcomas, many patients may live with the disease for many years. This may include patients with chronic slow growing tumors, which may recur multiple times over decades, such as a well differentiated liposarcoma of the retroperitoneum. This may also include patients with metastatic GIST who are living for years, in some cases more than a decade, on chronic anticancer therapy. These unique challenges of survivorship will continue to challenge our field as our treatments for cancer continue to improve and patients are living well with cancer.

In summary, sarcomas represent a biologically diverse set of diseases that may occur at a variety of primary locations, frequently requiring radical surgery, radiotherapy, and at times, systemic therapy, which in some cases may be required for years. This heterogeneity leads to unique challenges when focusing on survivorship, as each case of a patient with sarcoma is unique, and assessing each patient's needs is required to appropriately support patients following a diagnosis of a sarcoma.

Adjuvant Imatinib

Although surgery remains the mainstay of the treatment of primary localized GIST, at least 50% of the patients will develop disease recurrence with a median time to recurrence of two years for high risk disease.

The results of a phase III, double-blind, placebo-controlled trial of adjuvant imatinib after gross resection of primary localized GIST demonstrated an improvement in relapse free survival after one year of treatment.[38] Thus, imatinib was granted FDA approval for the treatment of GIST in the adjuvant setting, although the treatment duration has not been determined yet.

ROLE OF THE PCP

In each phase of the clinical history of a sarcoma patient, the primary care physician holds an important role.

Importantly, PCP should be aware of the possibility of sarcoma. Although rare in nature, 10,000 new cases of sarcoma are reported in the United States each year. Most patients present with a painless soft tissue mass. Although this presentation may be associated with a benign condition, the possibility of a sarcoma should be considered and referral for diagnosis and treatment is recommended.

In addition, both acute and late effects related to sarcoma treatment should be considered for patients treated for sarcoma. The exact risks for each patient will vary, however physical therapy, fertility counseling, cardiac, and renal monitoring should all be considered. Secondary malignancies, including leukemia should be screened for annually in appropriate patients.

The Childhood Cancer Survivorship Study suggests that second cancers, cardiovascular, renal and musculoskeletal disease and endocrinopathies were the most commonly reported health problems, and the incidence of chronic conditions increases over time and does not plateau.[39–41] Survivors from bone tumors and soft tissue sarcoma are among those with the highest incidence of moderate to severe health conditions when compared to other childhood cancer survivors.

CONCLUSION

Sarcomas represent a group of rare and heterogeneous diseases. In the last years, the improvements in surgical techniques and radiation therapy delivery strategies led to better local disease control rate, reducing, at the same time, amputations. Moreover, the introduction of multi agent chemotherapy regimens lead to improvement in overall survival in selected sarcoma histotypes. The introduction of imatinib and sunitinib allow patients with metastatic GIST to live with GIST as a chronic disease.

However, it is worth noting that some of these treatments increase the risk of late effects such as second cancers and cardiac diseases, major causes of late mortality, together with disease recurrence. Survivors of bone and soft tissue sarcoma may suffer from multiple severe health conditions, that impact, especially in the pediatric-young adult population, on their psychosocial and physical development, which ultimately reduce both their quality of life and life expectancy. It is therefore critical that risks associated with specific therapies be discussed with the patient and ongoing awareness of these challenges should be addressed with the patient and the care team. We strongly believe that the close monitoring of sarcoma survivors remains crucial to identify treatment late sequelae that are amenable of intervention.

REFERENCES

1. Singer, S., et al., Management of soft-tissue sarcomas: an overview and update. Lancet *Oncol*, 2000. 1: p. 75–85.

2. World Health Organization. Pathology and Genetics of Tumours of Soft Tissue and Bone. World Health Organization, 2002.

3. Fletcher, C.D., The evolving classification of soft tissue tumours: an update based on the new WHO classification. *Histopathology*, 2006. 48(1): p. 3–12.

4. van de Rijn, M. and J.A. Fletcher, Genetics of soft tissue tumors. *Annu Rev Pathol*, 2006. 1: p. 435–66.

5. Nesbit, M.E., Jr., et al., Multimodal therapy for the management of primary, nonmetastatic Ewing's sarcoma of bone: a long-term follow-up of the First Intergroup study. *J Clin Oncol*, 1990. 8(10): p. 1664–74.

6. Grier, H.E., et al., Addition of ifosfamide and etoposide to standard chemotherapy for Ewing's sarcoma and primitive neuroectodermal tumor of bone. *N Engl J Med*, 2003. 348(8): 694–701.

7. Link, M.P., et al., The effect of adjuvant chemotherapy on relapse-free survival in patients with osteosarcoma of the extremity. *N Engl J Med*, 1986. 314(25): 1600–1606.

8. Raney, R.B., et al., The Intergroup Rhabdomyosarcoma Study Group (IRSG): Major Lessons From the IRS-I Through IRS-IV Studies as Background for the Current IRS-V Treatment Protocols. Sarcoma. 2001. 5(1): 9–15.

9. Blay, J.Y. and A. Le Cesne, Adjuvant chemotherapy in localized soft tissue sarcomas: still not proven. *Oncologist*, 2009. 14(10): 1013–20.

10. Hosalkar, H.S. and J.P. Dormans, Limb sparing surgery for pediatric musculoskeletal tumors. *Pediatr Blood Cancer*, 2004. 42(4): 295–310.

11. Ferguson, P.C., Surgical considerations for management of distal extremity soft tissue sarcomas. *Curr Opin Oncol*, 2005. 17(4): 366–69.

12. Rosenberg, S.A., et al., The treatment of soft-tissue sarcomas of the extremities: prospective randomized evaluations of (1) limb-sparing surgery plus radiation therapy compared with amputation and (2) the role of adjuvant chemotherapy. Ann Surg, 1982. 196(3): 305–15.

13. Blaes, A.H., et al., Pathologic femur fractures after limb-sparing treatment of soft-tissue sarcomas. *J Cancer Surviv,* 4(4): 399–404.

14. Ness, K.K., et al., Physical performance limitations in the Childhood Cancer Survivor Study cohort. *J Clin Oncol,* 2009. 27(14): 2382–89.

15. Barr, R.D. and J.S. Wunder, Bone and soft tissue sarcomas are often curable—but at what cost?: a call to arms (and legs). *Cancer,* 2009. 115(18): 4046–54.

16. Parks, R., et al., Differences in activities of daily living performance between long-term pediatric sarcoma survivors and a matched comparison group on standardized testing. *Pediatr Blood Cancer,* 2009. 53(4): 622–28.

17. Albritton, K.H., Sarcomas in adolescents and young adults. *Hematol Oncol Clin North Am,* 2005. 19(3): 527–46, vii.

18. Von Hoff, D.D., et al., Daunomycin-induced cardiotoxicity in children and adults. A review of 110 cases. *Am J Med,* 1977. 62(2): 200–208.

19. Von Hoff, D.D., et al., Risk factors for doxorubicin-induced congestive heart failure. *Ann Intern Med,* 1979. 91(5): 710–17.

20. Myrehaug, S., et al., Cardiac morbidity following modern treatment for Hodgkin lymphoma: supra-additive cardiotoxicity of doxorubicin and radiation therapy. *Leuk Lymphoma,* 2008. 49(8): 1486–93.

21. Paulides, M., et al., Prospective longitudinal evaluation of doxorubicin-induced cardiomyopathy in sarcoma patients: a report of the late effects surveillance system (LESS). *Pediatr Blood Cancer,* 2006. 46(4): 489–95.

22. Schover, L.R., et al., Having children after cancer. A pilot survey of survivors' attitudes and experiences. *Cancer,* 1999. 86(4): 697–709.

23. Byrne, J., et al., Genetic disease in offspring of long-term survivors of childhood and adolescent cancer. *Am J Hum Genet,* 1998. 62(1): 45–52.

24. Longhi, A., et al., Fertility in male patients treated with neoadjuvant chemotherapy for osteosarcoma. *J Pediatr Hematol Oncol,* 2003. 25(4): 292–96.

25. Longhi, A., et al., Reproductive functions in female patients treated with adjuvant and neoadjuvant chemotherapy for localized osteosarcoma of the extremity. *Cancer,* 2000. 89(9): 1961–65.

26. Ginsberg, J.P., et al., Long-term survivors of childhood Ewing sarcoma: report from the childhood cancer survivor study. *J Natl Cancer Inst.* 102(16): 1272–83.

27. Kenney, L.B., et al., High risk of infertility and long term gonadal damage in males treated with high dose cyclophosphamide for sarcoma during childhood. *Cancer,* 2001. 91(3): 613–21.

28. Williams, D., P.M. Crofton, and G. Levitt, Does ifosfamide affect gonadal function? *Pediatr Blood Cancer,* 2008. 50(2): 347–51.

29. Widemann, B.C., et al., High-dose methotrexate-induced nephrotoxicity in patients with osteosarcoma. *Cancer,* 2004. 100(10): 2222–32.

30. Stohr, W., et al., Nephrotoxicity of cisplatin and carboplatin in sarcoma patients: a report from the late effects surveillance system. *Pediatr Blood Cancer,* 2007. 48(2): 140–47.

31. Stohr, W., et al., Ifosfamide-induced nephrotoxicity in 593 sarcoma patients: a report from the Late Effects Surveillance System. *Pediatr Blood Cancer,* 2007. 48(4): 447–52.

32. Lewis, M.J., et al., Ototoxicity in children treated for osteosarcoma. *Pediatr Blood Cancer,* 2009. 52(3): 387–91.

33. Hall, E.J. and C.S. Wuu, Radiation-induced second cancers: the impact of 3D-CRT and IMRT. *Int J Radiat Oncol Biol Phys,* 2003. 56(1): 83–88.

34. Dematteo, R.P., et al., Clinical management of gastrointestinal stromal tumors: before and after STI-571. *Hum Pathol,* 2002. 33(5): 466–77.

35. Dagher, R., et al., Approval summary: imatinib mesylate in the treatment of metastatic and/or unresectable malignant gastrointestinal stromal tumors. *Clin Cancer Res,* 2002. 8(10): 3034–38.

36. Quek, R., et al., Small molecule tyrosine kinase inhibitor and depression. *J Clin Oncol,* 2009. 27(2): 312–13.

37. Berman, E., et al., Altered bone and mineral metabolism in patients receiving imatinib mesylate. *N Engl J Med,* 2006. 354(19): 2006–13.

38. Ginsberg, J.P., et al., Adjuvant imatinib mesylate after resection of localised, primary gastrointestinal stromal tumour: a randomised, double-blind, placebo-controlled trial. *Lancet,* 2009. 373(9669): 1097–1104.

39. Oeffinger, K.C., et al., Chronic health conditions in adult survivors of childhood cancer. *N Engl J Med,* 2006. 355(15): 1572–82.

40. Hudson, M.M., et al., Health status of adult long-term survivors of childhood cancer: a report from the Childhood Cancer Survivor Study. *Jama,* 2003. 290(12): 1583–92.

41. Geenen, M.M., et al., Medical assessment of adverse health outcomes in long-term survivors of childhood cancer. *Jama,* 2007. 297(24): 2705–15.

26

HEAD AND NECK
CANCER SURVIVORSHIP

SEWANTI LIMAYE, MD, AND ROBERT HADDAD, MD

INTRODUCTION

Epidemiology, HPV, Prognosis

Head and neck cancer refers to a range of tumors that arise in the head and neck region, which includes the oral cavity, pharynx, larynx, nasal cavity, paranasal sinuses, and salivary glands. The worldwide incidence of head and neck cancer exceeds half a million cases annually, ranking it as the fifth most common cancer, and represents 6% of all cancers diagnosed annually.[1]

Smoking, chewing tobacco, betel nut chewing, and excessive alcohol consumption are considered to be the major risk factors. Human papilloma virus (HPV) has recently been associated with oropharyngeal squamous cell carcinoma. HPV16 has been recognized as the main causative agent. There is evidence that today, nearly 50% of all oropharyngeal cancers are associated with HPV. These cancers happen in younger patients and are known to have better prognosis than smoking related head and neck cancers.[2–7,33]

Treatment for head and neck cancer is complex due to the difference in management based on tumor sub-sites, aesthetic considerations, and the importance of maintaining organ functionality. A multidisciplinary approach is needed for management, which includes ear nose and throat surgery, medical and radiation oncology, dentistry, oral and maxillofacial surgery, plastic surgery, nutrition, physical and speech and swallow therapy, pain management, and often counseling services. Most of head and neck cancers are of the squamous cell type (HNSCC) and this chapter focuses on the survivorship issues involved with HNSCC.

Treatment and Prognosis Based on Stage and Location of Disease

Nearly one third of patients with HNSCC present with early stage (I and II) disease and are generally managed with single modality therapy involving either surgery or radiation. Five-year survival is high and falls between 60–90% depending on intensity of prior tobacco and alcohol exposure. Locally advanced

HNSCC (stages III, IVa, and IVb) has traditionally been associated with compromised five year survival of 40–60% despite multimodality therapy. Rates of survival have improved significantly secondary to growing association of HNSCC of oropharynx with HPV. This accounts for the changing epidemiology of oropharyngeal squamous cell carcinoma. HPV associated oropharyngeal carcinoma is usually locally advanced at presentation and may need tri-modality treatment. This includes chemotherapy, radiation therapy, and surgery. It defines a subset of patients with improved clinical behavior and treatment outcome.[8,9] The use of HPV status in clinical decision-making, however, remains investigational at this time.

Oral cavity cancers are best managed primarily with surgery. Adjuvant radiation with or without chemotherapy may be needed. Organ preservation is crucial in the management of locally advanced oropharyngeal and laryngeal cancers, and the treatment is usually concurrent chemoradiotherapy. Upfront chemotherapy, followed by definitive chemoradiotherapy, is also being utilized to reduce distant metastatic rates and to improve survival. Surgery is reserved as salvage for persistent or recurrent disease.[10–17] Locally recurrent disease may benefit from surgical salvage or reirradiation with concurrent chemotherapy.[18] Patients with stage IVc HNSCC or with distant metastasis are candidates for palliative chemotherapy with a median survival limited to one to two years.

Effect of Cancer Disparities on Survival

Cancer disparities have played an important role in cancer survival. Several reports have confirmed the effects of low socioeconomic status, gender, race or ethnicity, education, disability, geographic location, and sexual orientation on incidence, prevalence, morbidity, and mortality from cancer. These disparities have been reported in HNSCC as well.[19–27] A recently published report found no evidence of survival advantage for women as compared with men with HNSCC receiving similar multidisciplinary-directed care at a tertiary cancer center even when the analysis was restricted to individual sites (oral cavity, oropharynx, or larynx/hypopharynx).[28] In an analysis of 87 African American patients with HNSCC and a random sample of 261 white patients matched on age and smoking dose, black patients with cancers of the oral cavity and larynx were more likely diagnosed with advanced stages than whites, after adjusting for socioeconomic and insurance status and other confounding factors.[29] HPV status has been found to affect the survival disparities.[6,30,31] In a retrospective analysis of TAX324, oropharyngeal cancer in blacks was linked with worse overall survival than in whites. No black-white overall survival difference was noted in non-oropharyngeal patients, hence pointing towards the effect of HPV associated disease on survival.[31]

THE HEAD AND NECK CANCER SURVIVOR

Head and neck cancer survivors have issues related to the site of disease and the treatment they have received. The intensity of treatment, acute and chronic toxicities involved and aesthetics differences associated with the therapy bring it to the forefront of discussion of survivorship issues. Survivorship is defined as the physical, psychosocial, and economic issues of cancer from diagnosis until the end of life.[32] A survivor of head and neck cancer would be someone who was diagnosed with a cancer of the head and neck area and has undergone treatment. Head and neck survivorship rates have gone up steadily over the years with the advances in treatment and the decrease in smoking rates. There are more than half a million survivors of head and neck cancer in the United States today.[1] With increasing rates of HPV positive squamous cell carcinomas of head and neck area, and the improved prognosis associated with it, younger survivors are being seen and followed.[33]

SURVIVORSHIP ISSUES BASED ON LOCATION AND TREATMENT INVOLVED

Head and neck cancer survivorship issues vary in certain ways, based on the cancer subtype and the treatment involved. For patients with a history of oral cavity carcinoma who have had primary surgical management, recovery of the swallowing function and articulation is one of the main concerns. Patients with pharynx cancer (nasopharynx oropharynx and hypopharynx) have to deal with acute and chronic toxicities of radiation and chemotherapy.

Treatment for patients with laryngeal cancer patients often has the goal of organ preservation, but patients face issues with swallowing and phonation after undergoing chemoradiation. For the ones who require salvage laryngectomy after the primary concurrent therapy, mastering laryngeal prosthetic devices or electro larynx brings new challenges.

ACUTE TOXICITIES

Acute toxicities of head and neck cancer treatment would include the toxicities seen up to three to six months from completion of therapy. The primary treatment again determines the burden of the type of acute toxicity.

Acute Toxicities of Surgery

Surgical complications are linked to function and aesthetics. They are site-specific and could lead to significant psychological distress. However, with advances in reconstructive surgical techniques, focus on organ preservation, and growing awareness towards aggressive restorative speech and swallowing rehabilitation these issues are better managed today. Although partial glossectomy causes mild speech impairment or swallowing dysfunction, total or near total glossectomy could compromise function significantly.[34,35] The shift towards treating pharynx and larynx cancers with definitive chemoradiotherapy has been primarily for the sake of organ preservation. Patients who require radical tonsillectomy, base of tongue, or palate resection could develop swallowing dysfunction and chronic aspiration issues. Partial laryngectomy could also lead to chronic aspiration and the voice quality might not be restored completely.[36] Total laryngectomy is better from the aspiration perspective, but leads to major disability of lack of normal voice.[37] It could be quite challenging for patients who need to master the use of either a tracheoesophageal puncture or an electrolarynx for communication. Management of the neck could involve a neck dissection that could be radical and involve the resection of the spinal accessory nerve leading to shoulder weakness and pain, or, it could be modified neck dissection which is nerve sparing and usually does not cause significant disability. Complications of neck dissection are dependent upon the extent and type of dissection.[38–42] Early physical therapy should be instituted to prevent permanent disability once shoulder weakness has been recognized.[42] Bleeding and infection could occur but are not head and neck surgery specific.

Acute Toxicities from Radiation with or without Chemotherapy

Radiation with or without chemotherapy causes mucositis in almost all patients. Severe cases of mucositis require a feeding tube in more than half the patients going through concurrent treatment.[11,14–16] Amifostine and Palifermin have been studied in this setting to help reduce rates and intensity of mucositis, but the results have been modest at best.[47,48,49] Pain associated with mucositis can be debilitating if not managed well, leading to poor speech and swallow rehabilitation during and post-treatment. Weight loss is a common complication. Up to 10% of weight loss, even with the feeding tube, is expected. Excessive weight loss is often avoided with early feeding tube placement.[43,44] Radiation-induced dermatitis could add to the discomfort and change in appearance, which could be quite distressing. Pain management, nutritional support and follow up, speech and swallow therapy, and aggressive oral care are needed. Xerostomia, although considered to be a late complication, sets in during the second half of treatment and could be quite bothersome to patients.[45–51]

Acute Toxicities from Chemotherapy

Bolus Cisplatin has been used as a standard of care for radiation sensitization. Known side effects of Cisplatin are ototoxicity, nephrotoxicity, nausea, and peripheral neuropathy. It is known to contribute to the severity of mucositis and subsequent xerostomia.[14–16] With the inclusion of induction chemotherapy as another standard of care, toxicities related to the three drug combination regimen—Taxotere, Cisplatin, and 5-Fluorouracil have gained attention. Lowering of counts warranting antibiotic prophylaxis for febrile neutropenia, acute allergic reaction with taxanes, alopecia, mucositis, diarrhea, dehydration, and asthenia are well recognized.[12,13]

CHRONIC TOXICITIES: ISSUES OF THE HEAD AND NECK CANCER SURVIVOR: THE "NEW NORMAL"

Role of Quality of Life Assessment Tools in Measurement of Chronic Complications

Following the theme of the acute toxicities, the chronic toxicities of head and neck cancer treatment are dependent on the tumor site and the therapy given. Health-related quality of life (HRQOL) refers to the patient's perception of the impact of illness before, during, and after treatment. It includes somatic, functional, social, and psychological parameters of patient perception.[52-55] The head and neck specific QOL questionnaires could include questions related to pain, speech, chewing and swallowing, choking and aspiration, voice and articulation, dental health, trismus, xerostomia, sense of taste and smell, appearance and self-consciousness, maintenance of weight and feeding tube dependence, issues with sexuality, anxiety, and depression. There are several head and neck specific QOL tools that could help analyze the chronic complications of treatment. A few of these are mentioned here:

- University of Washington Quality of Life (UW-QOL)
- European Organization for Research and Treatment of Cancer Quality of Life Questionnaire—Head and Neck Specific Module (EORTC QLQ)-H&N35
- University of Michigan Head and Neck Quality of Life Questionnaire (HNQOLQ)
- Performance Status Scale for Head and Neck Cancer (PSS-HN).
- Functional Assessment of Cancer Therapy—Head and Neck (FACT-H&N)
- Head and Neck Radiotherapy Questionnaire (HNRQ)
- Quality of Life—Radiation Therapy Instrument (QOL-RTI)
- M.D. Anderson Dysphagia Inventory (MDADI)
- Sydney Swallow Questionnaire (SSQ)
- Swallowing Performance Status Scale (SPSS) Score
- Voice-Related QOL Measure (V-RQOL)

The QOL tools could help define the long-term complications better. In a study of patients with oral and oropharyngeal cancer at a one-year follow-up of tumor resection utilizing UW-QOL, the survivors presented significantly poorer overall and domain-specific ratings of quality of life. Chewing presented the largest reduction in score. Anxiety was the only domain that showed improvement at one year reflecting part resolution and part adjustment to the acute dysfunction involved with surgery.[35] Another study examined the long-term QOL of HNSCC survivors using EORTC- QLQ in a busy tertiary care center. The domains where most patients faired poorly included financial difficulties (54%), appetite loss (36%), fatigue (33%), cough (30%), dry mouth (64%), dental problems (42%), sticky saliva (40%), cough (39%), and problems with the mouth opening (32%). Patients with early-stage tumors and those treated with surgery alone had significantly better QOL scores when compared with advanced stage tumors and patients receiving either radiation alone or multimodality treatment, respectively.[56] Although the treatment received, affects QOL parameters, it has been hypothesized that baseline QOL and comorbidity could reflect on the QOL at one year from completion of treatment. This was analyzed in a study using UW-QOL tool and a strong relationship was noted between one-year UW-QOL scores and baseline UW-QOL scores.[57]

QOL tools could give alternative results, and could be confusing, requiring careful interpretation. Prophylactic feeding tube placement has been one such issue. There are studies that have indicated benefit in QOL measures with prophylactic feeding tube placement versus other studies that have shown worsening QOL scores with them.[44,57,58]

These tools could also help decide the appropriate management strategy in absence of difference in survival between two different standard treatment approaches. EORTC- QLQ was used for analyzing long-term quality of life after treatment for locally advanced oropharyngeal carcinoma with surgery and postoperative radiotherapy versus definitive concurrent chemoradiation. Surgical patients showed statistically higher problems with fatigue, pain, swallowing, social eating, and social contact. Chemoradiotherapy group reported significantly greater problems with teeth, dry mouth, and sticky saliva. The global QOL score was higher in chemoradiotherapy group. These results supported an organ preservation approach with chemoradiotherapy in patients with advanced oropharyngeal carcinoma.[59]

Specific Complications of Long-Term Head and Neck Cancer Survivors

Xerostomia

Xerostomia or dry mouth is seen to some extent in almost 100% of head and neck cancer survivors who have received radiation therapy as a part of their treatment and could compromise the quality of life of survivors. The degree of xerostomia depends on the area treated and dose received by the salivary glands. A dose of 40–50 Gy to the salivary glands is enough to cause permanent loss of saliva production. Intensity modulated radiation therapy (IMRT) utilizes three dimensional treatment planning, optimizing the amount of radiation given for local control but minimizing xerostomia by taking a parotid sparing approach.[60–66]

In a prospective, randomized, double-blind, placebo-controlled trial of patients who received at least 40 Gy of radiation to the head and neck, oral pilocarpine (5 mg three times a day), improved salivary production, and symptoms of dry mouth compared with placebo.[45]

Amifostine was evaluated in a multicenter, open label, randomized trial of patients who received definitive radiotherapy or postoperative adjuvant radiotherapy and total radiotherapy doses of at least 40 Gy. Patients were assigned to either radiation alone (cumulative dose of 50 to 70 Gy) or to the same radiation dose with amifostine (200 mg/m² intravenously daily 15 to 30 minutes before radiation). The incidence of grade 2 or higher acute and chronic xerostomia was significantly reduced in the amifostine arm and median salivary production was significantly improved. Nausea, vomiting, hypotension, and allergic reactions were significantly more common among patients treated with amifostine, although grade 3 toxicities were infrequent.[46] Benefit from the use of amifostine with IMRT is not known. Subcutaneous dosing is more convenient and was studied in a phase III trial.[50,51] Acupuncture has also seemed to benefit issues with xerostomia.[67-70]

Swallowing and Dysphagia

Rehabilitation and restoration of speech and swallowing are critical to quality of life of head and neck cancer survivors. Speech and swallowing impairment is seen in more than half of head and neck cancer patients even before the start of treatment.[71] The need for speech and swallowing rehabilitation therapy is often unexpected by the patient and their families. Pretreatment evaluation and counseling about the importance of speech and swallow rehabilitation could play a major role in improving compliance.

Swallowing has four discrete phases: oral preparatory, oral, pharyngeal, and esophageal phases. Various factors could affect different phases of swallowing, including loss of anatomic structure, xerostomia, problems with dentition and trismus, dysphagia and odynophagia, malnutrition and weight loss leading to lack of initiative, and depression. Several swallowing evaluation tools have been validated in studies and play an important role in following patients.[72-74] In a study using the MDADI questionnaire, it was reported that patients with primary tumors of the oral cavity and oropharynx had significantly greater swallowing disability with an adverse impact on their QOL compared with patients with primary tumors of the larynx and hypopharynx.[74]

Impaired speech and swallow function is common after oral or oropharyngeal surgery. Both the oral and the pharyngeal phase could be affected depending on the extent of surgery, type of reconstruction (if needed), and the type of adjuvant therapy given.[75] Swallowing dysfunction and aspiration could be seen to some extent in over 50% of patients undergoing partial laryngectomy.[76] Swallowing issues are minimal after total laryngectomy risk of aspiration low secondary to the separation of esophagus and trachea.

Impaired swallowing after radiation, with or without chemotherapy, has been linked to treatment associated fibrosis and xerostomia. A commonly recognized feature is the change in saliva that alters from thin secretions with a neutral pH to thick and acidic saliva production. Impaired pharyngeal motility, leading to retention of food in the pharynx, and decreased motility of the laryngeal complex, leading to higher risk of aspiration, are common presentations. While local control is improved with high dose bolus cisplatin and radiation, rates of dysphagia are also higher.[14] The total dose and volume of radiation given to supraglottic larynx and pharyngeal constrictor muscles has been shown to be a predictor of impaired swallowing and complications associated with it, like aspiration.[77,78] Intensity modulated therapy has shown to reduce the rates of dysphagia without compromising on local control by decreasing the volume and dose given to these structures.[79,80]

Videofluoroscopy, fiberoptic endoscopic evaluation of swallowing and barium swallow are a few diagnostic methods used for the evaluation of swallowing dysfunction. Swallowing exercises should be discussed and started before or with the start of radiotherapy and have been shown to enhance pharyngeal motility and help prevent aspiration. Emphasis on swallowing exercises is important at follow-up visits to promote compliance.[81,82] Patients with post-treatment esophageal stricture or esophageal stenosis benefit from endoscopic dilation. Combined antegrade and retrograde dilation has also been utilized for complete esophageal stenosis in post-treatment setting with good results.[83] Neuromuscular electrical stimulation has been utilized to build muscle strength, however, the results are conflicting.[84] Acupuncture has been shown to help improve dysphagia after chemoradiation as well.[85]

Speech and Voice Production

Speech and articulation could be significantly impaired after treatment for oral cavity cancer. In one recent report, speech intelligibility was found to be reduced for increasing tumor size, increasing resection volume and the floor of the mouth or alveolar crest cancers and cancers requiring mandibular resection.[86] Reduced speech intelligibility has been reported widely with total or partial glossectomy.[87,88] Speech therapy is required to improve speech intelligibility. Advances in reconstructive surgical techniques with tissue transfer, mandibular plates, and palatal prosthesis have helped improve speech intelligibility and swallowing mechanisms after surgery.[89–91] Voice and phonation issues affect patients with laryngeal cancer treated with chemoradiation and to larger extent patients who have had a laryngectomy. Voice therapy is of help in patients with hoarseness and problems with phonation after chemoradiation for glottic cancer.[92]

Speech rehabilitation after total laryngectomy could be challenging for the patient.[93] It could involve an artificial larynx, transesophageal puncture, or esophageal voice production. Artificial larynx or electrolarynx is an electronic device that produces vibration, which is transmitted through the oral cavity. Esophageal speech is the conventional voice restoration method utilizing quick air intake into the esophagus and using it for phonation. Tracheoesophageal puncture involves a small surgical fistula between trachea and esophagus with a unidirectional valve prosthesis that prevents the airway from food entry. This type of speech restoration is considered to be superior to any other kind.

Chronic Pain

Chronic pain after treatment, although not very common, can be debilitating. Multiple factors have been found to contribute to this issue. Neck stiffness from surgery and radiation, nerve regeneration, neuropathic and neuralgic pain, radionecrosis, and osteoradionecrosis could all lead to pain and discomfort. Any pain in the post-treatment setting warrants a full work up. Drugs like gabapentin and carbamazepine seem to help with the post-treatment neuralgia. Utilization of pain management services, incorporation of physical therapy, and active follow-up with dental services is extremely helpful. Acupuncture has also been known to help.[69]

Neck Stiffness

Neck stiffness is one of the common chronic sequelae of treatment and is seen with patients who have received neck radiation. It is present more in patients who have had both radiation and salvage neck dissection or neck dissection followed by adjuvant radiation with or without chemotherapy.[69,94]

Lymphedema

Lymphedema of the neck is common, although poorly recognized and reported. It could occur after surgery to the neck and face or after radiation to the head and neck area. Although the head and neck lymphedema generally resolves with time, it could be severe and lead to permanent neck stiffness and disfigurement. Early institution of lymphedema therapy known as complete decongestive therapy is needed and helpful in preventing chronic complications from it.

Dental Health

Dental care and follow up is extremely important after radiation to the head and neck area. Compromised dental health can be frustrating and impact the quality of life (QOL) of survivors. Worsening of dental health after treatment is common and is thought to be secondary to xerostomia, change is salivary pH to acidic, demineralization and decreased vascularity associated with radiation. Pre-treatment evaluation of teeth and all necessary extractions and restorations should be performed at least two weeks prior to starting radiation. Aggressive dental prophylaxis is needed to prevent tooth decay. At least twice a year cleaning is warranted in addition to daily use of fluoride trays or fluoride toothpaste. Restoration of dentition is important for edentulous patients after completion of therapy for nutritional and aesthetic reasons.

Osteoradionecrosis

Osteoradionecrosis could be seen in patients needing dental restorations or extractions in previously radiated area. Pre and post extraction hyperbaric oxygen has been utilized for prevention, however, with conflicting data. Treatment for osteoradionecrosis involves debridement, prolonged antibiotics, and hyperbaric oxygen. Some patients with extensive osteoradionecrosis require marginal or segmental mandibulectomy with reconstruction. Chondroradione-crosis may result from laryngeal radiation and could benefit from hyperbaric therapy.

Trismus

Trismus or lock jaw could occur in up to 35% of head and neck cancer patients following radiation and in patients treated with surgery. It is caused by inflammation and fibrosis of the pterygoid and masseter muscles.[95] Aggressive jaw exercises and passive motion applied several times per day helps to some extent. Rehabilitation devices like Therabite or Dynasplint have had good results.

Ototoxicity

Acute unilateral conductive hearing loss could result from serous otitis media from radiation. Myringotomy is helpful in such situations and might provide immediate relief. Cisplatin, used most commonly as a radiation sensitizer, could lead to irreversible sensory neural hearing deficit. The ototoxicity is dose dependent and leads to high frequency hearing loss. Pretreatment hearing analysis is warranted in any patient with baseline hearing issues. Close symptomatic monitoring during treatment and change of therapy to alternative agents when needed helps prevent significant hearing damage.

Neurotoxicity

Lhermitte's sign is a shock-like sensation radiating down the spine into the feet and is produced by neck flexion. It results from transient myelopathy from radiation or from high dose platinum therapy and is seen in nearly 10% of patients in the post-treatment period. This could be very distressing to the patient; however, is a self-resolving condition over a period of few months.

Peripheral neuropathy could be seen in patients who receive cisplatin after a cumulative dose of 300 mg/m². Careful patient selection is important to avoid exacerbating previously existing neuropathy from other causes. The neuropathy usually improves over time, albeit, complete resolution is not seen in general.

Cardiovascular Toxicity

Ischemic stroke is described as a late complication of neck irradiation. Carotid artery stenosis has been thought to contribute to this risk. Studies have shown correlation with definitive head and neck radiation and progressive carotid atherosclerotic plaque formation, especially over time. The carotid plaque score has been correlated with age, hyperlipidemia, and dose of radiation received.[104–106] Currently, there are no specific guidelines for surveillance of carotid artery stenosis and prospective studies are needed in the era of IMRT. Carotid artery rupture or carotid blowout syndrome and oropharyngocutaneous fistula are major complications mostly seen in patients undergoing a combination of both radiation and neck dissection. These are seen in tumors involving the carotid sheath or with gross involvement of soft tissue of the neck.

Hypothyroidism

Patients receiving neck radiation are at risk to develop primary hypothyroidism. The incidence goes up with passage of time and patients could become hypothyroid one to two years after completion of treatment. Survivors should be monitored for hypothyroidism with TSH levels drawn every 6–12 months.

Employment

Head and neck cancer and its treatment can be temporarily disabling. Patients who have undergone treatment qualify for short and long-term disability. Employment and return to work in survivors is linked to better QOL scores. In a recent study of survivors in the working age group of less than 65 years, median time of returning to work was six months. 71% of patients returned to work within six months after treatment. Oral dysfunction, loss of appetite, deteriorated social functioning, and high levels of anxiety were found to be barriers to their return to employment.[96]

Psychosocial Issues of the Survivors and Their Care Givers

Psychosocial adjustments of survivors and their caregivers are intimately linked to their QOL goals. Psychosocial issues like anxiety, mood disorder, fatigue, and depression are seen in considerable number of head and neck cancer survivors. In a recent study, approximately 43% of head and neck cancer survivors were found to have mild to moderate anxiety and nearly 37% had mild to moderate depression. The authors concluded that the treating clinicians should be trained to identify and correctly refer psychologically distressed patients to appropriate existing psychiatric services.[97] In another study evaluating the caregivers of head and neck cancer survivors 6–24 months post-treatment, moderate to severe distress was seen in 38% of caregivers.[98] Active counseling of the patient and family members during and after treatment play an important role in minimizing the psychosocial burden and help in rehabilitation.

Cosmesis

Facial disfigurement, loss or change of organ function, fear of recurrence and death, and revised self image could all prove challenging to adjustment.

Body image reintegration and adjustment is thought to happen over time and requires compassion, patience, and encouragement from family, friends, and the treating clinician.

Sexuality

Although sexuality is a key issue with head and neck cancer survivors, minimal attention has been given to it over time. Alterations in self image, disfigurement, change in oral sensation and odor, anxiety, and depression have been thought to contribute to this issue. Chemotherapy could lead to altered sensation, arousal, and erectile dysfunction in men. Addressing these issues early on is important in maintaining sexual harmony, especially with the epidemiological shift in age of presentation, with HPV associated head and neck cancer being seen in younger population. Issues related to transmission of HPV to a spouse or partner adds a significant burden to a relationship. A clear understanding of the issues related to HPV and its transmission is crucial. Vaccination strategies should be discussed with patients and their partners. A longitudinal study of nearly 300 HNC patients showed that they returned to baseline on nearly all aspects of QOL after 12 months post treatment, with only a few exceptions: dry mouth, sensory problems, and dissatisfaction with sexual function.[99]

Secondary Cancers

Second primary cancers have been reported in up to 20% of head and neck cancer survivors when these cancers were primarily related to smoking and alcohol abuse. Hypopharynx cancer is the most common head and neck site leading to distant recurrence. For oral cavity and oropharynx cancers, the site of recurrence is the head and neck area, verses hypopharynx and larynx cancers when the site of recurrence could be lung.[98] Nearly 10% of smoking-associated head and neck cancer patients will develop primary lung cancer in their lifetime. Second primary cancers after HPV associated head and neck cancers are extremely rare and possibly fall in the category of general population. With emerging data about difference in sexual practices of HPV positive patients, longitudinal follow-up and reporting of second primaries is warranted.[100,101]

Lifestyle Modification: Smoking and Alcohol Cessation

There is substantial proof to support the concept of smoking cessation to impact on mortality figures. Patients who continue smoking and drinking alcohol have been found to have worse local control and overall survival.[102] In a recently published report, less than 44% of smoking cancer patients quit smoking after their cancer diagnosis, and only 62% of smoking cancer patients received smoking cessation counseling from their physicians. Authors concluded that intervention programs are needed to help cancer survivors to quit smoking.[103] Patients should be counseled for smoking and alcohol cessation routinely and aggressively.

SURVEILLANCE PROPOSAL

Routine follow up is crucial after head and neck cancer treatment. A restaging PET scan is recommended at 12 weeks from completion of therapy to document remission. No further imaging is generally recommended unless indicated for symptomatic evaluation. Clinical follow-up of head and neck cancer is specialty specific because of difficult and inaccessible anatomy. Depending on the residual symptoms, patients should be followed every six weeks in the first year and have a detailed exam including a direct laryngoscopy or a fiberoptic exam. Patients should ideally be followed by all members of the multidisciplinary team, at least for the first few years. The intensity of these exams go down with passage of time, based on the NCCN guidelines (Table 26.1) since majority of recurrences occur in the first two to three years. Patients should learn to do self examinations of the neck and bring any persistent and bothersome symptoms like new onset hoarseness, cough, pain, hearing problems, or any palpable lumps to their physicians notice. The risk of recurrence, although low, persists for patients with history of (and continued) smoking; such patients should continue to be followed beyond the five year timeline.

At each follow up visit, attention should be paid to diet and nutrition, swallowing, xerostomia, speech, neck stiffness, dental health, general health, and follow-up with primary care, age appropriate screening of other malignancies and thyroid function. Improved awareness around psychosocial issues and sexuality is needed. With younger survivors in the HPV era, discussions around sexuality, fertility, and psychosocial well being are needed.

TABLE 26.1 SURVEILLANCE RECOMMENDATIONS FOR SURVIVORS OF HNSCC

Year	Clinical surveillance
1	Every two to three months
2	Every three to four months
3	Every three to four months
4	Every four to six months
5	Every four to six months
>5	Every six to twelve months

REFERENCES

1. Parkin DM, Bray F, Ferlay J, et al.: Global cancer statistics, 2002. *CA Cancer J Clin* 55:74–108, 2005.

2. Mehta V, Yu GP, Schantz SP: Population-based analysis of oral and oropharyngeal carcinoma: changing trends of histopathologic differentiation, survival and patient demographics. *Laryngoscope* 120:2203–12, 2010.

3. Nasman A, Attner P, Hammarstedt L, et al.: Incidence of human papillomavirus (HPV) positive tonsillar carcinoma in Stockholm, Sweden: an epidemic of viral-induced carcinoma? *Int J Cancer* 125:362–6, 2009.

4. Kreimer AR, Clifford GM, Boyle P, et al.: Human papillomavirus types in head and neck squamous cell carcinomas worldwide: a systematic review. *Cancer Epidemiol Biomarkers Prev* 14:467–75, 2005.

5. Dahlstrand H, Nasman A, Romanitan M, et al.: Human papillomavirus accounts both for increased incidence and better prognosis in tonsillar cancer. *Anticancer Res* 28:1133–8, 2008.

6. Ryerson AB, Peters ES, Coughlin SS, et al.: Burden of potentially human papillomavirus-associated cancers of the oropharynx and oral cavity in the U.S., 1998–2003. *Cancer* 113:2901–9, 2008.

7. Chaturvedi AK, Engels EA, Anderson WF, et al.: Incidence trends for human papillomavirus-related and -unrelated oral squamous cell carcinomas in the United States. *J Clin Oncol* 26:612–9, 2008.

8. Ang KK, Harris J, Wheeler R, et al.: Human papillomavirus and survival of patients with oropharyngeal cancer. *N Engl J Med* 363:24–35, 2010.

9. Lowy DR, Munger K: Prognostic implications of HPV in oropharyngeal cancer. *N Engl J Med* 363:82–4, 2010.

10. Haddad RI, Shin DM: Recent advances in head and neck cancer. *N Engl J Med* 359:1143–54, 2008.

11. Bonner JA, Harari PM, Giralt J, et al.: Radiotherapy plus cetuximab for squamous-cell carcinoma of the head and neck. *N Engl J Med* 354:567–78, 2006.

12. Posner MR, Hershock DM, Blajman CR, et al.: Cisplatin and fluorouracil alone or with docetaxel in head and neck cancer. *N Engl J Med* 357:1705–15, 2007.

13. Vermorken JB, Remenar E, van Herpen C, et al.: Cisplatin, fluorouracil, and docetaxel in unresectable head and neck cancer. *N Engl J Med* 357:1695–704, 2007.

14. Forastiere AA, Goepfert H, Maor M, et al.: Concurrent chemotherapy and radiotherapy for organ preservation in advanced laryngeal cancer. *N Engl J Med* 349:2091–8, 2003.

15. Bernier J, Domenge C, Ozsahin M, et al.: Postoperative irradiation with or without concomitant chemotherapy for locally advanced head and neck cancer. *N Engl J Med* 350:1945–52, 2004.

16. Cooper JS, Pajak TF, Forastiere AA, et al.: Postoperative concurrent radiotherapy and chemotherapy for high-risk squamous-cell carcinoma of the head and neck. *N Engl J Med* 350:1937–44, 2004.

17. Liu WS, Hsin CH, Chou YH, et al.: Long-term results of intensity-modulated radiotherapy concomitant with chemotherapy for hypopharyngeal carcinoma aimed at laryngeal preservation. *BMC Cancer* 10:102, 2010.

18. Sher DJ, Haddad RI, Norris CM, Jr., et al.: Efficacy and toxicity of reirradiation using intensity-modulated radiotherapy for recurrent or second primary head and neck cancer. *Cancer* 116:4761–8, 2010.

19. http://seer.cancer.gov/publications/disparities/:

20. http://crchd.cancer.gov/disparities/defined.html:

21. Bach PB, Schrag D, Brawley OW, et al.: Survival of blacks and whites after a cancer diagnosis. JAMA 287:2106–13, 2002.

22. Goodwin WJ, Thomas GR, Parker DF, et al.: Unequal burden of head and neck cancer in the United States. Head Neck 30:358–71, 2008.

23. Shiboski CH, Schmidt BL, Jordan RC: Racial disparity in stage at diagnosis and survival among adults with oral cancer in the U.S. Community Dent Oral Epidemiol 35:233–40, 2007.

24. Morse DE, Kerr AR: Disparities in oral and pharyngeal cancer incidence, mortality and survival among black and white Americans. *J Am Dent Assoc* 137:203–12, 2006.

25. Albain KS, Unger JM, Crowley JJ, et al.: Racial disparities in cancer survival among randomized clinical trials patients of the Southwest Oncology Group. *J Natl Cancer Inst* 101:984–92, 2009.

26. Murdock JM, Gluckman JL: African-American and white head and neck carcinoma patients in a university medical center setting. Are treatments provided and are outcomes similar or disparate? *Cancer* 91:279–83, 2001.

27. Settle K, Taylor R, Wolf J, et al.: Race impacts outcome in stage III/IV squamous cell carcinomas of the head and neck after concurrent chemoradiation therapy. *Cancer* 115:1744–52, 2009.

28. Roberts JC, Li G, Reitzel LR, et al.: No evidence of sex-related survival disparities among head and neck cancer patients receiving similar multidisciplinary care: a matched-pair analysis. *Clin Cancer Res* 16:5019–27, 2010.

29. Ragin CC, Langevin SM, Marzouk M, et al.: Determinants of head and neck cancer survival by race. Head Neck, 2010.

30. Schrank TP, Han Y, Weiss H, et al.: Case-matching analysis of head and neck squamous cell carcinoma in racial and ethnic minorities in the United States-Possible role for human papillomavirus in survival disparities. Head Neck, 2010.

31. Settle K, Posner MR, Schumaker LM, et al.: Racial survival disparity in head and neck cancer results from low prevalence of human papillomavirus infection in black oropharyngeal cancer patients. Cancer Prev Res (Phila) 2:776–81, 2009.

32. http://www.nccn.com/component/glossary/Glossary-1/S/Survivorship-188/

33. Gillison ML, Harris J, Westra W, et al.: Survival outcomes by tumor human papillomavirus (HPV) status in stage III-IV oropharyngeal cancer (OPC) in RTOG 0129. [Abstract] *J Clin Oncol 27* (Suppl 15): A-6003, 2009.

34. Mittal BB, Pauloski BR, Haraf DJ, et al.: Swallowing dysfunction—preventative and rehabilitation strategies in patients with head-and-neck cancers treated with surgery, radiotherapy, and chemotherapy: a critical review. *Int J Radiat Oncol Biol Phys* 57:1219–30, 2003.

35. Biazevic MG, Antunes JL, Togni J, et al.: Survival and quality of life of patients with oral and oropharyngeal cancer at 1-year follow-up of tumor resection. *J Appl Oral Sci* 18:279–84, 2010.

36. Lee NK, Goepfert H, Wendt CD: Supraglottic laryngectomy for intermediate-stage cancer: U.T.M.D. Anderson Cancer Center experience with combined therapy. Laryngoscope 100:831–6, 1990.

37. Weissler MC: Management of complications resulting from laryngeal cancer treatment. *Otolaryngol Clin North Am* 30:269–78, 1997.

38. Erisen L, Basel B, Irdesel J, et al.: Shoulder function after accessory nerve-sparing neck dissections. Head Neck 26:967–71, 2004

39. Cappiello J, Piazza C, Nicolai P: The spinal accessory nerve in head and neck surgery. Curr Opin Otolaryngol Head Neck Surg 15:107–11, 2007.

40. Ferlito A, Rinaldo A, Silver CE, et al.: Neck dissection: then and now. Auris Nasus Larynx 33:365–74, 2006.

41. Koybasioglu A, Tokcaer AB, Uslu S, et al.: Accessory nerve function after modified radical and lateral neck dissections. *Laryngoscope* 110:73–7, 2000.

42. McNeely ML, Parliament MB, Seikaly H, et al.: Effect of exercise on upper extremity pain and dysfunction in head and neck cancer survivors: a randomized controlled trial. *Cancer* 113:214–22, 2008.

43. Rutter CE, Yovino S, Taylor R, et al.: Impact of early percutaneous endoscopic gastrostomy tube placement on nutritional status and hospitalization in patients with head and neck cancer receiving definitive chemoradiation therapy. Head Neck, 2010.

44. Salas S, Baumstarck-Barrau K, Alfonsi M, et al.: Impact of the prophylactic gastrostomy for unresectable squamous cell head and neck carcinomas treated with radio-chemotherapy on quality of life: Prospective randomized trial. *Radiother Oncol* 93:503–9, 2009.

45. Johnson JT, Ferretti GA, Nethery WJ, et al.: Oral pilocarpine for post-irradiation xerostomia in patients with head and neck cancer. *N Engl J Med* 329:390–5, 1993.

46. Brizel DM, Wasserman TH, Henke M, et al.: Phase III randomized trial of amifostine as a radioprotector in head and neck cancer. *J Clin Oncol* 18:3339–45, 2000.

47. Borges L, Rex KL, Chen JN, et al.: A protective role for keratinocyte growth factor in a murine model of chemotherapy and radiotherapy-induced mucositis. *Int J Radiat Oncol Biol Phys* 66:254–62, 2006.

48. Spielberger R, Stiff P, Bensinger W, et al.: Palifermin for oral mucositis after intensive therapy for hematologic cancers. *N Engl J Med* 351:2590–8, 2004.

49. Stiff PJ, Emmanouilides C, Bensinger WI, et al.: Palifermin reduces patient-reported mouth and throat soreness and improves patient functioning in the hematopoietic stem-cell transplantation setting. *J Clin Oncol* 24:5186–93, 2006.

50. Bardet E, Martin L, Calais G, et al: Subcutaneous Compared With Intravenous Administration of Amifostine in Patients With Head and Neck Cancer Receiving Radiotherapy: Final Results of the GORTEC2000–02 Phase III Randomized Trial. *J Clin Oncol* 29:127–33, 2011

51. Haddad R, Sonis S, Posner M, et al: Randomized phase 2 study of concomitant chemoradiotherapy using weekly carboplatin/paclitaxel with or without daily subcutaneous amifostine in patients with locally advanced head and neck cancer. *Cancer* 115:4514–23, 2009

52. Cella DIaamip-oqollToP-O, Holland, JC, et al (Eds), Oxford University Press, New York 1998.

53. Schipper H, Levitt, M. Measuring quality of life: risks and benefits. Cancer Treat Rep 1985; 69:1115.

54. Specific Scales TaM, In: Quality of Life and Pharmacoeconomics in Clinical Trials (second edition), Spilker, B (Ed), Lippincott-Raven, Philadelphia 1996. pp 161–355.

55. Cella DFACITMMotFAoCITFS-VCoO, Research and Education, Evanston Northwestern Hospital Health Care and Northwestern University, November 1997.

56. Chaukar DA, Walvekar RR, Das AK, et al: Quality of life in head and neck cancer survivors: a cross-sectional survey. Am J Otolaryngol 30:176–80, 2009.

57. El-Deiry MW, Futran ND, McDowell JA, et al: Influences and predictors of long-term quality of life in head and neck cancer survivors. *Arch Otolaryngol Head Neck Surg* 135:380–4, 2009

58. Rogers LQ, Rao K, Malone J, et al: Factors associated with quality of life in outpatients with head and neck cancer 6 months after diagnosis. *Head Neck* 31:1207–14, 2009

59. Boscolo-Rizzo P, Stellin M, Fuson R, et al: Long-term quality of life after treatment for locally advanced oropharyngeal carcinoma: surgery and postoperative radiotherapy versus concurrent chemoradiation. *Oral Oncol* 45:953–7, 2009.

60. Lee NY, de Arruda FF, Puri DR, et al: A comparison of intensity-modulated radiation therapy and concomitant boost radiotherapy in the setting of concurrent chemotherapy for locally advanced oropharyngeal carcinoma. *Int J Radiat Oncol Biol Phys* 66:966–74, 2006.

61. Yao M, Karnell LH, Funk GF, et al: Health-related quality-of-life outcomes following IMRT versus conventional radiotherapy for oropharyngeal squamous cell carcinoma. *Int J Radiat Oncol Biol Phys* 69:1354–60, 2007.

62. Graff P, Lapeyre M, Desandes E, et al: Impact of intensity-modulated radiotherapy on health-related quality of life for head and neck cancer patients: matched-pair comparison with conventional radiotherapy. *Int J Radiat Oncol Biol Phys* 67:1309–17, 2007.

63. Lin A, Kim HM, Terrell JE, et al: Quality of life after parotid-sparing IMRT for head-and-neck cancer: a prospective longitudinal study. *Int J Radiat Oncol Biol Phys* 57:61–70, 2003.

64. Parliament MB, Scrimger RA, Anderson SG, et al: Preservation of oral health-related quality of life and salivary flow rates after inverse-planned intensity- modulated radiotherapy (IMRT) for head-and-neck cancer. *Int J Radiat Oncol Biol Phys* 58:663–73, 2004.

65. Kam MK, Leung SF, Zee B, et al: Prospective randomized study of intensity-modulated radiotherapy on salivary gland function in early-stage nasopharyngeal carcinoma patients. J Clin Oncol 25:4873–9, 2007.

66. Sher DJ, Balboni TA, Haddad RI, et al: Efficacy and Toxicity of Chemoradiotherapy Using Intensity-Modulated Radiotherapy for Unknown Primary of Head and Neck. *Int J Radiat Oncol Biol Phys*, 2010.

67. Lu W, Matulonis UA, Doherty-Gilman A, et al: Acupuncture for chemotherapy-induced neutropenia in patients with gynecologic malignancies: a pilot randomized, sham-controlled clinical trial. *J Altern Complement Med* 15:745–53, 2009.

68. Lu W, Rosenthal DS: Recent advances in oncology acupuncture and safety considerations in practice. *Curr Treat Options Oncol* 11:141–6, 2010.

69. Pfister DG, Cassileth BR, Deng GE, et al: Acupuncture for pain and dysfunction after neck dissection: results of a randomized controlled trial. *J Clin Oncol* 28:2565–70, 2010.

70. Wong RK, Sagar SM, Chen BJ, et al: Phase II Randomized Trial of Acupuncture-Like Transcutaneous Electrical Nerve Stimulation to Prevent Radiation-Induced Xerostomia in Head and Neck Cancer Patients. *J Soc Integr Oncol* 8:35–42, 2010.

71. Pauloski BR, Rademaker AW, Logemann JA, et al: Pretreatment swallowing function in patients with head and neck cancer. *Head Neck* 22:474–82, 2000.

72. Stenson KM, MacCracken E, List M, et al: Swallowing function in patients with head and neck cancer prior to treatment. *Arch Otolaryngol Head Neck Surg* 126:371–7, 2000.

73. Dwivedi RC, St Rose S, Roe JW, et al: Validation of the Sydney Swallow Questionnaire (SSQ) in a cohort of head and neck cancer patients. *Oral Oncol* 46:e10–4, 2010.

74. Chen AY, Frankowski R, Bishop-Leone J, et al: The development and validation of a dysphagia-specific quality-of-life questionnaire for patients with head and neck cancer: the M.D. Anderson dysphagia inventory. *Arch Otolaryngol Head Neck Surg* 127:870–6, 2001.

75. Pauloski BR, Logemann JA: Impact of tongue base and posterior pharyngeal wall biomechanics on pharyngeal clearance in irradiated postsurgical oral and oropharyngeal cancer patients. *Head Neck* 22:120–31, 2000.

76. Simonelli M, Ruoppolo G, de Vincentiis M, et al: Swallowing ability and chronic aspiration after supracricoid partial laryngectomy. *Otolaryngol Head Neck Surg* 142:873–8, 2010.

77. Caglar HB, Tishler RB, Othus M, et al: Dose to larynx predicts for swallowing complications after intensity-modulated radiotherapy. *Int J Radiat Oncol Biol Phys* 72:1110–8, 2008.

78. Eisbruch A, Schwartz M, Rasch C, et al: Dysphagia and aspiration after chemoradiotherapy for head-and-neck cancer: which anatomic structures are affected and can they be spared by IMRT? *Int J Radiat Oncol Biol Phys* 60:1425–39, 2004.

79. Feng FY, Kim HM, Lyden TH, et al: Intensity-modulated radiotherapy of head and neck cancer aiming to reduce dysphagia: early dose-effect relationships for the swallowing structures. *Int J Radiat Oncol Biol Phys* 68:1289–98, 2007.

80. Feng FY, Kim HM, Lyden TH, et al: Intensity-modulated chemoradiotherapy aiming to reduce dysphagia in patients with oropharyngeal cancer: clinical and functional results. *J Clin Oncol* 28:2732–8, 2010.

81. Kulbersh BD, Rosenthal EL, McGrew BM, et al: Pretreatment, preoperative swallowing exercises may improve dysphagia quality of life. *Laryngoscope* 116:883–6, 2006.

82. Carroll WR, Locher JL, Canon CL, et al: Pretreatment swallowing exercises improve swallow function after chemoradiation. *Laryngoscope* 118:39–43, 2008.

83. Goguen LA, Norris CM, Jaklitsch MT, et al: Combined antegrade and retrograde esophageal dilation for head and neck cancer-related complete esophageal stenosis. *Laryngoscope* 120:261–6, 2010.

84. Carnaby-Mann GD, Crary MA: Examining the evidence on neuromuscular electrical stimulation for swallowing: a meta-analysis. *Arch Otolaryngol Head Neck Surg* 133:564–71, 2007.

85. Weidong L, Posner MR, Wayne P, et al: Acupuncture for dysphagia after chemoradiation therapy in head and neck cancer: a case series report. *Integr Cancer Ther* 9:284–90, 2010.

86. Stelzle F, Maier A, Noth E, et al: Automatic Quantification of Speech Intelligibility in Patients After Treatment for Oral Squamous Cell Carcinoma. *J Oral Maxillofac Surg,* 2011.

87. Sun J, Weng Y, Li J, et al: Analysis of determinants on speech function after glossectomy. *J Oral Maxillofac Surg* 65:1944–50, 2007.

88. Bressmann T, Sader R, Whitehill TL, et al: Consonant intelligibility and tongue motility in patients with partial glossectomy. *J Oral Maxillofac Surg* 62:298–303, 2004.

89. Marunick M, Tselios N: The efficacy of palatal augmentation prostheses for speech and swallowing in patients undergoing glossectomy: a review of the literature. *J Prosthet Dent* 91:67–74, 2004.

90. Rieger J, Bohle Iii G, Huryn J, et al: Surgical reconstruction versus prosthetic obturation of extensive soft palate defects: a comparison of speech outcomes. *Int J Prosthodont* 22:566–72, 2009.

91. Keereweer S, de Wilt JH, Sewnaik A, et al: Early and long-term morbidity after total laryngopharyngectomy. Eur Arch Otorhinolaryngol 267:1437–44, 2010.

92. van Gogh CD, Verdonck-de Leeuw IM, Boon-Kamma BA, et al: The efficacy of voice therapy in patients after treatment for early glottic carcinoma. *Cancer* 106:95–105, 2006.

93. Hillman RE, Walsh MJ, Wolf GT, et al: Functional outcomes following treatment for advanced laryngeal cancer. Part I—Voice preservation in advanced laryngeal cancer. Part II—Laryngectomy rehabilitation: the state of the art in the VA System. Research Speech-Language Pathologists. Department of Veterans Affairs Laryngeal Cancer Study Group. *Ann Otol Rhinol Laryngol Suppl* 172:1–27, 1998.

94. Goguen LA, Chapuy CI, Li Y, et al: Neck dissection after chemoradiotherapy: timing and complications. *Arch Otolaryngol Head Neck Surg* 136:1071–7, 2010.

95. Sciubba JJ, Goldenberg D: Oral complications of radiotherapy. *Lancet Oncol* 7:175–83, 2006.

96. Verdonck-de Leeuw IM, van Bleek WJ, Leemans CR, et al: Employment and return to work in head and neck cancer survivors. *Oral Oncol* 46:56–60, 2010.

97. Veer V, Kia S, Papesch M: Anxiety and depression in head and neck out-patients. J *Laryngol Otol* 124:774–7, 2010.

98. Ross S, Mosher CE, Ronis-Tobin V, et al: Psychosocial adjustment of family caregivers of head and neck cancer survivors. *Support Care Cancer* 18:171–8, 2010.

99. Bjordal K, Ahlner-Elmqvist M, Hammerlid E, et al: A prospective study of quality of life in head and neck cancer patients. Part II: Longitudinal data. *Laryngoscope* 111:1440–52, 2001.

100. Morris LG, Sikora AG, Patel SG, et al: Second Primary Cancers After an Index Head and Neck Cancer: Subsite-Specific Trends in the Era of Human Papillomavirus-Associated Oropharyngeal Cancer. *J Clin Oncol*, 2010.

101. Dahlstrom KR, Li G, Tortolero-Luna G, et al: Differences in history of sexual behavior between patients with oropharyngeal squamous cell carcinoma and patients with squamous cell carcinoma at other head and neck sites. *Head Neck*, 2010.

102. Mayne ST, Cartmel B, Kirsh V, et al: Alcohol and tobacco use prediagnosis and postdiagnosis, and survival in a cohort of patients with early stage cancers of the oral cavity, pharynx, and larynx. *Cancer Epidemiol Biomarkers Prev* 18:3368–74, 2009.

103. Burke L, Miller LA, Saad A, et al: Smoking behaviors among cancer survivors: an observational clinical study. *J Oncol Pract* 5:6–9, 2009.

104. Carmody BJ, Arora S, Avena R, et al: Accelerated carotid artery disease after high-dose head and neck radiotherapy: is there a role for routine carotid duplex surveillance? *J Vasc Surg* 1999;30: 1045.

105. Dubec JJ,Munk PL, Tsang V et al: Carotid artery stenosis in patients who have undergone radiation therapy for head and neck malignancy. *Br J Radiol.* 1998 Aug; 71(848):872–75.

106. Chang YJ, Chang TC, Lee TH et al: Predictors of carotid artery stenosis after radiotherapy for head and neck cancers. *J Vasc Surg.* 2009 Aug; 50(2):280–85.

27

GYNECOLOGY SURVIVORSHIP

SUSANA CAMPOS, MD, MPH

INTRODUCTION

- It is estimated that there are 11.7 million cancer survivors. This represents approximately 4% of the population.
- The majority of cancer survivors are currently 65 years of age and older.
- Gynecological malignancies represent one of the most common cancer sites (9%)
- The majority of adults diagnosed with cancer will be alive in five years.
- Approximately 14% of the 11.7 million estimated cancer survivors were diagnosed 20 or more years ago. (Adapted from National Coalition for Survivorship Research www. cancer.gov/contact)

With improvements in early detection and multimodality therapy long term survival for patients with gynecological malignancies is possible. As outlined by the National Coalition for Survivorship Research[1] gynecological cancers represents 9% of cancer survivors. Gynecological neoplasms include a spectrum of malignancies that include carcinoma of the ovaries, uterus, cervix, fallopian tubes, peritoneum, vagina, and vulva. The vast majority of these cancers are uterine cancers (43,470 new cases each year)[2] while cancer of the cervix is the least common with only 12,000 new cases anticipated in 2010.[2] Despite a lower incidence, ovarian cancer has the highest mortality rate of any gynecologic cancer. In 2009, 21,550 new cases were estimated to have been diagnosed in the United States.[2] An estimated 21,880 new cases of this cancer will be diagnosed in the United States in 2010 and about 13,850 women will die of this disease.[2] With the exception of cervical cancer where the peak age of disease is 47 years of age the risk of gynecological cancers tends to increase with age. However, data has emerged noting that 3–17 % of all epithelial ovarian cancers occur in women less than 40 years of age.[3,4,5,6]

Risk factors associated with gynecological malignancies vary. In cervical cancer molecular and epidemiologic data indicate that the Human Papillomavirus is the principal cause of invasive cervical cancer,[7] while in uterine cancer risk factors include unopposed estrogen, diet, and hereditary factors.[8,9,10]

Ovarian cancer risk factors include advanced age, family history or hereditary cancer syndromes, nulliparity, estrogen replacement, talc powder, pelvic inflammatory disease, and possibly ovulation inducing agents.[11]

Effective screening tools exist for several malignancies including breast and colon cancer. The introduction of the Pap smear resulted in a significant reduction in the incidence cervical cancer. However, unlike other malignancies there is currently no reliable biomarker or radiographical modality that can detect early stage ovarian cancer. The Ca125 biomarker, a biomarker often used to track response to therapy, lacks sensitivity and as such is a poor biomarker.[12] Additionally, transvaginal ultrasonography is ineffective at detecting ovarian cancer early enough to improve clinical outcomes.[13] As such, ovarian cancer, unlike cervical and uterine cancer, is often diagnosed at advanced stages.

The principle modes of therapy in the management of gynecological cancers are similar and often include one or more treatment modalities, namely cytoreductive surgery, radiation therapy, and combination platinum and taxane based chemotherapy. Advances in all disciplines have been reported with the introduction of minimally invasive surgical techniques,[14,15] targeted radiation fields,[16–20] and also the introduction of novel schedules and routes of administration of cytotoxic agents.[21,22] Recent advances in the management of these once thought of as *terminal illnesses* has allowed the medical community to focus on survivorship, a term once used with trepidation but now currently embraced.

Survivorship research has emerged as a new discipline. As defined by the National Coalition for Survivorship,[1] cancer survivorship research is focused on the physical, psychosocial, and economic effects of cancer diagnosis and its treatment. Survivorship research focuses on all phases of treatment. It aims to research treatment-related outcomes such as late effects of treatment, causes of impaired quality of life, and also to navigate educational resources. An individual is considered a cancer survivor from the time of diagnosis, throughout life. The definition of a survivor not only pertains to the patients but is extended to include family members, friends, and caregivers (adapted from the National Coalition for Cancer Survivorship).

Several domains will be discussed in the following chapter. These include a discussion on the recent progress in treatment modalities that have had an effect on survivorship care, toxicities of local and systemic care, fertility, psychosocial parameters, and surveillance of disease.

PROGRESS IN DISEASE TREATMENTS AFFECTS SURVIVORSHIP CARE

Local Therapy

Over the last several years, significant progress has been made in the treatment of patients with gynecological cancers. Surgical techniques have evolved that have direct benefit to the patient diagnosed with gynecological malignancies. These procedures have resulted in smaller incisions, less blood loss, less postoperative pain, and a shorter hospital stay. These procedures encompass laparoscopic surgery assisted radical vaginal hysterectomies, radical vaginal trachelectomy, and laparoscopic hysterectomy. The Gynecologic Oncology Group (GOG) LAP 2 trial[23] was a large, randomized trial designed to determine equivalency outcomes of laparoscopically assisted vaginal hysterectomy/bilateral salpingo-oophorectomy (LAVH/BSO) with surgical staging when compared with traditional laparotomy with a total abdominal hysterectomy (TAH)/BSO with surgical staging in early-stage endometrial cancer. This study reported less morbidity in the laparoscopy groups. Of note patient's quality of life was assessed using the FACT-G at one week, six weeks, and at six months post surgery. FACT-G scores of patients that were scoped were significantly higher than patients who underwent an open laparotomy at six weeks.

In ovarian cancer, minimally invasive surgery has been used in various stages of the disease. Recently reported was a retrospective case control analysis[24] comparing perioperative outcomes and survival of patients with epithelial ovarian cancer undergoing robotic surgical treatments versus laparoscopy or laparotomy approach. There was a statistically significant difference in mean operating times between robotic, laparoscopic, and laparotomy procedures (p < 0.05), mean blood loss, and length of hospital stay. There was no difference in overall survival among the three approaches in patient care (p = .08).

In addition to conservative abdominal surgery, radiation techniques have improved over the last several years contributing to the well being of gynecological cancer survivors. Radiation therapy is an important integral component in the treatment of patients with both uterine and cervical cancer. Recently reported were the results of a clinic trial termed PORTEC II,[25] Post-Operative Radiation Therapy for Endometrial Carcinoma—a multicenter randomized phase III trial comparing external beam radiation and vaginal brachytherapy. In this study patients were randomized either to vaginal brachytherapy (VBT) or external beam radiation therapy (EBRT). Although local recurrences were higher in patients receiving only brachytherapy there was no statistically significant difference in overall survival thereby highlighting that in carefully selected patients toxicity can be minimized without effecting overall survival. Rates of acute grade 1–2 gastrointestinal toxicity were significantly lower in the VBT group than in the EBRT group at completion of radiotherapy (12.6% versus 53.8%).

In 1999, several randomized trials[26–30] led to the recommendation to consider concurrent platinum-based chemotherapy as primary therapy for patients with locally advanced cervical cancer. A disease free survival, as well as overall survival, was documented in these trials. However, improved clinical outcomes translated into acute and chronic adverse effects. These included nausea, vomiting, diarrhea, gastrointestinal consequences, bladder irritation, and bone marrow suppression. Long term consequences described include bowel obstruction and strictures, fistulization, insufficiency fractures, and lymph edema. Both short and long term have an impact on quality of life. Intensity modulated radiation therapy is currently being utilized in selected cohorts of patients with cervical cancer.[31,32,33,34] IMRT has the potential to mitigate the collateral effects of radiation therapy, and in some cases improve targeted tumor volumes, thereby optimizing tumor control. Numerous clinical trials have explored intensity modulated therapy in the management of patients with gynecological malignancies.[19,20,34] Several cooperative group trials (RTOG -0418, RTOG 0724, GOG 263) are exploring the role of pelvic IMRT in posthysterectomy setting for patients with endometrial or cervical carcinoma. Objectives of the RTOG-0408 include an analysis of reduction in short term bowel injury and the rates of loco-regional control and disease free survival. Trials are currently in progress and patients should be made aware of these findings so that they can actively participate in their treatment choices.

Systemic Therapy

Platinum and taxane therapy is the backbone of therapy in patients with advanced ovarian, cervical, and uterine cancer. Newer agents including both cytotoxic as well as biological agents[35-39] have recently been introduced that have unique side effects. A careful understanding of these toxicities when individualizing treatment is of paramount importance. These agents can have cumulative as well as irreversible side effects affecting the long term quality of life of patients treated for gynecological malignancies. These include fatigue, pain, nausea, hypertension, renal dysfunction, hypersensitivity reactions, rash, alopecia, cardiac arrhythmias, bowel complications, and most commonly peripheral neuropathy. Although there is a potential for multiple side effects associated with the armamentarium of therapeutic agents the most common side effects include neuropathy, gastrointestinal disturbances, and fatigue.

Systemic Therapy: Neurological Consequences of Therapy

Neuropathy is a common and debilitating complication of cancer and its treatment. The onset can be sudden and surface post chemotherapy or can slowly progress over time. For most regimens neuropathy increases with the dose and duration of therapy and is abrogated by the withdrawal of the offending agent. A notable exception is the platinum agents, the mainstay of therapy for most gynecological cancers, for which symptoms may progress for weeks to months after the treatment completion. This is often termed "a coasting effect." The incidence of neuropathy can also increase with the particular combination of agents and the schedule of specific chemotherapeutic agents. Recently published were the results of GOG 172[22] which reported a progression free survival as well as an overall survival of patients with the use of intraperitoneal cisplatin and paclitaxel chemotherapy. Wenzel and colleagues[40] reported the first analysis of the quality of life (QOL) results in GOG 172 using the FACT-O, GOG-NTX (neurotoxicity scale) and pain measure.

Patients receiving intraperitoneal therapy reported significantly worse neuro-toxicity three to six weeks after completing chemotherapy and one year later. Additionally, a dose dense approach of weekly chemotherapy has been associated with greater antitumor potency. Recently, a Japanese (JGOG) study[21] demonstrated the superiority of dose dense weekly paclitaxel in combination with three weekly carboplatin when compared with conventional treatment in the first line treatment of advanced ovarian cancer. The dose dense arm was associated with significantly improved median progression free survival (28.0 months versus 17.2 months; HR 0.71) and a three year overall survival rate (72.1% versus 65.1); HR0.75. Weekly paclitaxel chemotherapy has been associated with an increase in neuropathy.[41] As such, clinicians in addition to patients must be made aware of this trade off—namely improved progression free survival and overall survival coupled with the potential for increase toxicity.

In addition to toxicity, which can impair QOL, neuropathy can also result in treatment delays, dose reductions, or discontinuation of therapy, which in turn can affect overall prognosis. Effectively managing and controlling the consequences of this adverse effect requires early recognition and treatment of symptoms. A careful assessment of all potential etiologies is imperative. A careful history and physical is important prior to commencing therapy, as a select group of patients may have additional conditions that predispose them to heighten neurological consequences. Potential factors include a personal and family history of hereditary neuropathy (Charcot-Marie Tooth disease), diabetes, HIV, and alcohol use. Physical exam should increase sensory assessment, deep tendon reflexes, assessment of motor weakness, and autonomic symptoms such as constipation, orthostatic hypotension, and urinary dysfunction.[42]

Several agents are being explored that may help alleviate and or prevent these symptoms.[42] Patients should be advised as to the pro and cons of these agents as these agents themselves can at times have significant side effects. Agents with positive findings in randomized clinic trials include Vitamin E, Calcium/Magnesium supplementation, Glutamine, Glutathione, and N-acetylcysteine. Agents that are currently being investigated in ongoing Phase III trials include Vitamin B12/Vitamin B6 (NCT 00659269), Acetyl-L-carnitine (NCT 00775645), and Alpha Lipoic Acid (NCT 00705029). Common agents for pain management in neuropathy include (1) Duloxetine (potential side effects include nausea, xerostomia, constipation, and diarrhea (2) Gabapentin (potential side effects include somnolence, dizziness, GI symptoms, mild edema, cognitive impairment, gait disturbances (3) 5% Lidocaine (potential side effects include rash/erythema) (4) Opioids (potential side effects include constipation, nausea, vomiting, sedation, confusion, and respiratory depression), pregabalin (potential side effects include dizziness, somnolence, xerostomia, edema, blurred vision), Tramadol (potential side effects include dizziness, constipation, nausea, somnolence, and tricyclic) antidepressants (potential side effects include anticholinergic effects, interactions with drug metabolism).

Systemic and Local Therapy: Gastrointestinal Consequences of Therapy

Gastrointestinal distress is common in patients with gynecological malignancies prior to diagnosis, during treatment, and after the completion of therapy. Patients often present with abdominal bloating, constipation, diarrhea, and/or early satiety. Complicating a patient's course is the treatment modalities often employed in the management of the disease. Cytoreductive surgery can be complicated by constipation, nausea, and bowel dysfunction. Cytotoxic therapies, especially the platinum agents (cisplatin), are considered highly emetogenic and often require numerous antiemetic regimens which in turn often result in constipation, diarrhea increased flatulence, abdominal bloating, and nausea. Autonomic dysfunction can also be associated with antineoplastic agents and can be associated with constipation and bloating. Bevacizumab, a novel monoclonal antibody directed at the vascular endothelial growth factor, has been associated with improved progression free survival[35,36] in the upfront management of patients with ovarian cancer. This agent also is known to have activity in patients with recurrent ovarian,[43-47] uterine,[39] and cervical cancer.[48] However, collateral damage associated with these antiangiogenic therapies, including bowel perforations[49] or anastomotic leakage, can have a significant emotional impact on a patient's life. Personalized oncological care in this patient population (i.e. avoiding the use of this agent in patients with the following characteristics: acute diverticulitis, intra-abdominal abscess, gastrointestinal obstruction, tumor at the perforation site, abdominal carcinomatosis, previous abdominal pelvic radiotherapy) is yet another tool that contributes to that of survivorship care.

Radiation therapy, the principal modality utilized in both in cervical and uterine cancer (rarely in ovarian cancer), can be associated with chronic diarrhea, incontinence, benign postoperative adhesions, adhesions resulting in bowel obstructions, chronic radiation enteritis, indigestion, and pain. The nutritional status of patients suffering from radiation enteritis can be severely compromised due to alteration of nutrient absorption secondary to mucosal damage. Investigators[50] have tried to outline predicative factors for the development of late side effects. Researchers have reported that cumulative acute symptoms are more predictive of late symptoms. The association was noted to be independent of the radiotherapy dose delivered.

Symptoms of bowel dysfunction are associated with poor body image, malnutrition, and interference with social functioning. A careful review of symptoms with patients during and after treatment may allow early interventions such as a referral to the nutritional services or to the gastrointestinal discipline to explore other causes of gastrointestinal distress.

In addition to a proactive approach at the initiation of therapy, advanced gynecological patients often face significant gastrointestinal difficulty in the later stages of their disease. Bowel obstructions are common in patients with advanced ovarian cancer. Numerous investigators[51,52] have studied the role of long acting octreotide for the treatment and symptomatic relief of bowel obstructions in advanced ovarian cancer. Partnering with pain and palliative teams in institutions may afford advanced gynecological patients additional support.

Systemic Therapy: Fatigue

Although fatigue is commonly reported in cancer patients it is rarely investigated and often these symptoms are neglected. Fatigue is a widespread and highly significant symptom in ovarian carcinoma survivors. Ovarian carcinoma survivors suffering from fatigue reported low QOL, high rates of anxiety and depression, and low social support.[53] It is often attributed to the treatment related consequences of therapy but more often than not has at its root a multifactorial cause. Possible factors include anemia, concurrent medications, weight loss, changes in metabolism, endocrine disorders, emotional distress, disturbed sleep habits, a decline in physical activity, pain, poor nutrition, and dehydration. Recently novel therapeutics in the management of ovarian cancer has been associated with significant fatigue. Oral vascular endothelial growth factor receptor inhibitors have been showed to affect the endocrine axis causing at times significant alterations in thyroid function which result in significant fatigue[37,38] Patients participating in these clinical trials should be well informed on the potential side effects of these novel agents as it can result in a significant burdenon quality of life.

Several disciplines have reported a strong benefit of physical activity and quality of life. Currently a trial is being conducted to examine the impact of exercise on the QOL in ovarian cancer survivors. Investigators propose to evaluate, in 230 sedentary women diagnosed with Stage I-III ovarian cancer, the impact of a six-month, moderate-intensity, aerobic exercise intervention on QOL. Women will be randomized to an exercise program or attention control group. Women randomized to exercise will participate in 150 minutes of aerobic exercise per week (e.g., five 30-min sessions/wk). The investigators will conduct baseline and six-month clinic visits to evaluate the effect of exercise on QOL. Additional information on current studies addressing the role of physical activity can be found on the National Coalition Survivorship website.[1]

Loss of Fertility: A Consequence of Both Local and Systemic Therapy

Preservation of fertility is one of many factors facing young patients diagnosed with gynecological neoplasms. Surgical techniques, (i.e. radical trachelectomy in cervical cancer) endocrine treatment in early endometrial cancer, and fertility sparing surgery in early stage ovarian neoplasms have improved QOL in patients facing loss of reproductive function. However, despite the emergence of a new discipline coined *Oncofertility*, informational gaps remain. These include the lack of disease specific guidelines for the prevention of gonadic failure, the lack of coordination among various subspecialty clinicians caring for these women,[54,55] the lack of scientific data surrounding the risk of specific therapeutics on gonadal failure, the risk of infertility interventions in disease recurrences, and the lack of methods to reduce the incidence and gravity of reproductive distress. In the gynecological discipline, concern centers on the uncertain efficacy of fertility options that exist given the extensive surgery often rendered, the uncertain detrimental effects of chemotherapy to remaining reproductive organs, and the timing and execution of fertility workup relative to disease requiring treatment. Given that fertility is an important late and long-term issue for cancer survivors the oncofertility program of any institution is one that must involve collaboration between the survivorship program, the Department of Reproductive Endocrinology and Psycho-oncology.

Psychosocial and Sexual Aspects Facing Gynecological Cancer Survivors

Survivors of gynecological malignancies face not only the potential physical consequences of therapy but also are faced with an array of emotional challenges that may persist years after diagnosis.[56,57] These challenges include anxiety, anger, depression, fear of social relationships, and fear of follow-up of diagnostic testing. In addition, matters of sexuality and intimacy after gynecological cancers are of paramount importance to patients, yet there is a body of literature that suggests that these needs are not being appropriately addressed by health care providers. One report[58] noted that only 21% of health care providers discussed sexual matters. Reasons varied as to why there was a lack of communication. Often health care providers noted that it was an embarrassment; there was limited time or a low priority at diagnosis and during treatment.

Numerous investigators[59-64] have addressed the psychosocial management of patients with gynecological cancers. Focus has centered on parameters such as vasomotor symptoms, loss of fertility, altered body image, sexual function, relationships with family, friends and work colleagues, daily functioning, financial concerns, and spiritual well being. Investigators have tried to assess whether there is a difference in the psychosocial issues that patients face with early stage gynecological malignancies versus advanced stage disease. Recently researchers[65] described the QOL, consequences of treatment, complementary therapy use, and factors correlating with psychological state in 58 survivors of early-stage ovarian cancer. Survivors were interviewed using standardized measures to assess physical, psychological, social, and sexual functioning; impact of cancer on socioeconomic status; and complementary therapy use. Although survivors reported good physical QOL scores, menopausal and intimacy issues dominated their concerns. Less than 10% of survivors reported either an interest in sex or were sexually active. A small fraction of patients required treatment for family/personal problems and antianxiety medications. The majority of survivors reported fear of cancer recurrence and anxiety when their CA125 was tested. Better mental health was significantly related to less fatigue (Functional Assessment of Cancer Therapy [FACT]-fatigue, r = 0.61, P < 0.0001), less pain (European Organization for Research and Treatment of Cancer [EORTC], r = −0.54, P 0.0001), fewer stressful life events (Life Event Scale, r = −0.44, P > 0.001), and greater social support (MOS Social Support Survey, r = 0.41, P < 0.01). The authors concluded that early-stage ovarian cancer survivors had few physical complaints and unmet needs, but psychological distress was evident in a subset of survivors. Kornblith et al.[66] characterized the QOL of ovarian cancer patients over a one-year period of time. This study focused on understanding the extent of physical and well as psychological distress coupled with the medical and sociodemographic factors that were predictive of distress. In this study one third of the patients presented with symptoms of anxiety and depression of moderate to severe intensity. Wenzel et al.[56] described the physical, psychosocial, social, and spiritual well being associated with long-term ovarian survivors. The authors highlighted that abdominal, gynecological, and neurotoxicity symptoms influenced overall physical well being in survivorship. Sexual dysfunction was relatively prevalent. Specifically highlighted were problems with libido, arousal, orgasm, and intercourse. Interestingly, emotional well being ratings in this GOG study were more variable. The study highlighted that of the 20% of the patient population that experienced distress, fear centered on future diagnostic tests and recurrences. The authors did capture information on the evidence of resilience and growth as results of ovarian cancer experience and specifically commented on the importance of spirituality and confidence.

A persistent theme among many QOL studies in survivors of gynecological malignancies pertains to matters of sexuality and intimacy.[64] The National Health and Social Life survey suggested that among women affected by some form of female sexual dysfunction a substantially higher incidence occurs in women dealing with gynecological cancers. Women report symptoms of Female Sexual Arousal Disorder (FSAD), defined as a persistent or recurrent inability of a woman to achieve or maintain an adequate lubrication-swelling response during sexual activity. This lack of physical response may be acquired as a consequence of surgery or treatment and has both physiological and psychological causes. FSAD results in sexual avoidance and disruptive interactions with partners. Health care providers should focus on providing patients and their partners alternative therapy such as psychotherapy in hopes of restoring intimacy. Additionally, health care providers should communicate information regarding patient/family support groups, workshops, and advocacy groups. Numerous organizations including the American Cancer Society, the National Ovarian Cancer Coalition, and Gilda's Club offer services to patients, friends, and family members of cancer survivors.

SURVEILLANCE RECOMMENDATIONS

QOL studies have highlighted that the fear of future diagnostic tests and procedures dominate many patients' emotional state. However, equally concerning is the fear of recurrence. The Ca125 biomarker is often utilized to tract response to induction therapy for ovarian cancer but is also used to monitor for recurrences. This biomarker—although not always accurate—has tremendous impact on a patient's QOL. Recently Rustin and colleagues[67] reported a randomized study that emphasized the futility of this marker. Patients with an elevated marker were randomized to either continued observation or immediate treatment. The authors reported no overall survival advantage to early intervention in patients with a rising Ca125. Although some individuals have embraced the result of this study, others, both health care providers as well as patients, have highlighted the limitations of the study such as the limited course of treatments employed in the recurrent setting coupled with the characteristics of the patient population. Others have highlighted that the limitations of this study lie not in the biomarker itself but in the absence of satisfactory agents for patients with recurrent ovarian cancer. In the interim surveillance recommendations should be personalized to the individual. The NCCN guidelines[68,69,70] provide modules that guide the health care provider in achieving a balance between careful monitoring for recurrence and appropriate utilization of diagnostic procedures.

CONCLUSIONS

Research dedicated to Cancer Survivorship is a new discipline and one that must be met with enthusiasm and participation from multiple disciplines. Physical and psychosocial domains should both be explored. A personalized therapeutic approach to patients in their early stages or late stages of disease will ensure that survivorship needs are tailored. Through the past and current work of patients and health care providers the term survivorship has entered and will remain in the vocabulary of the gynecological discipline.

REFERENCES

1. National Cancer Institute. Cancer Survivorship Research: http://www.cancer.gov/contact.

2. Jemal A, Siegel R, Ward E, et al. Cancer Statistics,2009. *CA Cancer J Clin.* 59(4):225–49,2009.

3. Duska, LR Chang, Y, Flynn, CE, et al. Epithelial ovarian carcinoma in the reproductive age group. *Cancer* 85: 2623–29,1999.

4. Plaxe, SC, Braly, PS, Freddo, JL, et al. Profiles of women age 30–39 and age less than 30 with epithelial ovarian cancer. *Obstet Gynecol* 81: 651–54, 1993.

5. Rodríguez, M, Nguyen, HN, Averette, HE, et al. Epithelial ovarian malignancies in women less than 25 or equal to 25 years of age. *Cancer* 73: 1245–50, 1994.

6. Swerenton, KD, Hislop, TG, Spinally, J, et al. Ovarian carcinoma: a multivariate analysis of prognostic factors. *Obstetric Gynecology* 65: 264–7,1985.

7. Ibeanu OA. Molecular Pathogenesis of Cervical Cancer. *Cancer Biol Ther.* 1;11(3), 2011.

8. Meyer LA, Broaddus RR, Lu KH. Endometrial cancer and Lynch syndrome: clinical and pathologic considerations. *Cancer Control.* 16(1):14–22, 2009.

9. Linkov F, Edwards R, Balk J, et al. Endometrial hyperplasia, endometrial cancer and prevention: gaps in existing research of modifiable risk factors. *Eur J Cancer* 44(12):1632–44,2008.

10. Fader AN, Arriba, LN, Frasure HE, et al. Endometrial cancer and obesity: epidemiology, biomarkers, prevention and survivorship. *Gynecol Oncol.* 114(1):121–7, 2009.

11. Grant DJ, Moorman PG, Akushevich L. Primary peritoneal and ovarian cancers: an epidemiological comparative analysis. *Cancer Causes Control* 21(7):991–8, 2010.

12. Hakama M, Stenman UH, Knekt P. CA 125 as a screening test for ovarian cancer. *J Med Screen* 3(1):40–2, 1996.

13. Stirling D, Evans DG, Pichert G, et al. Screening for familial ovarian cancer: failure of current protocols to detect ovarian cancer at an early stage according to the International Federation of Gynecology and Obstetrics system. *J Clin Oncol.* 23(24):5588–5596, 2005.

14. Nezhat C, Saberi NS, Shahmohamady B, et al. Robotic-assisted laparoscopy in gynecological surgery. *JSLS* 10(3):317–320,2006.

15. Geisler JP, Orr CJ, Khurshid N, et al. Robotically assisted laparoscopic radical hysterectomy compared with open radical hysterectomy. *Int J Gynecolo Cancer* 20 (3): 438–42, 2010.

16. Portelance L, Chao KS, Grigsby PW, et al. Intensity-modulated radiation therapy (IMRT) reduces small bowel, rectum, and bladder doses in patients with cervical cancer receiving pelvic and paraarotic irradiation. *Internal Journal of Radiation Oncology Bio Phys* 51:261–266, 2001.

17. Roeske JV, Lujan A, Rotmensch J, et al. Intensity modulated whole pelvic radiation therapy in patients with gynecological malignancies. *Int J Radia Oncol Bio Phys* 48:1613–1621, 2000.

18. Lujan AE, Mundt AJ, Yamada SD, et al. Intensity–modulated radiotherapy as a means of reducing dose to bone marrow in gynecologic patients receiving pelvic radiotherapy. *Int J Radia Oncol Bio Phys* 57:516–521, 2003.

19. Mundt AJ, Lujan AE, Rotmensch J, et al. Intensity–modulated whole pelvic radiotherapy in women with gynecologic malignancies. *Int J Radiatr Oncol Bio Phys* 52: 1330–1337, 2002.

20. Mundt AJ, Mell LK, Roeske J, et al. Preliminary outcome and toxicity report of external-field, intensity modulated radiation therapy. *Int J Radiat Oncol Biol Phys* 56:1354–1360, 2003.

21. Katsumata N, Yasuda M, Takahashi F et al. Dose-dense paclitaxel once a week in combination with carboplatin every 3 weeks for advanced ovarian cancer: a phase 3, open-label, randomized controlled trial. *Lancet* 17;374(9698):1331–8, 2009.

22. Armstrong DK, Bundy B, Wenzel L, et al. Gynecologic Oncology Group. Intraperitoneal cisplatin and paclitaxel in ovarian cancer. *N Engl J Med.*54:34–43, 2006.

23. Walker JL, Piedmonte M, Spirtos N, et al. Surgical Staging of uterine cancer: randomized phase II trial of laparoscopy vs. laparotomy- A Gynecological Oncology Group Study (GOG): Preliminary results. *J Clin Oncol.* 10;27(32):5331–6, 2009.

24. Magrina JF, Zanagnolo V, Noble BN, et al. Robotic approach for ovarian cancer: Perioperative and survival results and comparison with laparoscopy and laparotomy. *Gynecol Oncol.* 2010.

25. Nout RA, Smit VT, Putter H, et al. Vaginal brachytherapy versus pelvic external beam radiotherapy for patients with endometrial cancer of high-intermediate risk

(PORTEC-2): an open-label, non-inferiority, randomized trial. *Lancet* 375 (9717):816–23, 2010.

26. Whitney CW, Sause W, Bundy BN, et al. Randomized comparison of fluorouracil plus cisplatin versus hydroxyurea as an adjunct to radiation therapy in stage IIB-IVA carcinoma of the cervix with negative para-aortic lymph nodes: a Gynecologic Oncology Group and Southwest Oncology Group study *J Clin Oncol.* 17(5):1339–48, 1999.

27. Rose PG, Bundy BN, Watkins EB, et al. Concurrent cisplatin-based radiotherapy and chemotherapy for locally advanced cervical cancer. *N Engl J Med.* 340(15):1144–53,1999.

28. Keys HM, Bundy BN, Stehman FB, et al. Cisplatin, radiation, and adjuvant hysterectomy compared with radiation and adjuvant hysterectomy for bulky stage IB cervical carcinoma. *N Engl J Med.* 340(15):1154–61, 1999.

29. Peters, WA, Liu PY, Barrett RJ, et al. Concurrent chemotherapy and pelvic radiation therapy compared with pelvic radiation therapy alone as adjuvant therapy after radical surgery in high-risk early-stage cancer of the cervix. *J Clin Oncol.* Apr;18(8):1606–13, 2008.

30. Eifel PJ, Winter K, Morris M, et al. Pelvic irradiation with concurrent chemotherapy versus pelvic and para-aortic irradiation for high risk cervical cancer: An update of RTOG 90–01. *J Clin Oncol* 22:872–880, 2004.

31. Sanghani M, Mignano J. Intensity modulated radiation therapy: a review of current practice and future directions. Intensity Modulated Radiation therapy: A review of current practice and future directions. *Technol Cancer Res Treat.* 5(5):447–50, 2006.

32. Yang R, Xu S, Jiang W, et al. Dosimetric comparison of postoperative whole pelvic radiotherapy for endometrial cancer using three-dimensional conformal radiotherapy, intensity-modulated radiotherapy, and helical tomotherapy. *Acta Oncol.* 49(2):230–6, 2010.

33. Loiselle C, Koh WJ. The Emerging Use of IMRT for Treatment of Cervical Cancer. *Journal of the National Comprehensive Cancer Network* 8 (12): 1425–1433, 2010.

34. Gerszten K, Colonello K, Heron DE, et al. Feasibility of concurrent cisplatin and extended- field radiation therapy (EFRT) using intensity—modulated radiotherapy (IMRT) for carcinoma of the cervix. *Gynecol Oncol* 102:182–188, 2006.

35. Burger RA, Brady MF, Bookman MA et al. Phase III Trial of Bevacizumab in the Primary Treatment of Advanced Epithelial Ovarian, Primary Peritoneal or Fallopian Tube Cancer: A Gynecologic Oncology Group (GOG) Study *J Clin Oncol.* 28(7s): Abstract #LBA1, 2010.

36. Perren T, et al on behalf of GCIG ICON7 collaborators. ICON7 A randomized, two arm, multi-centre Gynaecologic Cancer InterGroup phase III trial of adding bevacizumab to standard chemotherapy (carboplatin and paclitaxel) in first line treatment of patients with epithelial ovarian cancer. ESMO 2010.

37. Matulonis UA, Berlin S, Ivy P, et al. Cediranib, an oral inhibitor of vascular endothelial growth factor receptor kinases, is an active drug in recurrent epithelial ovarian, fallopian tube and peritoneal cancer. *Journal of Clinical Oncology.* 27(33):5601–5606, 2009.

38. Hirte HW, Vidal L, Fleming GF, et al. A phase II study of cediranib (AZD2171) in recurrent or persistent ovarian, peritoneal or fallopian tube cancer. Final results of a PMH, Chicago and California consortia trial. *Journal of Clinical Oncology.* 26(298S) abstract 5521, 2008.

39. Aghajanian C, Sill MW, Darcy K, et al. A phase II evaluation of bevacizumab in the treatment of recurrent or persistent endometrial cancer: A Gynecologic Oncology Group (GOG) study. *J Clin Oncol* 27:15s, 2009 (suppl; abstr 5531).

40. Wenzel LB, Huang HQ, Armstrong DK, et al. Baseline quality of life (QOL) as a predictor of tolerance to intraperitoneal (IP) chemotherapy for advanced epithelial ovarian cancer (EOC): A Gynecological Oncology Group (GOG) study. *Journal of Clinical Oncology* SCO Annual Meeting Proceedings 24 (June 20 Supplement):5007, 2006.

41. Beuselinck B, Wildiers H, Wynendale W et al. Weekly paclitaxel versus weekly docetaxel in elderly or frail patients with metastatic breast carcinoma: a randomized phase-II study of the Belgian Society of Medical Oncology Crit Rev Oncol Hematol. 75(1):70–7, 2010.

42. Stubblefield MD, Burstein HJ, Burton AW, et al. NCCN Task Force: Management of Neuropathy in Cancer. *Journal of the National Comprehensive Cancer Network.* 7 Supplement 5 S1-S26, 2009.

43. Burger R, Sill M, Monk B, et al. Phase II Trial of Bevacizumab in Persistent or Recurrent Epithelial Ovarian Cancer or Primary Peritoneal Cancer. A Gynecological Oncology Group Study. *J Clin Oncol* 25 (33): 5165–5171, 2007.

44. Cannistra S, Matulonis U, Penson R, et al. Phase II Study of Bevacizumab in Patients with Platinum–Resistant Ovarian Cancer or Peritoneal Serous Cancer. *J Clin Oncol* 25(33): 5180–5186, 2007.

45. Garcia A, Hirte H, Fleming G, et al. Phase II Clinical Trial of Bevacizumab and Low- Dose Metronomic Oral Cyclophosphamide in Recurrent Ovarian Cancer: A Trial of the California, Chicago and Princess Margaret Hospital Phase II Consortia. *J Clin Oncol.* 26 (1):76–82, 2008.

46. Wright J, Hageman A, Rader J, et al. Bevacizumab Combination Therapy in Recurrent Platinum Refractory Epithelial Ovarian Carcinoma or Peritoneal Serous Cancer. *Cancer* 25(33):5180–5186, 2007.

47. Chua J, Siege KV, Downs LS, et al. Bevacizumab plus cyclophosphamide in heavily pretreated patients with recurrent ovarian cancer. *Gynecol Onc* 107: 326–330, 2007.

48. Monk BJ, Still MW, Burger RA, et al. Phase II trial of bevacizumab in the treatment of persistent or recurrent cervical cancer. *Gynecol Oncol* 103:489–493, 2006.

49. Simpkins F, Belinson J, Rose P, et al. Avoiding bevacizumab related gastrointestinal toxicity for recurrent ovarian cancer by careful patient screening. *Gynecol Oncol* 107:118–123, 2007.

50. Wedlacke LJ, Thomas K, Lalji, A, et al. Predicting late effects of pelvic radiotherapy: is there a better approach? *Int J Radiat Oncol Bio Phys* 78(4):1163–70, 2010.

51. Matulonis UA, Seiden MV, Roche M, et al. Long-acting octreotide for the treatment and symptomatic relief of bowel obstruction in advanced ovarian cancer. *J Pain Symptom Manage.* 30(6):563–9, 2005.

52. Ripamonti C, Panzeri C, Groff L, et al. The role of somatostatin and octreotide in bowel obstruction: pre-clinical and clinical results Tumori. 87(1):1–9, 2001.

53. Holzner B, Kemmler G, Meraner V, et al. Fatigue in Ovarian Carcinoma Patients, A Neglected Issue? *Cancer* 97 (6): 1564–1572, 2003.

54. Duffy CM, Allen SM, Clark, MA. Discussions regarding reproductive health for young women with breast cancer undergoing chemotherapy. *Journal of Clinical Oncology,* 23(4), 766–773, 2005.

55. Quinn, GP, Vadaparampil, ST, Lee, JH, et al. Physician Referral for Fertility Preservation in Oncology Patients: A National Study of Practice Behaviors, *Journal of Clinical Oncology,* 27(35), 5952–5957, 2009.

56. Wenzel LB, Donnelly JP, Fowler JM., et al. Resilience, Reflection and Residual Stress in Ovarian Cancer Survivorship: A Gynecological Oncology Group Study. *Psycho-Oncology* 11:142–153, 2002.

57. Penson RT, Wenzel LB, Vergote I, et al. Quality of Life Considerations in Gynecologic *Cancer.* 95 Suppl 1:S247–57,. 2006.

58. Stead, ML, Brown, JM, Fallowfield, L, et al. Lack of communication between healthcare professionals and women with ovarian cancer about sexual issues. *British Journal of Cancer,* 88:666–671, 2003.

59. Fitch M. Psychosocial Management of Patients with Recurrent Ovarian Cancer: Treating the Whole Patient to Improve Quality of Life. *Seminars in Oncology Nursing* 19 (3): 40–53, 2004.

60. Levine EG, Silver B, et al. A Pilot Study: Evaluation of a Psychosocial Program for Women with Gynecological Cancers. *Journal of Psychosocial Oncology* 25 (3):75–98, 2007.

61. Houck K, Avis NE, Gallant JM, et al. Quality of Life in Advanced Ovarian Cancer: Identifying Specific Concerns. *Journal of Palliative Medicine* 2(4):397–402, 1999.

62. von Gruenigen V, Huang HQ, Gil KM, et al. Assessment of Factors that Contribute to Decreased Quality of Life in Gynecologic Oncology Group Ovarian Cancer Trials. *Cancer* 115: 4857–4864, 2009.

63. von Gruenigen V, Huang HQ, Gil KM, et al. A Comparison of Quality of Life Domains and Clinical Factors in Ovarian Cancer Patients: A Gynecologic Oncology Group 39(5):839–846, 2010.

64. Ratner ES, Foran KA, Schwartz PE, et al. Sexuality and Intimacy in Gynecological Cancer. *Maturitas* 66:23–26, 2010.

65. Matulonis UA, Kornblith A, Lee H, et al. Long-term adjustment of early-stage ovarian cancer survivors. *Int J Gynecol Cancer* 18(6):1183–93, 2008.

66. Kornblith AB, Thaler HT, Wong G, et al. Quality of life in women with ovarian cancer. *Gynecol Oncol* 59:231–242, 1995.

67. Rustin GJ, van der Burg ME, Griffin CL, et al. Early versus delayed treatment of relapsed ovarian cancer (MRC OV05/EORTC 55955): a randomised trial. *Lancet.* 376(9747):1155–63, 2010.

68. Morgan RJ Jr, Alvarez RD, Armstrong DK, et al. Epithelial Ovarian Cancer. *J Natl Compr Canc Netw.* 9(1):82–113, 2011.

69. Greer BE, Koh WJ, Abu-Rustum NR. Cervical Cancer. *J Natl Compr Canc Netw.* 8(12):1388–416, 2010.

70. Greer BE, Koh WJ, Abu-Rustum N, et al. Uterine Neoplasms. Clinical Practice Guidelines in Oncology. *J Natl Compr Canc Netw.* 7(5):498–531, 2009.

28

HODGKIN'S DISEASE SURVIVORSHIP

KAREN WINKFIELD, MD, PHD, AND ANDREA NG, MD

INTRODUCTION

It is estimated that more than 8,000 men and women in the United States will be diagnosed with Hodgkin's lymphoma (HL) in 2010.[1] The incidence of HL shows two peaks: the first in young adulthood (age 15–35) and the second in those over 55 years old (Figure 28.1).[1] Improved staging as well as advances in systemic therapy and radiation techniques have resulted in steady improvements in overall survival in the last several decades (Figure 28.2). The young age at diagnosis combined with improved survival make it imperative to provide long-term follow-up of survivors to monitor for and effectively treat any late toxicity that may be associated with HL treatments. Studies of long-term survivors of HL have shown that while the cumulative incidence of cancer-specific mortality levels off over time, treatment-related deaths continue to rise.[2–5] The two leading causes of death in HL survivors are second malignancies and cardiovascular disease. Other late complications that can substantially reduce quality of life include non-coronary atherosclerotic disease, pulmonary disease, and endocrine dysfunction, such as hypothyroidism and infertility. Understanding therapy-related complications and the impact lifestyle choices may have can inform decisions regarding patient counseling and the appropriate strategies to be employed in the long-term care of survivors.

THERAPEUTIC ADVANCEMENTS

For many decades, extended-field radiation therapy alone was standard of care for patients with early stage HL.[6] Treatment fields were large and encompassed the site of disease at presentation as well as adjacent nodal areas. A standard mantle field encompasses the submandibular, cervical, supraclavicular, infraclavicular, axillary, mediastinal, subcarinal, and hilar lymph nodes. Radiation doses often exceeded 40 Gy. Chemotherapy had traditionally been used in the treatment of more advanced stages of HL, but were eventually incorporated into the treatment of early stage disease.[7,8] Tables 28.1

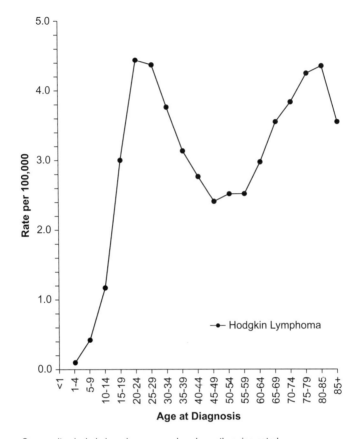

Cancer sites include invasive cases only unless otherwise noted.
Incidence source: SEER 13 areas (Sanfrancisco, Connecticut, Detroit, Hawaii, Iowa,
New Mexico, Seattle, Utah, Atlanta, San Jose-Monterey, Los Angeles, Alaska Native
Registry and Rural Georgia).

Figure 28.1. SEER Crude Incidence Rates, 1992–2007. (Adapted from www.seer
.cancer.gov.)

and 2 summarize the toxicities associated with radiation therapy and various
chemotherapeutic regimens for HL.

With the advent of combined modality therapy for early-stage disease,
fewer cycles of chemotherapy, smaller radiation treatment fields, and lower
radiation doses have been adopted. Following results of a recent randomized
trial, two cycles of ABVD (Doxorubicin [Adriamycin], Bleomycin, Vinblas-
tine, Dacarbazine) followed by 20 Gy of involved-field radiation therapy is
now the standard of care for selected patients with early-stage, favorable-
prognosis HL.[9] Efforts are ongoing to further reduce the radiation field size
from involved-field radiation therapy to involved-node radiation therapy.[10] It
is hoped that treatment reduction in carefully-selected, favorable patients will
reduce the risks of some of the long-term toxicities in current long-term HL
survivors.

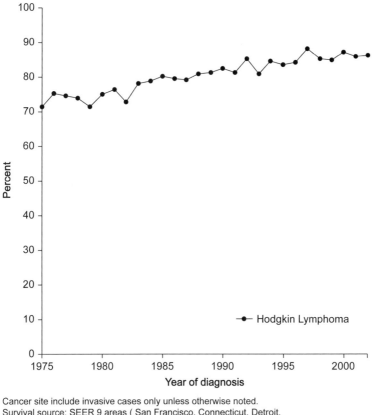

Cancer site include invasive cases only unless otherwise noted.
Survival source: SEER 9 areas (San Francisco, Connecticut, Detroit,
Hawaii, Iowa, New Mexico, Seattle, Utah, and Atlanta).
The 5-year survival estimates are calculated using monthly intervals.

Figure 28.2. SEER Relative Survival Rates, 1975–2002. (Adapted from www.seer
.cancer.gov.)

TABLE 28.1 TOXICITIES ASSOCIATED WITH RADIATION THERAPY FOR HODGKIN'S
LYMPHOMA

Acute and Subacute Complications	Temporary Local Alopecia
	Temporary Local Skin Reaction
	L'hermitte's Syndrome
	Radiation Pneumonitis
	Xerostomia/Dental Caries
	Hypothyroidism
Long-Term Complications	Second Malignancy
	Cardiac Disease
	Non-Coronary Vascular Disease
	Pulmonary Dysfunction
	Sterility (if pelvic irradiation)
	Esophageal dismotility (rare)
	Cervicoscapular muscular atrophy (rare)

TABLE 28.2 FIRST-LINE CHEMOTHERAPEUTIC REGIMENS USED IN TREATMENT OF CLASSICAL HODGKIN'S LYMPHOMA AND TOXICITIES

Regimen	Drugs Included	Acute Side Effects	Long-Term Toxicities
MOPP	Mechlorethamine Vincristine Prednisone Procarbazine	Fatigue Nausea/vomiting Alopecia Myelosuppresion Infection	Infertility Leukemia Solid tumors: (Lung cancer, gastric cancer)
Stanford V	Doxorubicin (Adriamycin) Mechlorethamine Vincristine Vinblastine Bleomycin Etoposide Prednisone	Fatigue Nausea/vomiting Alopecia Myelosuppre-sion Infection	Does not appear to be associated with leukemia and infertility risks; long term cardiopulmonary risk unknown
ABVD	Doxorubicin (Adriamycin) Bleomycin Vinblastine Dacarbazine	Fatigue Nausea/vomiting Alopecia Myelosuppre-sion Infection Peripheral neuropathy Bleomycin lung toxicity	Does not appear to be associated with leukemia and infertility risks; data on long-term cardiac risks emerging
BEACOPP (baseline or dose-escalated and variants)	Bleomycin Etoposide Adriamycin Cyclophosphamide Vincristine Procarbazine Prednisone	Fatigue Nausea/vomiting Alopecia Myelosuppre-sion Infection Peripheral neuropathy Bleomycin lung toxicity	Infertility Leukemia Long-term cardiopul-monary and solid tumor risks unknown

LONG-TERM TREATMENT SEQUELAE

Second Malignancy

Example: A.B. is a 51-year-old woman who presented at age 19 with a left neck mass. An excisional biopsy revealed Hodgkin's lymphoma, the nodular sclerosing type. A chest x-ray showed mediastinal adenopathy extending above the aortic arch and below the carina. Staging laparotomy, including splenectomy and liver biopsy, was performed. No subdiaphragmatic disease was noted. She completed a course of radiation to a total dose of 40 Gy to a mantle field (mediastinum, bilateral axillae, and neck) and para-aortic lymph nodes. No chemotherapy was given. She tolerated treatment well and had no evidence of recurrent disease. She has been followed by mammogram testing since the age of 30. A recent screening mammogram demonstrates a

7 mm nodule in the upper outer quadrant of the right breast; biopsy confirms invasive ductal carcinoma.

Second malignancies following treatment of HL are the leading cause of death in HL survivors, and include solid tumors, NHL, and leukemia. Solid tumors account for 70–80% of all second malignancies after HL, and are direct effects of the use of radiation and chemotherapy for treatment of HL.[4,11–13] The most common solid tumors after HL include cancers of the breast, lung, and gastrointestinal tract.[14] Much of the data regarding the development of second malignancies after treatment of HL are based on treatment regimens that have since been modified. However, HL survivors who are now middle-aged may have completed therapy decades ago during an age when larger radiation fields, higher radiation doses, and more toxic chemotherapeutic regimens were utilized. Additionally, while therapeutic improvements are expected to result in fewer second malignancies, the data from trials evaluating modern treatment regimens is not fully matured. Therefore, all HL survivors should have adequate screening programs in place.

Breast Cancer

The incidence of breast cancer is significantly higher in HL patients, particularly those who received radiation as part of their treatment.[15] The latency period for the development of breast cancer is about 10–15 years following treatment of HL.[15] Women diagnosed with and treated for HL at a young age (age < 35) have a significantly higher risk of developing breast cancer than women diagnosed over the age of 35.[4,15–18] Higher doses of radiation and large treatment fields also increase the risk of developing breast cancer.[5,16,18] One study showed that mantle field irradiation was associated with a 2.7-fold increased risk of breast cancer compared with mediastinal irradiation alone.[19] Similarly, a meta-analysis found that extended field-radiotherapy was associated with a significantly higher breast cancer risk than involved-field radiotherapy (odds ratio = 3.25, $p = 0.04$).[20] Patients who experience early menopause due either to chemotherapy or pelvic irradiation have a reduced breast cancer risk from other HL survivors, indicating that hormonal exposure is a modifier of breast cancer risk following treatment of HL.[5,18,21]

Lung Cancer and Malignancies of the Gastrointestinal Tract

Use of radiation therapy, alkylating chemotherapy, and smoking are all associated with an increased risk of lung cancer in HL patients.[11,22,23] A significant dose-response relationship for the development of lung cancer has been demonstrated for both the use of radiation and chemotherapy,[11,23] and smoking was found to have a multiplicative effect on treatment-related lung cancer in patients treated with both radiotherapy and alkylating chemotherapy.[22] While solid tumors of the esophagus, stomach, colorectum, pancreas, and liver are significantly increased after HL when compared to the general population,[11,12,14,22] the absolute risk of developing a gastrointestinal cancer is still quite low (less than 5/10,000 person years). In general, chemotherapy did not seem to increase the risk of solid tumors in the gastrointestinal tract, although doses of procarbazine >13,000mg did result in a significant increase in risk of gastric cancer compared to patients with lower doses.[24] As with both breast and lung cancer, increasing radiation dose to the gastrointestinal tract results in an increased risk of second malignancy.[24]

Leukemia

The risk of developing leukemia following treatment for HL is related to the use of alkylating chemotherapy, and increases in a dose-dependent manner with relative risk increasing with the number of chemotherapy cycles used.[25,26] The current standard chemotherapy for HL, ABVD, does not appear to be associated with risk of leukemia,[27] although there is a leukemia risk with dose-escalated BEACOPP, which has been shown to be superior to standard-dose chemotherapy in advanced-stage HL[28] (see Table 28.2).

Cardiovascular Morbidity

Example (con'd): During initial evaluation, A.B. reveals that at age 39 she experienced a sudden, temporary loss of vision in her left eye. A bilateral carotid ultrasound revealed diffuse atherosclerosis with 40–60% stenosis of the left carotid artery and 20–40% stenosis on the right. She was placed on Coumadin, aspirin, and metoprolol. Three years later, she developed exertional chest pain. Cardiac catheterization showed total occlusion of the left subclavian artery, 90% occlusion of the left main coronary artery, and 50% occlusion of the right coronary artery. She underwent triple bypass surgery and stenting of the left subclavian artery.

Coronary Artery Disease and Valvular Dysfunction

Cardiac mortality is the leading non-cancer cause of death in long-term HL survivors. Chemotherapy and radiation therapy both contribute to cardiac toxicity. HL survivors experience a three to five-fold risk of coronary artery disease when compared to the general population.[29,30] Cardiac toxicity from radiation therapy is related to radiation dose and includes pericardial disease, cardiomyopathy, conduction defects, valvular defects, and coronary artery disease.[31] The risk of radiation-induced valvular dysfunction, including stenosis and aortic regurgitation, increases with time from treatment, and may not be detected by physical exam alone.[32]

Doxorubicin-based chemotherapy alone has been associated with increased cardiac mortality, although studies showing this effect are limited by small numbers of patients and short follow-up time.[20,33,34] Patients with advanced stages of HL are treated aggressively with more cycles of chemotherapy, and therefore cumulative doses of doxorubicin are higher. However, the competing risk of cancer-specific mortality may confound the results of these smaller studies. Cardiac morbidity increases with the use of combined modality therapy. Studies show that hospitalization due to cardiac morbidity increases with doxorubicin plus mediastinal radiation when compared to patients treated with radiation alone.[29,30] Traditional cardiac risk factors, including hyperlipidemia, hypertension, diabetes mellitus, and smoking, are additional modifiers that contribute to the risk of treatment-related cardiac disease after HL.[29,30,35]

Noncoronary Atherosclerotic Vascular Disease

Mantle field and neck irradiation for HL have been associated with a two to five-fold risk of stroke compared to the normal population.[19,36,37] In one study, the incidence was 2% at 5, 3% at 10, and 7% at 20 years.[35] However, the absolute excess risks are low, estimated at 0.1% per person per year. Routine duplex screening of the carotid arteries is therefore likely of low yield. As with other long-term sequelae, there is significant radiation dose response relationship in the development of noncoronary atherosclerotic vascular disease.[35] As with coronary artery disease, traditional risk factors for stroke such as smoking, diabetes, and hypertension further added to the risk of cerebrovascular accidents in HL survivors.[19]

Endocrine Dysfunction

Hypothyroidism is observed in up to 60% of HL survivors who had radiation as part of their treatment regimen.[17,38,39] The risk of thyroid dysfunction is related to the dose of radiation delivered.[39,40] Thyroid stimulating hormone levels should be included as part of routine follow-up blood tests in patients who have received neck irradiation to detect subclinical cases of hypothyroidism.

Infertility is a major concern for both men and women of childbearing age who are undergoing treatment for HL. The risk of infertility is primarily related to exposure to alkylating chemotherapy, but can be related to pelvic radiation as well. Loss of fertility was a significant side effect of treatment with MOPP.[41,42] Use of ABVD in early stage disease has resulted in improved fertility rates in HL survivors. Although ABVD is associated with azoospermia, the majority of men show recovery of spermatogenesis following treatment.[43] Female gonadal function also appears to be preserved after treatment with ABVD.[44] The more intense chemotherapeutic regimens utilized in advanced stages of HL are still associated with increased sterility. In particular, BEA-COPP and its variants have been shown to induce continuous amenorrhea in more than 50% of women treated with eight cycles of chemotherapy.[45] Most men develop azoospermia following treatment with BEACOPP on sperm function. In one study, only 10% of patients had recovery of spermatogenesis after a median period of 3.6 years.[46]

TABLE 28.3 CURRENT FOLLOW-UP RECOMMENDATIONS FOR SURVIVORS OF
HODGKIN'S LYMPHOMA (ADAPTED)

Late Effects	Follow-Up Recommendations
Breast cancer	- Annual breast examination - Annual screening mammogram 8 years after treatment or by age 40 - Consider breast magnetic resonance imaging screening as an adjunct to mammogram - Consider referral to high-risk breast clinic for discussion of chemoprevention
Lung cancer	- Smoking cessation
Skin cancer	- Annual skin examination - Sun safety practice
Cardiac disease	- Referral to cardiologist for baseline evaluation 10 years after treatment - Resting and stress echocardiogram (frequency depending on baseline findings and existence of other cardiac risk factors) - Reduction of traditional risk factors (lipid screening, blood pressure control, smoking cessation, physical activity, healthy diet)
Non-coronary vascular disease	- Annual examination for carotid bruits; obtain carotid ultrasound if suspicious clinical findings - Reduction of traditional risk factors (lipid screening, blood pressure control, smoking cessation, physical activity, healthy diet)
Infertility	- Referral to reproductive endocrinologist as needed
Hypothyroidism	- Annual thyroid examination - Annual thyroid function tests

Men and women of child-bearing age should be adequately counseled regarding endocrine dysfunction and fertility issues before treatment for HL is initiated. If indicated, referral to a fertility specialist is encouraged.

FOLLOW-UP GUIDELINES

In the first five years of post-treatment surveillance after HL, the focus is on the detection of relapsed HL and to manage acute and subacute side effects of treatment. The follow-up includes physical exams, blood tests, and radiographic tests. The current National Comprehensive Cancer Network (NCCN) practice guidelines suggest restaging with CT-based imaging every 6 to 12 months for the first two to three years, and then annually up to five years.[47] Annual blood pressure, serum glucose, and lipid screening are also recommended.

After five years, the attention shifts towards screening for and management of late effects of therapy. Table 28.3 summarizes recommendations on follow-up for long-term HL survivors. Annual mammogram should begin no later than 8 to 10 years after treatment, or at age 40, whichever comes first. Chemoprevention strategies with the use of anti-estrogens such as tamoxifen or raloxifene have been explored in high risk populations.[48-50] Referral to a high-risk clinic for counseling regarding chemoprevention may be of benefit in women at increased breast cancer risk due to their treatment history and other risk factors. Breast MRI as an adjunct to mammogram is recommended by the American Cancer Society for women with history of chest irradiation between ages 10–30. However, clinical data on its utility in the HL survivor population is unknown. The potential increased sensitivity needs to be weighed against increased false positive findings leading to unnecessary biopsies and anxiety.

The optimal cardiac screening tests and screening intervals are unknown. Evaluation by cardiac specialists is strongly encouraged in patients who are 10 years or longer out from chest irradiation. The NCCN recommends that a baseline stress test or echocardiogram be considered at 10 years.

LIFESTYLE MODIFICATIONS

HL survivors can improve their outcomes by maintaining a healthy lifestyle. Minimizing traditional risk factors for cardiovascular disease is essential. Survivors should be encouraged to address any current cardiac risk factors that they have, including hypertension, diabetes, obesity, physical inactivity, and smoking. Smoking cessation will reduce the risk of lung cancer, cardiac disease, and stroke. HL survivors should undergo routine skin examination and encouraged to adopt sun-safety practice to reduce skin cancer risks. To address chronic health conditions, referral to medical specialists may be required. However, survivors can improve their overall health by avoiding poor health habits, including smoking or overeating, and maintaining excellent health habits such as weight control and exercise. Lifestyle modifications along with regular lipid, cardiac, and cancer screening are critical to prolonging overall survival of HL survivors.

COORDINATED CARE

As previously noted, most of the complications of treatment are closely related to the extent of treatment exposure. Given the high cure rate of HL, especially for patients with early-stage disease, considerable effort has been directed at treatment reduction in recent years, including reduction in radiation field size and dose, omission of radiotherapy, and reduction of the number of cycles of chemotherapy.[9,10] However, many treatment-related complications are associated with long latency periods, some of which may take decades for manifestation. Extended follow-up is therefore needed to fully document the long-term consequences of modern therapy for HL.

HL survivors and their oncologists are encouraged to maintain relationships with the primary care physicians through the course of treatment and during long-term follow-up. Although much of the follow-up care for HL survivors will be provided by specialists, the primary care provider is an important ally during survivorship and should be aware of the screening recommendations and the results of tests performed.

REFERENCES

1. SEER database. Accessed September 29, 2010.

2. Cosset JM, Henry-Amar M, Meerwaldt JH. Long-term toxicity of early stages of Hodgkin's disease therapy: the EORTC experience. EORTC Lymphoma Cooperative Group. *Ann Oncol.* 1991;2 Suppl 2:77–82.

3. Hoppe RT. Hodgkin's disease: complications of therapy and excess mortality. *Ann Oncol.* 1997;8(Suppl 1):115–118.

4. Ng AK, Bernardo MV, Weller E, et al. Second malignancy after Hodgkin disease treated with radiation therapy with or without chemotherapy: long-term risks and risk factors. *Blood.* Sep 15 2002;100(6):1989–1996.

5. van Leeuwen FE, Klokman WJ, Stovall M, et al. Roles of radiation dose, chemotherapy, and hormonal factors in breast cancer following Hodgkin's disease. *J Natl Cancer Inst.* Jul 2 2003;95(13):971–980.

6. Duhmke E, Franklin J, Pfreundschuh M, et al. Low-dose radiation is sufficient for the noninvolved extended-field treatment in favorable early-stage Hodgkin's disease: long-term results of a randomized trial of radiotherapy alone. *J Clin Oncol.* Jun 1 2001;19(11):2905–2914.

7. Connors JM. State-of-the-art therapeutics: Hodgkin's lymphoma. *J Clin Oncol.* Sep 10 2005;23(26):6400–6408.

8. Macdonald DA, Connors JM. New strategies for the treatment of early stages of Hodgkin's lymphoma. *Hematol Oncol Clin North Am.* Oct 2007;21(5):871–880.

9. Engert A, Plütschow A, Eich HT, Lohri A, Dörken B. Reduced Treatment Intensity in Patients with Early-Stage Hodgkin's Lymphoma. *N Engl J Med.* 2010;363:640–652.

10. Girinsky T, van der Maazen R, Specht L, et al. Involved-node radiotherapy (INRT) in patients with early Hodgkin lymphoma: concepts and guidelines. *Radiother Oncol.* Jun 2006;79(3):270–277.

11. Dores GM, Metayer C, Curtis RE, et al. Second malignant neoplasms among long-term survivors of Hodgkin's disease: a population-based evaluation over 25 years. *J Clin Oncol.* Aug 15 2002;20(16):3484–3494.

12. Swerdlow AJ, Barber JA, Hudson GV, et al. Risk of second malignancy after Hodgkin's disease in a collaborative British cohort: the relation to age at treatment. *J Clin Oncol.* 2000;18(3):498–509.

13. van Leeuwen FE, Klokman WJ, Veer MB, et al. Long-term risk of second malignancy in survivors of Hodgkin's disease treated during adolescence or young adulthood. *J Clin Oncol.* 2000;18(3):487–497.

14. Hodgson DC, Gilbert ES, Dores GM, et al. Long-term solid cancer risk among 5-year survivors of Hodgkin's lymphoma. *J Clin Oncol.* Apr 20 2007;25(12):1489–1497.

15. Hancock SL, Tucker MA, Hoppe RT. Breast cancer after treatment of Hodgkin's disease. *J Natl Cancer Inst.* Jan 6 1993;85(1):25–31.

16. Inskip PD, Robison LL, Stovall M, et al. Radiation dose and breast cancer risk in the childhood cancer survivor study. *J Clin Oncol.* Aug 20 2009;27(24):3901–3907.

17. Robison LL, Bhatia S. Late-effects among survivors of leukemia and lymphoma during childhood and adolescence. *Br J Haematol.* Aug 2003;122(3):345–359.

18. Travis LB, Hill DA, Dores GM, et al. Breast cancer following radiotherapy and chemotherapy among young women with Hodgkin disease. *Jama.* Jul 23 2003;290(4):465–475.

19. De Bruin ML, Dorresteijn LD, van't Veer MB, et al. Increased risk of stroke and transient ischemic attack in 5-year survivors of Hodgkin lymphoma. *J Natl Cancer Inst.* Jul 1 2009;101(13):928–937.

20. Franklin J, Pluetschow A, Paus M, et al. Second malignancy risk associated with treatment of Hodgkin's lymphoma: meta-analysis of the randomized trials. *Ann Oncol.* Dec 2006;17(12):1749–1760.

21. Hill DA, Gilbert E, Dores GM, et al. Breast cancer risk following radiotherapy for Hodgkin lymphoma: modification by other risk factors. *Blood.* Nov 15 2005;106(10):3358–3365.

22. van Leeuwen FE, Klokman WJ, Stovall M, et al. Roles of radiotherapy and smoking in lung cancer following Hodgkin's disease. *J Natl Cancer Inst.* 1995;87(20):1530–1537.

23. Willemze R, Jaffe ES, Burg G, et al. WHO-EORTC classification for cutaneous lymphomas. *Blood.* Feb 3 2005.

24. van den Belt-Dusebout AW, Aleman BM, Besseling G, et al. Roles of radiation dose and chemotherapy in the etiology of stomach cancer as a second malignancy. *Int J Radiat Oncol Biol Phys.* Dec 1 2009;75(5):1420–1429.

25. Kaldor JM, Day NE, Clarke EA, et al. Leukemia following Hodgkin's disease. *N Engl J Med.* Jan 4 1990;322(1):7–13.

26. van Leeuwen FE, Chorus AM, van den Belt-Dusebout AW, et al. Leukemia risk following Hodgkin's disease: relation to cumulative dose of alkylating agents, treatment with teniposide combinations, number of episodes of chemotherapy, and bone marrow damage. *J Clin Oncol.* 1994;12(5):1063–1073.

27. Schonfeld SJ, Gilbert ES, Dores GM, et al. Acute myeloid leukemia following Hodgkin lymphoma: a population-based study of 35,511 patients. *J Natl Cancer Inst.* Feb 1 2006;98(3):215–218.

28. Engert A, Diehl V, Franklin J, et al. Escalated-dose BEACOPP in the treatment of patients with advanced-stage Hodgkin's lymphoma: 10 years of follow-up of the GHSG HD9 study. *J Clin Oncol.* Sep 20 2009;27(27):4548–4554.

29. Aleman BM, van den Belt-Dusebout AW, De Bruin ML, et al. Late cardiotoxicity after treatment for Hodgkin lymphoma. *Blood.* Mar 1 2007;109(5):1878–1886.

30. Myrehaug S, Pintilie M, Tsang R, et al. Cardiac morbidity following modern treatment for Hodgkin lymphoma: supra-additive cardiotoxicity of doxorubicin and radiation therapy. *Leuk Lymphoma.* Aug 2008;49(8):1486–1493.

31. Gaya AM, Ashford RF. Cardiac complications of radiation therapy. *Clin Oncol (R Coll Radiol).* May 2005;17(3):153–159.

32. Heidenreich PA, Hancock SL, Lee BK, Mariscal CS, Schnittger I. Asymptomatic cardiac disease following mediastinal irradiation. *J Am Coll Cardiol.* Aug 20 2003;42(4):743–749.

33. Swerdlow AJ, Higgins CD, Smith P, et al. Myocardial infarction mortality risk after treatment for Hodgkin disease: a collaborative British cohort study. *J Natl Cancer Inst.* Feb 7 2007;99(3):206–214.

34. Myrehaug S, Pintilie M, Yun L, et al. A population-based study of cardiac morbidity among Hodgkin lymphoma patients with pre-existing heart disease. *Blood.* Jul 1.

35. Hull MC, Morris CG, Pepine CJ, Mendenhall NP. Valvular dysfunction and carotid, subclavian, and coronary artery disease in survivors of Hodgkin lymphoma treated with radiation therapy. *Jama.* Dec 3 2003;290(21):2831–2837.

36. Bowers DC, McNeil DE, Liu Y, et al. Stroke as a late treatment effect of Hodgkin's Disease: a report from the Childhood Cancer Survivor Study. *J Clin Oncol.* Sep 20 2005;23(27):6508–6515.

37. Morris B, Partap S, Yeom K, Gibbs IC, Fisher PG, King AA. Cerebrovascular disease in childhood cancer survivors: A Children's Oncology Group Report. *Neurology.* Dec 1 2009;73(22):1906–1913.

38. Hancock SL, Cox RS, McDougall IR. Thyroid diseases after treatment of Hodgkin's disease. *N Engl J Med.* Aug 29 1991;325(9):599–605.

39. Weiss LM, Movahed LA, Warnke RA, Sklar J. Detection of Epstein-Barr viral genomes in Reed-Sternberg cells of Hodgkin's disease. *N Engl J Med.* Feb 23 1989;320(8):502–506.

40. Constine LS, Donaldson SS, McDougall IR, Cox RS, Link MP, Kaplan HS. Thyroid dysfunction after radiotherapy in children with Hodgkin's disease. *Cancer.* Feb 15 1984;53(4):878–883.

41. De Bruin ML, Huisbrink J, Hauptmann M, et al. Treatment-related risk factors for premature menopause following Hodgkin lymphoma. *Blood.* Jan 1 2008;111(1):101–108.

42. van der Kaaij MA, Heutte N, Le Stang N, et al. Gonadal function in males after chemotherapy for early-stage Hodgkin's lymphoma treated in four subsequent trials by the European Organisation for Research and Treatment of Cancer: EORTC Lymphoma Group and the Groupe d'Etude des Lymphomes de l'Adulte. *J Clin Oncol.* Jul 1 2007;25(19):2825–2832.

43. Anselmo AP, Cartoni C, Bellantuono P, Maurizi-Enrici R, Aboulkair N, Ermini M. Risk of infertility in patients with Hodgkin's disease treated with ABVD vs MOPP vs ABVD/MOPP. *Haematologica.* Mar-Apr 1990;75(2):155–158.

44. Hodgson DC, Pintilie M, Gitterman L, et al. Fertility among female Hodgkin lymphoma survivors attempting pregnancy following ABVD chemotherapy. *Hematol Oncol.* Mar 2007;25(1):11–15.

45. Behringer K, Breuer K, Reineke T, et al. Secondary amenorrhea after Hodgkin's lymphoma is influenced by age at treatment, stage of disease, chemotherapy regimen, and the use of oral contraceptives during therapy: a report from the German Hodgkin's Lymphoma Study Group. *J Clin Oncol.* Oct 20 2005;23(30):7555–7564.

46. Sieniawski M, Reineke T, Nogova L, et al. Fertility in male patients with advanced Hodgkin lymphoma treated with BEACOPP: a report of the German Hodgkin Study Group (GHSG). *Blood.* Jan 1 2008;111(1):71–76.

47. NCCN Clinical Practice Guidelines for Hodgkin Lymphoma v.2.2010.

48. Cummings SR, Eckert S, Krueger KA, et al. The effect of raloxifene on risk of breast cancer in postmenopausal women: results from the MORE randomized trial. Multiple Outcomes of Raloxifene Evaluation. *Jama.* Jun 16 1999;281(23):2189–2197.

49. Fisher B, Costantino JP, Wickerham DL, et al. Tamoxifen for prevention of breast cancer: report of the National Surgical Adjuvant Breast and Bowel Project P-1 Study. *J Natl Cancer Inst.* Sep 16 1998;90(18):1371–1388.

50. Veronesi U, Maisonneuve P, Costa A, et al. Prevention of breast cancer with tamoxifen: preliminary findings from the Italian randomized trial among hysterectomised women. Italian Tamoxifen Prevention Study. *Lancet.* Jul 11 1998;352(9122):93–97.

29

Non–Hodgkin's Lymphoma Survivorship

Matthew S. Davids, MD, Richard N. Boyajian, NP, and David C. Fisher, MD

Introduction

Non-Hodgkin lymphomas (NHL) are a diverse group of lymphoproliferative disorders with a wide range in their clinical course. While the more indolent forms of NHL, such as follicular lymphoma, are unlikely to be cured with conventional therapy, aggressive NHL subtypes, such as diffuse large B cell lymphoma (DLBCL) can increasingly be cured with intensive chemotherapy sometimes in combination with radiotherapy. Approximately 65,000 people were diagnosed with NHL in the United States in 2010, and the incidence of the disease is on the rise.[1] In fact, the incidence of NHL has approximately doubled since the 1970s, with a continued 1–2% increase per year in the 2000s. These increases have been seen predominantly in high-grade, potentially curable subtypes.[2] With a median age at diagnosis of 67, NHL is often a disease of middle-aged and older adults, yet as the life expectancy of the general population continues to increase, NHL survivors now commonly live for many years after completing curative therapy. The age-specific (crude) incidence rates for NHL are depicted in Figure 29.1.

NHL survivors often must deal with long-lasting toxicities of intensive therapy. Second malignancies, cardiovascular disease, infertility, and other endocrine dysfunction, as well as cognitive sequelae, are all commonly seen in this population. In this chapter, we will briefly review recent therapeutic advancements in NHL and then describe the commonly observed long-term toxicities in survivors of these treatments. Through a deepened understanding of these late treatment effects, we can begin to more effectively counsel our patients on the risks they face and the lifestyle modifications and other interventions that can reduce the ill effects of these complications. Effectively managing these consequences of therapy may improve the quality of life (QOL) of NHL survivors, and has the potential to prolong their survival even further.

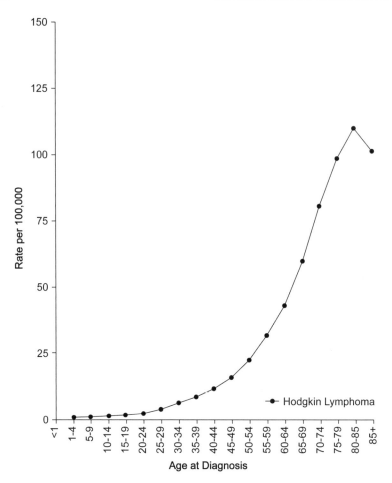

Cancer sites include invasive cases only unless otherwise noted.
Incidence source: SEER 13 areas (San Francisco, Connecticut, Detroit, Hawaii, Iowa, New Mexico, Seattle, Utah, Atlanta, San Jose-Monterey, Los Angeles, Alaska Native Registry and Rural Georgia).
Rates are per 100,000.
Data points were not shown for rates that were based on less than 16 cases.

Figure 29.1. SEER Crude Incidence Rates, 1992–2007. (Adapted from www.seer .cancer.gov.)

THERAPEUTIC ADVANCEMENTS

Aggressive, high grade NHL used to be uniformly lethal within weeks to months after diagnosis. The advent of modern chemotherapy in the 1940s and 1950s provided hope that the disease could potentially be curable. Indeed, NHL was one of the first malignancies to be successfully cured with combination chemotherapy alone. Early nitrogen mustard and alkylator-based combinations were highly toxic, and only cured a small number patients. In the 1970s, the CHOP (cyclophosphamide, doxorubicin, vincristine, and prednisone) combination was pioneered at the NCI, and was able to improve cure rates while reducing toxicities. With the addition of the monoclonal antibody rituximab in the late 1990s, the standard first-line therapy for aggressive NHL used today, CHOP-R, was established.

Using a typical eight cycle course of CHOP-R chemotherapy in advanced DLBCL, the five year overall survival rate is now on the order of 60%.[3] In limited-stage DLBCL, three cycles of CHOP followed by involved-field radiotherapy has been able to achieve a five year overall survival rate of 82%,[4] and the addition of rituximab to this regimen has likely pushed survival rates over 90%. These therapeutic advancements have helped the number of survivors of DLBCL and other aggressive NHL subtypes to grow steadily in recent years.

Though the strides made in improving NHL cure rates have been significant, a substantial minority of patients ultimately died of the disease. Much attention has been paid to improving cure rates and developing new regimens that are effective in these patients with relapsed disease. The challenges facing NHL survivors has, in general, been less well studied. Though fortunate to have been cured, NHL survivors must deal with a diverse array of long-term sequelae with the potential to negatively impact both their quality of life and ultimately their survival. Toxicities of radiotherapy and front-line chemotherapy are summarized in Tables 29.1 and 29.2, respectively.

TABLE 29.1 TOXICITIES ASSOCIATED WITH RADIATION THERAPY FOR NON-HODGKIN'S LYMPHOMA

Acute and Subacute Complications	Temporary Local Alopecia
	Temporary Local Skin Reaction
	L'hermitte's Syndrome
	Radiation Pneumonitis
	Xerostomia/Dental Caries
	Hypothyroidism
Long-Term Complications	Second Malignancy
	Cardiac Disease
	Non-Coronary Vascular Disease
	Pulmonary Dysfunction
	Sterility (if pelvic irradiation)
	Esophageal dysmotility (rare)
	Cervicoscapular muscular atrophy (rare)

TABLE 29.2 TOXICITIES OF THE MOST COMMON FIRST-LINE CHEMOTHERAPEUTIC
REGIMEN USED IN THE TREATMENT OF AGGRESSIVE NON-HODGKIN'S LYMPHOMA

Regimen	Drugs Included	Acute Side Effects	Long-Term Toxicities
CHOP-R	Cyclophosphamide	Fatigue	Second malignancies:
	Doxorubicin	Nausea/Vomiting	(leukemia and solid
	Vincristine	Alopecia	tumors)
	Prednisone	Myelosuppresion	Congestive heart
	Rituximab	Infection	failure
		Peripheral	Stroke
		neuropathy	Progressive
		Constipation	multifocal leukoen-
		Infusion reactions	cephalopathy (rare)

LONG-TERM TREATMENT SEQUELAE

Second Malignancies

Case Example: RR was 56 years old in 2002 when he was diagnosed with stage III, grade 3B follicular lymphoma. He received 8 cycles of CHOP and Rituxan, achieved a complete remission, and then received consolidation with autologous stem cell transplantation using high dose Cytoxan, BCNU, and etoposide conditioning. He remained in remission, but in 2009, he noticed new fatigue and recurrent sinus infections. His blood counts began to gradually drop, and he became mildly leukopenic, anemic, and thrombocytopenic. Bone marrow biopsy revealed a hypercellular marrow with numerous dysplastic forms and less than 5% blasts, and cytogenetics revealed monosomy 7. He was diagnosed with myelodysplastic syndrome, refractory anemia subtype, and referred for a reduced intensity allogeneic stem cell transplantation.

As illustrated in the case, perhaps no treatment complication is more devastating to an NHL survivor both physically and psychologically than the development of a second malignancy. Though often mentioned upfront as a risk by the treating oncologist, most patients when faced with a new diagnosis of cancer pay little attention to the small possibility of developing a future malignancy. It may be hard for a cancer patient to imagine that chemotherapy and radiation, the very treatments used to cure cancer, may also play a role in causing a new cancer to develop.

Yet the development of a second malignancy is unfortunately a common problem in NHL survivors. A cohort of 2,456 NHL patients under the age of 60 were found to have developed 123 second malignancies (5% of the cohort), with a 15-year cumulative risk of 11.2%.[5] By comparing rates seen in the study to rates in the general population, the standard incidence ratio (SIR) of three cancers in particular were found to be elevated: leukemia (SIR

8.8, 17 cases), lung cancer (SIR 1.6, 28 cases), and colon cancer (SIR 1.4, 10 cases). The relative risks were highest for patients who were younger at the time of treatment.

In a large study, 28,131 NHL patients from the Swedish Cancer Registry were found to have a SIR for all solid tumors of 1.65 (2,290 patients) and for hematologic malignancies of 5.36 (369 patients).[6] Of the 25 solid tumor sites evaluated, the SIR was elevated in all but nine of the sites. Younger patients were again found to be at higher cumulative risk, as the SIR for solid tumors increased up to 30 years after NHL diagnosis, with a peak between years 21 to 30 after diagnosis. Interestingly, women and men not receiving chemotherapy without radiation were found to be at slightly decreased risk for developing breast and prostate cancer, respectively. However, women who do go on to develop breast cancer after being cured of lymphoma may have a poorer prognosis than patients with de novo breast cancer. In a study of 53 women who developed breast cancer following lymphoma, 18 (34%) of whom had NHL, women who previously had lymphoma had a five-year DFS 54.5% versus 91% for matched controls, and a five-year OS of 86.6% versus 98.6% for controls, both of which were statistically significant.[7] The authors hypothesize that women with a previous lymphoma diagnosis may have been undertreated for their breast cancer, particularly with regard to irradiation.

In the largest study published to date, 77,876 NHL patients reported through the NCI's Surveillance, Epidemiology, and End Results (SEER) Program were followed, and 5,638 patients developed secondary malignancies, significantly more than the endemic rate (O/E, 1.14).[8] Patients receiving radiotherapy as part of their NHL treatment were at particularly high risk of developing sarcomas, breast cancers, and mesothelioma.

These risks of secondary malignancy are not unique to patients with advanced stage NHL. In a small retrospective study, four patients were found to have developed squamous cell carcinoma of the head and neck after receiving radiotherapy to this area as part of definitive therapy for localized, early-stage NHL.[9] This study highlights the need for close surveillance for second malignancies even for survivors of localized NHL.

Cardiovascular

As cardiovascular disease is the leading cause of death for all Americans, parsing out the increased risk for NHL survivors compared to the normal population can be challenging. In a study looking at 141 survivors of both NHL and Hodgkin lymphoma, only one patient developed long-term clinically significant congestive heart failure, though evidence of subclinical cardiomyopathy was detected on echocardiogram in 39 patients.[10] More recent studies suggest that the long-term clinically significant cardiovascular risks of undergoing chemotherapy and/or radiotherapy for NHL may be more substantial than was previously appreciated in earlier studies.

Case Example: M.A. was 65 years old in 2005 when he was diagnosed with stage IV DLBCL. He was treated with six cycles of R-CHOP chemotherapy, with a total cumulative dose of Adriamycin of 300 mg/m^2, and he achieved a complete remission. He continued to follow with his oncologist and in a survivorship clinic for the next five years. In 2010, he mentioned that although he was able to climb up and down from the cellar to the attic several times a day, he had noticed new dyspnea on exertion, but he attributed this to old age. He had a history of borderline HTN and prior smoking. An echocardiogram was performed and revealed an ejection fraction (EF) of 35% with global LV hypokinesis, consistent with congestive heart failure. He was referred to a cardiologist, who started him on an ACE inhibitor and beta-blocker. Although his EF remains mildly decreased, over time M.A. has noticed a significant improvement in his exercise tolerance.

In a large European study looking at cardiovascular risk for patients treated for aggressive NHL in the 1980s and 1990s, 476 patients who had received at least six cycles of doxorubicin-based chemotherapy were examined.[11] NHL survivors had an absolute cumulative incidence of cardiac disease that was 12% above that of the general population at five years, and 22% above at 10 years. Survivors were at particularly high risk for congestive heart failure (CHF) (SIR 5.4), with a smaller but still significant increase in the risk of stroke (SIR 1.8). Patients receiving radiotherapy (>40 Gy) were at particularly high risk of stroke. Interestingly, risk of coronary artery disease (CAD) was similar to that of the general population. In line with this observation is that most of the cases of CHF observed were found to be due to non-ischemic cardiomyopathy and rhythm disturbances much more frequently than CAD. This study also identified key risk factors for the development of cardiovascular events in NHL survivors. Pre-existing hypertension, young age at NHL diagnosis, need for salvage treatment, and amount of radiotherapy all correlated with an increased risk of the subsequent development of cardiac disease. Those patients receiving lower amounts of radiation (<40 Gy) and those not receiving mediastinal radiation appeared to be at the lowest risk of future cardiotoxicity.

In addition to these long-term cardiac toxicities, anthracycline-based chemotherapy has also been shown to have toxicity soon after completing NHL treatment. A retrospective study of 135 consecutive NHL patients undergoing CHOP in the 1990s found that 27 (20%) of patients developed a cardiac event within one year of treatment.[12] Fourteen of these patients had clinical signs of CHF, and three patients died suddenly from presumed cardiac causes. Cumulative dose of doxorubicin > 200 mg/m^2 and age > 50 appeared to be the most significant risk factors for an event on multivariate analysis.

Infertility and Endocrine Dysfunction

Given that the NHL patient population is generally middle-aged or elderly, the effects of treatment on fertility are not problematic for many survivors.

Case Example: D.B. was a 26 year-old newlywed in 2010 when she was diagnosed with stage IA anaplastic large cell lymphoma, ALK negative. It was recommended that she receive six cycles of CHOP chemotherapy and then proceed to consolidation with high dose autologous stem cell transplantation. After a discussion with her oncologist regarding the rate of infertility post-transplantation, she decided to postpone CHOP for three weeks in order to have urgent in vitro fertilization. She received an FSH injection, followed later by an HCG injection to stimulate her ovaries to produce and release a large number of eggs. The eggs were then surgically harvested and fertilized in a Petri dish with her husband's donated sperm to create several embryos. The highest quality embryos were then frozen for future use. D.B. was anxious about the delay in the treatment of her aggressive lymphoma, but this delay did not negatively impact her outcome. She had more peace of mind knowing that despite receiving aggressive therapy that she would likely be able to become pregnant using one of the frozen embryos, giving her the chance to have her own family.

However, for younger patients treated for NHL, decreased fertility following treatment is a major concern. As highlighted in the case, patients receiving high dose chemotherapy for stem cell transplantation, as well as those receiving salvage chemotherapy regimens, are at risk for infertility. This risk increases the older a patient is at the time of treatment.

In contrast to salvage and transplantation regimens, patients undergoing frontline chemotherapy for NHL can generally be reassured that their risk for infertility is low. A study of 36 Israeli women treated for aggressive NHL found that although half of the patients had amenorrhea during treatment, all but two patients recovered menses in the first remission, typically in the first three months after completing chemotherapy.[13] Eighteen patients (50%) became pregnant during the first remission. Those women who were given fertility-preserving measures such as GnRH agonists or OCPs were not found to improve recovery of regular menstruation or increase rates of pregnancy compared to those women treated without these interventions.

Another study looked at the effects of an intensified chemotherapy regimen with high-dose cyclophosphamide (so-called Mega-CHOP) in 13 consecutive women under age 40 with aggressive NHL.[14] Similarly, they found no significant effect of this regimen on fertility, with only one case of premature ovarian failure, and eight patients conceiving spontaneously and delivering healthy babies.

Male NHL survivors may also be concerned about the effects of chemotherapy and radiation on their fertility. A recent study from Norway looked at nearly 300 men under the age of 50 who were survivors of either NHL or HL and were treated with a variety of chemotherapy regimens.[15] Patients with NHL treated with CHOP-based chemotherapy were not at significantly increased risk of endocrine hypogonadism, as determined by abnormal LH, FSH, and testosterone levels. About 20% of these patients did have abnormal hormonal levels, but this was not significantly different than a group of patients receiving either no chemotherapy or receiving ABVD chemotherapy for Hodgkin lymphoma. NHL patients requiring more intensive regimens such as autologous stem cell transplantation did have about double the risk of endocrine hypogonadism at about 40%. Spermatic function and fertility were not specifically assessed in this study. Men above the age of 50 were about five times as likely as men less than 40 to show evidence of endocrine hypogonadism.

Less is known about other endocrinopathies resulting from treatment of NHL. Radiation to the neck and mediastinum can lead to hypothyroidism, and a small subgroup of NHL patients undergoing stem cell transplantation with TBI conditioning were reported to suffer from growth hormone deficiency, hypogonadism, insulin resistance, and dyslipidemia.[16] The incidence of these endocrine abnormalities in NHL survivors not requiring more intensive therapies is not well-described.

Cognitive

Neurologic complications due to treatment of other NHL subtypes are rare, but potentially serious. A much publicized recent concern has been the development of progressive multifocal leukoencephalopathy (PML) in a small subset of NHL survivors treated with rituximab. A recent report found 52 patients with lymphoproliferative disorders who developed PML following rituximab-based therapies.[17] This condition typically develops soon after completing therapy, with a median time from last rituximab dose to PML diagnosis of 5.5 months. Although still a very rare complication of rituximab use, the lethality of this condition is high, with a 90% case-fatality rate and a median time to

---

Case Example: K.M. was 56 years-old in 2005 when he was diagnosed with follicular lymphoma. He was originally treated with eight cycles of single agent Rituxan. He achieved a partial remission, but one year later, he required combination chemotherapy with Rituxan, Cytoxan, Vincristine, and prednisone (R-CVP). After completing R-CVP, he was given maintenance Rituxan every two to three months. About 18 months into maintenance Rituxan, his family members began to see behavioral changes, including slurred speech and confusion. K.M. also experienced vertigo, as well as left-arm numbness and tingling. A brain MRI identified abnormalities within the periventricular white matter, including a multifocal infarct on the right side. Initially, he was diagnosed with subacute thromboembolic infarcts; however, over the next two weeks, his symptoms worsened, and his speech progressively deteriorated. A second MRI indicated enlargement of cerebral sulci and cisterns. A cerebrospinal fluid (CSF) sample was obtained, and polymerase chain reaction (PCR) analysis was positive for JC virus, consistent with a diagnosis of progressive multifocal leukoencephalopathy (PML). The patient died from PML about three months later.

death of only two months after PML diagnosis. No clear risk factors for the development of PML have been identified.

Patients treated for primary CNS lymphoma (PCNSL) are at high risk of neurologic complications following treatment, particularly in the elderly. In a study of 28 PCNSL patients who had completed whole brain radiotherapy and/or high-dose methotrexate, mild to moderate impairments were found in multiple cognitive domains.[18] Deficits in memory, attention, and executive domains were particularly prominent. Patients who underwent WBRT had more pronounced deficits than those who had chemotherapy alone. In a follow-up prospective study, a similar group of patients were found to have some recovery of executive domain function at two years, but they continued to have persistent difficulties with verbal memory and motor speed.[19]

NHL survivors are also at risk for psychiatric complications following the completion of treatment. For example, in a survey of 886 NHL survivors who were on average 10 years post-diagnosis, 39% reported symptoms of post-traumatic stress disorder (PTSD), and 8% actually met diagnostic criteria for PTSD.[20] Younger, non-white patients with less education were more likely to experience these symptoms.

RISKS FOLLOWING AUTOLOGOUS STEM CELL TRANSPLANTATION

NHL survivors requiring autologous stem cell transplantation (ASCT) experience many of the same late effects as those receiving only conventional therapy, but they are also at risk for additional complications. In a study that included 184 NHL patients who were compared to sibling controls, ASCT survivors reported a higher frequency of cataracts, dry mouth, osteoporosis, neurosensory impairments, inability to attend work or school, and poor overall health.[21] Those receiving total body irradiation (TBI) had a higher risk of cataracts (odds-ratio [OR] 4.9) and dry mouth (OR 3.4) compared to those not receiving TBI. Females were more likely to report osteoporosis (OR 8.7) and abnormal balance, tremor, or weakness (OR 2.4). ASCT recipients also reported higher rates of CHF, exercise induced shortness of breath, and deep venous thrombosis.

FOLLOW-UP GUIDELINES

For the first five years after completing therapy for NHL, guidelines exist for surveillance of patients in complete remission, both to monitor for disease recurrence and also for sequelae of treatment. Recent National Comprehensive Cancer Network (NCCN) guidelines suggest office visits every three to six months and CT-based imaging every six months for the first two to three years, then annually for up to five years.[22] Once patients reach the five-year mark, they are often told that they have been cured of NHL. From this point forward, it becomes less clear how intensively they need to be followed. Currently, a growing trend has been for patients to transition back to their primary care physician, who often oversees this portion of the care. Given the increasing prevalence of NHL, it is therefore imperative that internists be aware of the potential late complications of NHL treatment.

Table 29.3 outlines some suggested approaches to monitoring for late toxicities of NHL treatment. No uniform guidelines exist for how to monitor NHL patients for the risks of second malignancy. Although checking periodic CBCs to screen for leukemia or MDS, performing chest x-rays to look for lung cancer or mesothelioma, or increasing the frequency of colonoscopy to rule out colorectal cancer all would seem like reasonable strategies to pursue, little data exist to support the benefit of these approaches. The American Cancer Society recommends breast MRI as an adjunct to mammogram for women younger than age 30 with a history of chest irradiation.

TABLE 29.3 CURRENT FOLLOW-UP RECOMMENDATIONS FOR SURVIVORS OF NON-HODGKIN'S LYMPHOMA

Late Effects	Follow-up Recommendations
Breast cancer	- Annual screening mammogram - Consider breast magnetic resonance imaging screening as an adjunct to mammogram - Consider referral to high-risk breast clinic for discussion of chemoprevention
Lung cancer	- Smoking cessation
Skin cancer	- Annual skin examination - Sun safety practice
Cardiac disease	- Referral to cardiologist for baseline evaluation after treatment - Resting and stress echocardiogram (frequency depending on baseline findings and existence of other cardiac risk factors) - Reduction of traditional risk factors (lipid screening, blood pressure control, smoking cessation, physical activity, healthy diet)
Non-coronary vascular disease	- Annual examination for carotid bruits; obtain carotid ultrasound if suspicious clinical findings - Reduction of traditional risk factors (lipid screening, blood pressure control, smoking cessation, physical activity, healthy diet)
Infertility	- Referral to reproductive endocrinologist as needed
Hypothyroidism	- Annual thyroid examination - Annual thyroid function tests
Cognitive	- Referral to a neurologist and/or psychiatrist for early intervention

Adapted from www.seer.cancer.gov.

As with second malignancies, the optimal frequency and intensity of monitoring for cardiovascular events in NHL survivors is undefined. Particularly those patients who underwent radiation should consider following with a cardiologist, particularly once they are more than 10 years out from their treatment. At a minimum, patients should be instructed not to ignore persistent troubling symptoms, and to bring them to the attention of their physician without delay. Physicians must be aware of their patients' history of NHL, and should not hesitate to pursue additional testing should suspicion of a late complication arise.

LIFESTYLE MODIFICATIONS

The cardiovascular sequelae of NHL treatment can be mitigated through active lifestyle modifications. Reducing or eliminating co-morbid conditions, such as obesity, diabetes, hypertension, and hyperlipidemia is important. Smokers should be encouraged to quit, both to reduce the risk of cardiac disease and of lung cancer. Resources should be provided to NHL survivors who smoke to educate them about the behavioral and pharmacologic interventions that can assist with smoking cessation efforts.

Engaging in regular physical activity appears to be particularly critical in helping NHL survivors to be healthy. Two recent studies have demonstrated that those NHL survivors who met public health guidelines of 150 minutes or more of moderately vigorous exercise per week had significantly better health-related quality of life than those who were sedentary.[23,24] Health-related quality of life was also found to have a positive correlation with getting at least some exercise. Therefore, we should be encouraging at least some exercise in all NHL survivors, and we can inform them that the more exercise they get, the better chance they have of improving their quality of life.

COORDINATED CARE

During treatment, NHL patients become accustomed to working closely with a multidisciplinary team that often includes medical oncologists, radiation oncologists, mid-level practitioners, nurses, and others. Ideally, the patient's primary care physician will continue to be involved with their care during treatment, as they often have a long-standing relationship with the patient that pre-dates their lymphoma diagnosis. Maintaining this relationship becomes particularly important after the patient completes treatment.

Typically, the medical oncologist will continue to follow the patient closely for several years after finishing therapy, and subsequently the patient transitions back to the primary care physician as their main provider. Often, there can be miscommunication during this transition period between well-meaning providers. Establishing a survivorship care plan is one way to facilitate communication and allocation of responsibility during this time period.[25]

Oncologists and primary care physicians should also be aware of the high prevalence of mental health issues faced by NHL survivors. For example, early identification of patients at risk for developing PTSD symptoms can facilitate referral to mental health professionals to initiate treatment.[20] Interventions such as this can aid greatly in patients' ability to return as closely as possible to the quality of life they enjoyed before their NHL diagnosis and treatment.

REFERENCES

1. SEER Database.

2. Muller AM, Ihorst G, Mertelsmann R, Engelhardt M. Epidemiology of non-Hodgkin's lymphoma (NHL): trends, geographic distribution, and etiology. Ann Hematol. 2005 Jan;84(1):1–12.

3. Feugier P, Van Hoof A, Sebban C, Solal-Celigny P, Bouabdallah R, Ferme C, et al. Long-term results of the R-CHOP study in the treatment of elderly patients with diffuse large B-cell lymphoma: a study by the Groupe d'Etude des Lymphomes de l'Adulte. *J Clin Oncol.* 2005 Jun 20;23(18):4117–26.

4. Miller TP, Dahlberg S, Cassady JR, Adelstein DJ, Spier CM, Grogan TM, et al. Chemotherapy alone compared with chemotherapy plus radiotherapy for localized intermediate- and high-grade non-Hodgkin's lymphoma. *N Engl J Med.* 1998 Jul 2;339(1):21–6.

5. Mudie NY, Swerdlow AJ, Higgins CD, Smith P, Qiao Z, Hancock BW, et al. Risk of second malignancy after non-Hodgkin's lymphoma: a British Cohort Study. *J Clin Oncol.* 2006 Apr 1;24(10):1568–74.

6. Hemminki K, Lenner P, Sundquist J, Bermejo JL. Risk of subsequent solid tumors after non-Hodgkin's lymphoma: effect of diagnostic age and time since diagnosis. *J Clin Oncol.* 2008 Apr 10;26(11):1850–7.

7. Sanna G, Lorizzo K, Rotmensz N, Bagnardi V, Cinieri S, Colleoni M, et al. Breast cancer in Hodgkin's disease and non-Hodgkin's lymphoma survivors. *Ann Oncol.* 2007 Feb;18(2):288–92.

8. Tward JD, Wendland MM, Shrieve DC, Szabo A, Gaffney DK. The risk of secondary malignancies over 30 years after the treatment of non-Hodgkin lymphoma. *Cancer.* 2006 Jul 1;107(1):108–15.

9. Toda K, Shibuya H, Hayashi K, Ayukawa F. Radiation-induced cancer after radiotherapy for non-Hodgkin's lymphoma of the head and neck: a retrospective study. *Radiat Oncol.* 2009;4:21.

10. Hequet O, Le QH, Moullet I, Pauli E, Salles G, Espinouse D, et al. Subclinical late cardiomyopathy after doxorubicin therapy for lymphoma in adults. *J Clin Oncol.* 2004 May 15;22(10):1864–71.

11. Moser EC, Noordijk EM, van Leeuwen FE, le Cessie S, Baars JW, Thomas J, et al. Long-term risk of cardiovascular disease after treatment for aggressive non-Hodgkin lymphoma. *Blood.* 2006 Apr 1;107(7):2912–9.

12. Limat S, Demesmay K, Voillat L, Bernard Y, Deconinck E, Brion A, et al. Early cardiotoxicity of the CHOP regimen in aggressive non-Hodgkin's lymphoma. *Ann Oncol.* 2003 Feb;14(2):277–81.

13. Elis A, Tevet A, Yerushalmi R, Blickstein D, Bairy O, Dann EJ, et al. Fertility status among women treated for aggressive non-Hodgkin's lymphoma. *Leuk Lymphoma.* 2006 Apr;47(4):623–7.

14. Dann EJ, Epelbaum R, Avivi I, Ben Shahar M, Haim N, Rowe JM, et al. Fertility and ovarian function are preserved in women treated with an intensified regimen of cyclophosphamide, adriamycin, vincristine and prednisone (Mega-CHOP) for non-Hodgkin lymphoma. *Hum Reprod.* 2005 Aug;20(8):2247–9.

15. Kiserud CE, Fossa A, Bjoro T, Holte H, Cvancarova M, Fossa SD. Gonadal function in male patients after treatment for malignant lymphomas, with emphasis on chemotherapy. *Br J Cancer.* 2009 Feb 10;100(3):455–63.

16. Steffens M, Beauloye V, Brichard B, Robert A, Alexopoulou O, Vermylen C, et al. Endocrine and metabolic disorders in young adult survivors of childhood acute lymphoblastic leukemia (ALL) or non-Hodgkin lymphoma (NHL). *Clin Endocrinol* (Oxf). 2008 Nov;69(5):819–27.

17. Carson KR, Evens AM, Richey EA, Habermann TM, Focosi D, Seymour JF, et al. Progressive multifocal leukoencephalopathy after rituximab therapy in HIV-negative patients: a report of 57 cases from the Research on Adverse Drug Events and Reports project. *Blood.* 2009 May 14;113(20):4834–40.

18. Correa DD, DeAngelis LM, Shi W, Thaler H, Glass A, Abrey LE. Cognitive functions in survivors of primary central nervous system lymphoma. *Neurology.* 2004 Feb 24;62(4):548–55.

19. Correa DD, Rocco-Donovan M, DeAngelis LM, Dolgoff-Kaspar R, Iwamoto F, Yahalom J, et al. Prospective cognitive follow-up in primary CNS lymphoma patients treated with chemotherapy and reduced-dose radiotherapy. *J Neurooncol.* 2009 Feb;91(3):315–21.

20. Smith SK, Zimmerman S, Williams CS, Preisser JS, Clipp EC. Post-traumatic stress outcomes in non-Hodgkin's lymphoma survivors. *J Clin Oncol.* 2008 Feb 20; 26(6):934–41.

21. Majhail NS, Ness KK, Burns LJ, Sun CL, Carter A, Francisco L, et al. Late effects in survivors of Hodgkin and non-Hodgkin lymphoma treated with autologous hematopoietic cell transplantation: a report from the bone marrow transplant survivor study. *Biol Blood Marrow Transplant.* 2007 Oct;13(10):1153–9.

22. NCCN Clinical Practice Guidelines for non-Hodgkin Lymphoma v.1.2011.

23. Bellizzi KM, Rowland JH, Arora NK, Hamilton AS, Miller MF, Aziz NM. Physical activity and quality of life in adult survivors of non-Hodgkin's lymphoma. *J Clin Oncol.* 2009 Feb 20;27(6):960–6.

24. Vallance JK, Courneya KS, Jones LW, Reiman T. Differences in quality of life between non-Hodgkin's lymphoma survivors meeting and not meeting public health exercise guidelines. *Psychooncology.* 2005 Nov;14(11):979–91.

25. Grunfeld E, Earle CC. The interface between primary and oncology specialty care: treatment through survivorship. *J Natl Cancer Inst Monogr.*2010(40):25–30.

30

Survivorship in Acute Myeloid Leukemia

Deepa Jeyakumar, MD,
and Kenneth Miller, MD

Introduction

Acute myeloid leukemia (AML) is a diverse group of malignant stem cell disorders characterized by clonal proliferation and accumulation of precursors of either myeloid, erythroid, megakaryocytic, or monocytic cell lineages. The proliferation of these neoplastic cells ultimately leads to inhibition of normal hematopoietic precursors and results in the clinical manifestations of the leukemias.

AML is primarily a disease of elderly individuals.[1] According to projections based on the Surveillance, Epidemiology, and End Result (SEER) database,[2] there will be 12,330 Americans diagnosed with acute myelogenous leukemia in 2010 with a median age of diagnosis of 67 years. In children less than 15 years of age, AML comprises 15–20% of all cases of leukemia, with a peak incidence of three to four years of age. The incidence of leukemia increases with age, with a peak incidence between 75 and 84 years (Figure 30.1).

Prognostic Indicators

AML is a clinically heterogeneous disease with marked differences in survival following treatment. Leukemogenesis is thought to be a multi-step process that involves damage to the hematopoietic progenitor cell at multiple stages.[3] In the past decade, advances in the molecular pathogenesis of AML have changed our understanding of the biology of AML and the use of allogeneic stem cell transplantation. The genetic events in the development of AML suggest that there are at least three types of mutations.[4] Type 1 mutations confer proliferative and survival advantages to the hematopoietic progenitors but do not affect differentiation. An example of Type 1 mutations would be FLT3 mutation which leads to proliferation of leukemia cells. Type 2 mutations impair hematopoietic differentiation. An example of a Type 2 mutation would be PML/RARα as seen in Acute Promyelocytic Leukemia (APL), which causes

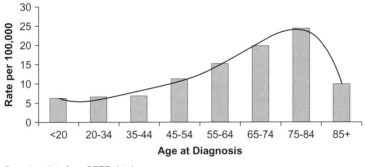

Based on data from SEER database

Figure 30.1. Incidence of Leukemia versus Age at Diagnosis.

an arrest in hematopoietic differentiation leading to accumulation of promyelocytes. Type 3 mutations are changes that contribute to leukemic growth by modulating an interdependent network of epigenetic controls essential for regulating cellular growth and maturation. An example of the Type 3 mutations includes somatic mutations in a gene encoding a DNA methyltransferase in patients with AML and normal cytogenetics.[5]

AML is more appropriately thought of as a group of disorders that have a heterogeneous clinical course with varying prognoses. The prognostic factors are based on the patient's age, blast (leukemic) cell morphology, and genetic abnormalities. It is useful to distinguish these subgroups of patients to determine their prognoses and to guide therapy. The prognosis of patients with acute myeloid leukemia can be divided by AML-related factors and patient-related factors.

AML-Related Factors

The diagnosis of AML requires greater than 20% circulating blasts on either peripheral blood smear or bone marrow. The diagnosis of AML can also be made when the blast percentage is less than 20% and certain disease-specific chromosomal abnormalities are found. In particular, the cases of AML that do not require greater than 20% circulating blast count are AML with t(8;21), inv(16) or t(16:16), or some cases of erythroleukemia. Mutations in t(8;21) and t(16:16) affect core binding transcription factors (CBFs): AML1 and CBFβ. The other exception is AML with t(15;17), also known as acute promyelocytic leukemia (APML). This group of AMLs is defined by their recurrent genetic abnormalities, and the clinical course of these subtypes of AML is generally associated with a younger age at diagnosis and a more favorable prognosis.[6]

Cytogenetic analysis and molecular mutations are an important part of the diagnosis and contribute to determining the treatment plan. The importance of cytogenetics over morphology is reflected in the new World Health Organization (WHO, 2008) classification system for acute myeloid leukemias (Table 30.1).[6]

TABLE 30.1 CORRELATION OF CYTOGENETICS AND MOLECULAR GENETIC DATA
IN AML WITH CLINICAL OUTCOMES

Genetic groups	Subsets
Favorable	t(8;21)(q22;q22); RUNX1-RUNXIT1 inv(16)(p13;1q22) or t(16;16)(p13;q22); CBFB-MYH11 mutated NPM1 without FLT3-ITD (normal karyotype) mutated CEBPA (normal karyotype)
Intermediate-1	Mutated NPM1 and FLT3-ITD (normal karyotype) Wild-type NPM1 and FLT3-ITD (normal karyotype) Wild-type NPM1 without FLT3-ITD (normal karyotype)
Intermediate-2	t(9;11)(p22;q23); MLLT3-MLL cytogenetic abnormalities not classified as favorable or adverse
Adverse	inv3(q21q26.2) or t(3;3)(q21;q26.2); RPN1-EV11 t(6;9)(p23;q34); DEK-NUP214 t(v;11)(v;q23); MLL rearranged −5 or del(5q); −7 or abnl(17p); complex karyotype

Adapted from Dohner, H, Estey EH, Amadori S, et al. Diagnosis and management of acute
myeloid leukemia in Adults: recommendations from an international expert panel, on behalf of
the European LeukemiaNet. *Blood.* 2010; 115: 453–474.[7]

Molecular genetic testing can help to further determine the clinical course
of the normal karyotype leukemia including mutations in the FLT3 (fms-
related tyrosine kinase 3) gene, the NPM1 (nucleophosmin) gene, and the
CEBPA (CCAAT/enhancer binding protein [C/EBP] alpha) gene.

Impact of Cytogenetic Analysis

Acute myeloid leukemias are frequently classified into three categories by
the cytogenetic changes: favorable (good)-risk, adverse (poor)-risk, and intermediate-risk (Table 30.2).[7]

Favorable—risk leukemias. Favorable risk leukemias represent approximately 25% of all AML. These leukemias tend to occur in younger patients
and generally have a better prognosis.

Adverse (Poor)—risk leukemias. Adverse (poor) risk leukemias include leukemias with deletions in one or more chromosomes or complex karotypic
abnormalities. AMLs with deletions in chromosome 5 or 7 typically occur in
patients with a history of antecedent myelodysplastic syndrome (MDS) and/or
a history of prior chemotherapy. AMLs with complex karotypes are typically
defined as the presence of more than three mutations. Finally, monosomal
karyotype leukemias are defined as having either two autosomal monosomies
or one autosomal monosomy with one structural abnormality.[8] This group
of disorders has a particularly unfavorable prognosis with a four-year overall
survival of 4%. The subset of adverse-risk leukemias carries a poor prognosis,
which should guide the choice of therapy.

TABLE 30.2 CORRELATION OF CYTOGENETICS WITH CLINICAL OUTCOMES

Risk Status	Cytogenetics
Good Risk	t(8;21) inv(16) t(16;16) t(15;17)
Intermediate Risk	Normal Cytogenetics +8 t(3;5)
Poor Risk	Complex cytogenetic abnormalities (>3 abnormalities) -5,5q- -7,7q- Other 11q23 abnormalities

Intermediate—risk leukemias. The intermediate-risk leukemias are the largest and most diverse group of leukemias and have normal karyotypes. These AMLs represent 40–48% of all leukemias and are heterogeneous with a very variable clinical course. With recent advances in molecular genetic testing, these leukemias can now be further subclassified. This subclassification is particularly helpful for determining what therapies may be needed post-remission.

Impact of Molecular Genetics

Cytogenetic analysis has helped predict the clinical course of favorable- and adverse-risk leukemias. (Table 30.2) However, the clinical course of normal karyotype leukemias is heterogeneous. The identification of various molecular mutations has helped differentiate subsets of leukemias that have distinct clinical courses. AMLs with mutations in the FLT3 (fms-related tyrosine kinase 3) gene, the NPM1 (nucleophosmin) gene, and the CEBPA (CCAAT/enhancer binding protein [C/EBP] alpha) gene have distinct clinical entities. Mutations in NPM1 with the absence of FLT3 mutation were also found to be associated with a favorable prognosis. Therefore, AMLs with CEBPA and/or NPM1 mutations are associated with improved outcomes. Alternatively, AMLs with mutations in FLT3 are associated with inferior outcomes (Table 30.3).

Determination of the mutation status is particularly important in intermediate-risk (normal cytogenetics) AML patients, since subsequent therapies including allogeneic stem cell transplantation may be considered based on the results of testing for FLT3, NPM1, EVI1, and CEBPA mutations. However, while prognostically important, it remains unclear how this information should ultimately be applied to the individual patient. Testing for FLT3, NPM1, and CEBPA mutations may help in counseling patients on the need for more intensive therapy or an allogeneic hematopoietic stem cell transplant. However, at this time, further studies are needed before gene mutation analysis can be used to

TABLE 30.3 PROGNOSTIC SUBGROUPS OF AML BASED ON PRESENTING
MOLECULAR ABNORMALITIES

Risk	Molecular Abnormalities
Good Risk	Normal cytogenetics with NPM1[a] Mutation Or CEBPA[b] mutation without FLT3-ITD[c]
Intermediate Risk	c-Kit and t(8;21) or Inv 16, t(16;16)
Poor Risk	High EVI1[d] expression, Normal cytogenetics with FLT3- ITD in the absence of NPM1 mutation

[a] NPM1 is a nucleolar phosphoprotein. Mutations in NPM1 lead to delocalization of the protein to the cytoplasm. Leukemias with NPM1 mutations are associated with better outcomes and present with higher WBC count.

[b] CEBPA is a transcription factor involved in normal myelopoiesis. CEBPA mutations are present in 10% of leukemias and more common among leukemias with normal karyotype. Mutations lead to expression of a truncated protein or occur within the carboxy-terminus, disrupting regions required for dimerization and/or DNA binding. CEBPA mutations are associated with leukemias with a more favorable outcome.

[c] FLT3 is a receptor for tyrosine kinase expressed on hematopietic progenitors. It is mutated in approximately one third of leukemias, particularly in normal karyotype leukemias. There are two types of mutations in FLT3: internal tandem duplication (ITD) and mutations in the tyrosine kinase domain TKD. The mutations lead to in-frame insertions within the juxtramembrane region of the receptor. Mutation in FLT3 is associated with leukemias that present with higher WBC count and worse outcomes. New treatment are being developed that will target these mutations to which may improve outcomes in these high risk patients.

[d] EVI1 is an oncogene on chromosome 3 which is involved in cell proliferation and cell differentiation. It appears to be involved in with other abnormalities in leukemic cell transformation. It is associated with a very aggressive for of AML with a poor prognosis.

determine whether a young patient in first complete remission should undergo an allogeneic stem cell transplant versus standard consolidation chemotherapy alone.

Other Disease-Related Factors

Important biological factors that contribute to the prognosis of AML include the white blood cell count upon presentation and extramedullary disease. A white blood cell count greater than 100,000 is considered an unfavorable risk factor, while a white blood cell count less than 10,000 is considered a favorable risk factor.

Patient-Related Factors

Some of the patient-related factors that contribute to an increased risk of leukemia include inherited and acquired genetic disorders, therapy-related exposures, and finally the age of the patient at diagnosis.

AML Related to Inherited Genetic Disorders

There are a variety of inherited genetic disorders that predispose the patient to the development of acute myeloid leukemia to various degrees. These include Down Syndrome, Bloom Syndrome, Klinefelter Syndrome, Patau Syndrome, Ataxia-Telangiectasia, Neurofibromatosis, Shwachman syndrome, Kostmann Syndrome, Fanconi anemia, and Li-Fraumeni Syndrome, among others.[3]

AML Related to Acquired Genetic Disorders

Finally, there are a variety of acquired genetic disorders that predispose the patient to the development of AML. The acquired genetic disorders include myelodysplastic syndrome, myeloproliferative neoplasms, aplastic anemia, paroxysmal noctural hemoglobulinuria, multiple myeloma, and nonseminomatous mediastinal germ cell tumors.

Secondary AML describes a subset of AML that develops in the context of prior MDS, myeloproliferative neoplasm (MPN) or secondary to proven leukemogenic exposure. De novo AML is defined as AML that develops in patients who have no clinical history of prior MDS, MPN or exposure to potential leukemogenic therapy or agents. This distinction is critical because secondary AMLs frequently have a distinct clinical course with a poor prognosis.

Secondary AMLs that develop in the context of an antecedent MDS typically have mutations in chromosome 5 and or 7. The risk of AML in the context of an antecedent MDS is highly variable and depends on the severity of MDS. In low-risk MDS, the risk of conversion to AML is less than 10% in 10 years. In high-risk MDS, the risk of developing AML approaches almost 50% in one year. The risk of AML in the context of an antecedent MPN is dependent on the type of MPN and the stage of the disease.

Therapy-Related AMLs

Secondary AMLs that develop after exposure to chemotherapy are known as therapy-related AMLs. Therapy-related AMLs represent 5 to 10% of all AMLs. Two potential leukemogenic agents that carry an increased risk of AML are alkylating agents or topoisomerase-II inhibitor agents. Patients who develop alkylating agent-associated AML usually have a history of antecedent MDS. Mutations in chromosomes 5 and 7 are typically found on cytogenetic analysis. The peak incidence of AML in these patients is 5 to 7 years after exposure. Patients who develop AML related to topoisomerase II inhibitor therapy usually do not have a history of antecedent MDS. Mutations in the MLL gene or 11q23 can be found on cytogenetic analysis. Topoisomerase II inhibitor therapy has been associated with AML and rarely APL. While therapy-related AML tend to have a poorer prognosis than de novo AML, therapy-related APL does not carry a worse prognosis than de novo APL.

Impact of Age

Age is an independent poor prognostic factor. Since the incidence of AML increases with age, it is primarily a disease of elderly individuals. Older patients appear to have a biologically different disease than younger patients. While the dividing line between younger and older patients is arbitrary, most studies consider AML in patients over the age of 60 as elderly AML. Older patients have a decreased frequency of favorable cytogenetic abnormalities and a higher incidence of poor prognostic cytogenetics. Age over 60 years is associated with a significantly poorer prognosis as well as lower complete remission rate, overall survival, remission duration, and relapse-free survival. Therefore, the combination of age over 60 years old and intermediate cytogenetics has a synergistic negative effect on relapse-free survival.[9]

TREATMENT REGIMENS

The standard treatment of AML has not meaningfully changed in the past 30 years and includes the use of an anthracycline and cytarabine. Therapies are divided into two distinct and interdependent phases: remission induction and post-remission therapies.

Remission Induction Therapy

In patients under the age of 60 years, the first phase is the induction therapy, which usually involves three days of an anthracycline and seven days of continuous infusion cytarabine ("3+7"). The aim of the remission induction regimen is to induce a complete remission (CR). Remission induction therapy (also known as induction therapy) is given initially to eradicate the majority of leukemic blasts (<5%) and to enable normal hematopoiesis.[10] In younger patients, attaining a CR is necessary for a prolonged survival and is the primary endpoint for all induction regimens. Attempts to improve on the "3+7" with the addition of other agents or dose intensification have produced variable, controversial, and inconsistent results.[11] Despite advances in the biology of AML, little has changed in the prior therapy. The overall remission rate for patients under the age of 60 years ranges from 50–75% and has changed little over the last two decades. Subsequently, post-remission therapy is employed to minimize the chances of recurrence of the leukemia and potentially offer the patient a cure of AML. The prognostic factors that are important are noted in Table 30.4.

Alternative Treatment Regimens

Other strategies for inducing remission include decitabine and azacitadine, which are members of a group of hypomethylating agents. These strategies can be particularly effective in patients with a history of antecedent MDS or older patients. When the patient is felt to be unfit for intensive chemotherapy,

TABLE 30.4 PROGNOSTIC FACTORS IN AML

Prognostic Factor	Impact on Prognosis
Auer Rods	Favorable
Cytogenetic Abnormalities	Variable
Age ≥ 60 years	Adverse
Monocytic Morphology	Adverse
Prior MDS or MPN	Adverse
Performance status > 2	Adverse
Presenting WBC > 20,000cmm	Adverse
Extramedullary Disease	Adverse
Courses to Attain a CR > 1	Adverse
Increased LDH	Adverse
CD 34 immunophenotype	Adverse
Flt 3 ITD mutation	Adverse
DNA methyltransferase (DMMT3A) mutations	Adverse

the goals of therapy frequently shift to palliation. Since decitabine is generally well tolerated, this regimen can be particularly well suited for older patients.

Post-Remission Therapies

Post-remission therapies include consolidation, maintenance, autologous stem cell transplantation and allogeneic stem cell transplantation, and are summarized in Table 30.5. The goal of these strategies is to prolong remission duration by eliminating minimal residual disease (MRD). The decision of which regimen to choose is a complex one requiring analysis of the patient's ability to tolerate the therapy as well as the biology of the leukemia. The decision of the most appropriate post-remission therapy is dependent on the patient's prognosis and remains controversial.

For younger patients with poor-risk cytogenetics or adverse prognostic features, allogeneic stem cell transplant from a related or unrelated donor is recommended. The prognosis for younger patients is markedly improved by the use of an allogeneic stem cell transplant in first remission and is generally accepted as a standard of care.

Consolidation/Maintenance

Typically, a consolidative regimen includes high-dose cytarabine (HiDAC). The doses range from $1-3$ grms/m^2 for $6-12$ doses. The period of neutropenia is variable and increases with each cycle. Patients over the age of 60 can be particularly sensitive to side effects and can rarely tolerate full doses. It is

TABLE 30.5 TREATMENT STRATEGIES IN AML

Treatment Strategies	Potential (Typical) Treatment Options
Induction (or Remission Induction) therapy	"3 + 7"
Consolidation	High dose Ara-C; Decitabine; Immunotherapy
Intensification	Brief course of Re-induction-like regimens
Maintenance therapy	Prolonged low dose therapy
Autologous Stem Transplant	dose intensification for select patients
Allogeneic Stem Cell Transplant	Related Donor; Unrelated Donor; Umbilical Cord Blood

most active in younger patients. Patients with favorable cytogenetics benefit most from HiDAC consolidation.

The role of maintenance, low dose chemotherapy, in most forms of AML is controversial. In older patients with AML, maintenance has been shown in some studies to improve disease free survival but not overall survival. Therefore, maintenance chemotherapy is generally not recommended.

Transplantation

Autologous transplantation remains an alternative to allogeneic transplantation due to its lower morbidity and mortality rates in the correct clinical scenario. Autologous transplantation is associated with a transplant-related mortality rate of less than 5% and few long term side effects.

Autologous transplantation appears to be an option in patients who are in first CR and have favorable-risk cytogenetics. However, the relapse rate remains high even many years later and therefore autologous transplantation cannot be considered curative for most patients. The overall benefit of autologous transplant is considered controversial.

Allogeneic Stem Cell Transplantation

Allogeneic transplantation remains the treatment of choice for young patients with high-risk or intermediate-risk AML. However, the use of an allogeneic stem cell transplant must be balanced against the morbidity, mortality, and potential long-term complications of the transplantation. The immediate risks of allogeneic transplantation include the risk of the conditioning regimens and prolonged immune suppression. The long-term toxicities are related to prolonged immune suppression, graft-versus-host disease, and cardiovascular, pulmonary toxicities, and sterility. These toxicities are summarized in Table 30.6.

Allogeneic stem cell transplantation is the treatment of choice in patients in their first CR with adverse cytogenetics or other prognostic factors. In addition,

TABLE 30.6 VARIOUS NON-INFECTIOUS TOXICITIES OF ALLOGENEIC TRANSPLANTATION

Organ System	Immediate	Late
Cardiovascular		Cardiomyopathy Congestive heart failure Valvular dysfunction arrhythmia
Pulmonary	Respiratory failure related to Engraftment syndrome	Bronchiolitis obliterans (BO) Bronchiolitis obliterans organizing pneumonia (BOOP) Idiopathic pneumonia syndrome (IPS)
Hepatobiliary	Veno-occlusive disease/sinusoidal obstructive syndrome	Chronic cholestasis related to chronic GvHD
Endocrine		Hypothyroidism Diabetes mellitus
Musculoskeletal		Osteopenia Avascular necrosis of joints Contractures of joints related to chronic GvHD
Ophthalmologic		Cataracts Dry eyes related to chronic GvHD or TBI
Dermatologic	Variable from maculopapular rash to desquamation related to acute GvHD	Hypopigmentation and scleroderma-tous changes related to chronic GvHD
Genitourinary		Infertility
Other		Secondary malignancies

allogeneic stem cell transplantation is the treatment of choice in patients who have relapsed and are in a second CR. The use of an allogeneic transplant is not recommended for patients with favorable cytogenetics in first complete remission, but remains the treatment of choice for younger patients with intermediate- and high-risk disease. The risks of the transplant and its impact on quality of life should be clearly discussed with the patient and his or her family.

OUTCOMES IN ELDERLY AML

Advanced age is a major adverse prognostic factor in AML (Figure 30.2). There are many factors that contribute to the poor prognosis of elderly AML including increased frequency of adverse cytogenetic abnormalities, comorbidities, as well as performance status. Furthermore, our understanding of the treatment of elderly AML is also limited by selection bias since the patients that are enrolled in clinical trials tend to be healthier or have an improved

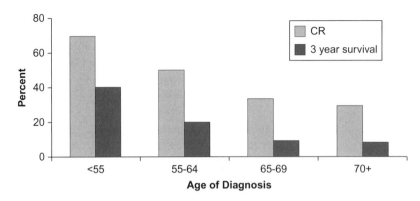

Figure 30.2. Complete Remission Rate and Three-Year Overall Survival versus Age.

performance status, which might overestimate the actual outcome of this subset of patients.[12,13,14]

The frequency of leukemias with adverse karyotype increases with age. In patients less than 56, 17% had favorable karyotypes and 35% had leukemias with adverse karyotypes. In contrast, in patients older than 75, only 4% and 51% had favorable versus unfavorable cytogenetics, respectively. The finding of multiple high-risk, poor prognostic variables in elderly patients with AML is reflected in their poor overall survival after standard intensive induction therapy. Elderly patients may attain a complete remission with intensive chemotherapy, but unlike younger patients, this does not correlate with an improved overall survival and disease-free survival. Therefore, before starting treatment the patient's potential for improved overall and disease-free survival should be factored in when determining treatment regimens. Moreover, elderly patients with a prior MDS and complex cytogenetic abnormalities do not appear to benefit from standard induction regimens.[15,16] Additionally, the assessment of the patient's performance status significantly determined the risk of early death as defined as death within 30 days of induction chemotherapy. The contribution of poor performance status did not affect early death in patients younger than 56 years but in patients older than 75, the early death rate was 14% in people with ECOG PS 0 and rose dramatically to 50% in people with ECOG PS 2, and peaked at 82% in people with ECOG PS 3. The ability of older patients to survive induction chemotherapy appears highly dependent on their pretreatment performance status.[17]

The optimal therapy for patients over the age of 60 years remains controversial. The correlation of complete remission rate and overall survival is not as strongly related in the older patient with AML. In a randomized trial of patient age 65 and older with AML, intensive chemotherapy was associated with a higher rate of CR but more early deaths led to similar overall survival compared to supportive care.[18] Despite significant advances made in supportive measures over more than the past decade, these results were confirmed in the randomized trial which demonstrated the survival benefit of decitabine over intensive chemotherapy in a subset of patients with AML.[15] The older patient without adverse cytogenetics and good performance status may benefit from intensive chemotherapy.

Complete remission and overall survival in elderly patients with AML appear to be highly dependent on performance status and age.

In the final analysis, the management of older patients with AML is controversial and needs to be individualized. We believe that the discussions with the patient should focus on survivorship and quality of life and not complete remission rates. In addition, the endpoint of CR may not be the most important outcome of interest in evaluating trials for elderly patients with AML. While many older patients may be fit for intensive standard induction chemotherapy, the decision must be individualized based on the patient's cytogenetics, performance status, comorbidities, and preferences. Given that the most important outcome of interest is overall survival, and various agents are able to provide some benefit in overall survival while not complete remission rate, the decision to forgo intensive chemotherapy in older patients with AML is reasonable. Moreover, while the diagnosis of AML suggests a sense of urgency to start therapy, there is time to assess prognostic factors and quality of life issues before deciding on the treatment options.

Sequelae of AML and Its Treatment

Short-Term Toxicities

Intensive chemotherapy requires a prolonged hospitalization of four to six weeks for induction chemotherapy. During intensive chemotherapy, the patient experiences a prolonged period of neutropenia associated with increased susceptibility to infection. A complete review of infection for which the neutropenic patient is at risk is beyond the scope of this chapter.

At the time of diagnosis, AML is associated with a significant negative impact on the patient's quality of life. Over the first six months, the quality of life of older patients who receive intensive chemotherapy or best supportive care remains stable, and treatment of intensive chemotherapy does not necessarily worsen quality of life compared with best supportive care.[19] A preliminary study suggests that, one year after chemotherapy alone, most patients show an improvement in their quality of life.[20]

Fatigue

The most common symptom of patients with AML is fatigue, as is the case with most cancers. Fatigue has been found to be inversely correlated with global health, major domains of quality of life and self-reported ADLs in older adults with AML.[21] AML may cause physiological changes related to anemia as well as psychological consequences related to depression. However, even when accounting for the effects of anemia and depression, patients may still have significant fatigue, reinforcing that fatigue can have a variety of causes. Preliminary evidence has implicated various cytokines in fatigue related to AML.[22] Furthermore, fatigue may also be a consequence of treatment. Regardless of the origins of fatigue, an observation study has suggested that fatigue was the most common symptom and was present at the time of diagnosis. At the completion of induction chemotherapy and one year later, fatigue improved.[23]

Prolonged periods of bed rest during the hospitalization lead to functional declines. Two studies have evaluated the benefits of light aerobic exercise on fatigue and depressive symptoms.[24,25]

Neurologic Complications

Cytarabine has been associated with neurologic sequelae, particularly when given at higher doses. These sequelae usually occur during the infusion or a few days after the infusion. The consequences range from ataxia, dysarthria, confusion, lethargy, and dysphagia. The risk factors from this toxicity are age greater than 40 as well as renal and/or liver compromise.[26]

Long-Term Toxicities of Intensive Chemotherapy

There is limited published experience on the long-term complications of chemotherapy with long-term survivors of AML who have been treated with intensive chemotherapy alone. The primary long-term complications of intensive chemotherapy alone for AML include cardiac complications, secondary myelodysplastic syndrome/AML, and infertility.

Cardiac Complications

The prototype of chemotherapy, which is potentially cardiotoxic, is anthracycline. It is characterized by a dose-dependent progressive decrease in systolic left ventricular function. The mechanism is thought to be related to direct myocardial injury due to formation of free radicals. A total dose of 400 mg/m^2 of doxorubicin is associated with a 0.14% risk of congestive heart failure, while a total dose of 550 mg/m^2 of doxorubicin is associated with a 7% risk of congestive heart failure. In addition to cardiomyopathy, other manifestations of late cardiotoxicity include overt congestive heart failure, valvular dysfunction, and arrhythmia. Finally, the age and gender of the patient can be important in prognosticating risk of cardiac toxicity. Advanced age and male gender are associated with increased risk of cardiac toxicity.

Secondary Myelodysplastic Syndrome/AML

One devastating complication after treatment for leukemia is development of a different therapy-related AML. In one study, up to 6.5% of patients treated for acute promyelocytic leukemia developed a therapy-related MDS/AML.[27]

There have been case reports describing the development of therapy-related MDS/AML in the setting of prior AML treatment with different cytogenetic abnormalities.[28]

Infertility

Infertility has been reported as a major complication of induction and consolidative chemotherapy alone. Infertility can be permanent in middle aged patients.[29]

Complications of Allogeneic Stem Cell Transplantation

Long term survivors of AML frequently have survived after allogeneic stem cell transplantation since it remains the only potentially curable treatment. However, there is significant morbidity and mortality associated with this treatment. The initial toxicity of stem cell transplantation is related to the conditioning regimen, infections related to prolonged neutropenia, engraftment failure and graft-versus-host disease (GvHD). The initial goal of transplantation is long-term survival. Bhatia et al. reported that 80% of those who survive the first two years post-transplant are expected to be long-term survivors. [30]

Once the patient survives the first two years, the goals of therapy shift to management of potential long-term toxicities. Much of our knowledge about the long-term toxicities of allogeneic stem cell transplantation is derived from the Bone Marrow Transplantation Survivor Study, a retrospective cohort study of participants who received hematopoietic cell transplantation between 1974 and 1998 and survived for more than two years. Using this database, Bhatia et al. reported that the leading causes of late death after allogeneic stem cell transplantation are relapse of the leukemia and chronic GvHD at 29% and 22%, respectively.[30] Other causes of late death after allogeneic stem cell transplantation include late infection in the absence of chronic GvHD (11%), secondary malignancy (7%), pulmonary complications (5%), and cardiac complications (3%).

Complications of transplantation can be divided into early and late complications. The late complications can be subdivided into delayed (which is between three months and two years), late (two to 10 years) and very late (beyond 10 years). The various complications have summarized in Table 30.6.

Cardiac and Cardiovascular Complications

Late cardiac and cardiovascular events may occur years after transplantation. They may be related to gender, age at transplantation, traditional cardiovascular risk factors, and GvHD. Bhatia et al. found that the risk of premature death due to cardiac complications was 2.3-fold increased compared with the general population.[30] In a retrospective analysis of 265 long-term survivors, the cumulative incidence of an arterial event defined as cerebrovascular disease, coronary artery disease and peripheral artery disease was 22% at 25 years.[31] When adjusted for age, patients treated with allogeneic transplantation had a seven-fold increased relative risk of an arterial event at 15 years.

The cardiovascular damage seen in allogeneic stem cell survivors is thought to be related to a chronic inflammatory state. Furthermore, there could be endothelial damage related to condition regimen with or without total body irradiation (TBI). Finally, the endothelial cells may be a site of GvHD. Finally, allogeneic stem cell transplant survivors are not immune to common diseases that plague the general population, including diabetes, hypertension and hyperlipidemia. Baker et al. reported that the odds ratio of development of diabetes in long-term survivors is 3.9 when compared with their siblings, $p = 0.04$.[32] Baker et al. also reported a 2.0 fold increased risk of developing hypertension in survivors when compared with their siblings.[33] Taskinen et al. proposed that additional risk factors particular to this population are post-transplant endocrine dysfunction, prolonged treatment with immunosuppressive medications, and sedentary lifestyle.[34] Finally, a rare cause of cardiac dysfunction is cardiac GvHD. In a series of 11 patients with cardiac GvHD, Rackley et al. reported that the arterial obstruction was found to be due to intimal proliferation rather than typical atherosclerosis. Two patients in that series died of myocardial infarction.[35]

Thus, with identification of these possible cardiac toxicities, appropriate recommendations for this group have not yet been finalized. Initial recommendations for screening for late cardiac complications after hematopoietic stem cell transplantation survivors include treatment of cardiovascular risk factors include diabetes, hypertension, hyperlipidemia, and smoking cessation.[36] The use of afterload reducers for anthracycline-induced late cardiomyopathy is unclear and remains an area of active research.

Pulmonary Complications

There are infectious complications related to immunocompromised state as well as noninfectious complications. Noninfectious pulmonary complications include bronchiolitis obliterans (BO), bronchiolitis obliterans organizing pneumonia (BOOP), and idiopathic pneumonia syndrome (IPS).[37] These events typically occur between three months and two years after transplantation. In a retrospective analysis, the two-year cumulative incidence of delayed onset noninfectious pulmonary complications was 10% among 438 patients who survived more than three months and was 15.6% among those with chronic GvHD.[38] The presence of pulmonary complications was associated with a 15-fold increased risk of late death compared with the baseline population.[33] The causes of pulmonary complications were interstitial pneumonitis (BOOP) (58%) and pulmonary fibrosis (BO) (25%). One can speculate that the interstitial pneumonia is related to BOOP or infection and that the pulmonary fibrosis is related to bronchiolitis obliterans.

Bronchiolitis obliterans is strongly associated with chronic GvHD and can be a pulmonary manifestation of chronic GvHD. Bronchiolitis obliterans is a nonspecific inflammatory injury affecting primarily small airways. Initially, the damage appears to be more obstructive on pulmonary function testing. However, in the more advanced stage, often there can be both obstructive and restrictive changes on pulmonary function testing. The median onset is one year post-transplantation, and the main symptoms are dry cough, progressive dyspnea, and wheezing. Initial chest X-ray may be normal. However, in more advanced phases, hyperinflation may be present. Bronchiolitis obliterans can be clinically diagnosed by a FEV1/FVC ratio < 0.7 or FEV1 < 75% with evidence of air trapping or small airway thickening or bronchiectasis on high-resolution CT and the absence of infection in the respiratory tract. Biopsy is not always necessary for diagnosis. Treatments include high-dose corticosteroids, and the addition of cyclosporine and other immunosuppressants can be required. Prevention of Pneumoncystis jirovecii and superinfection is also critical. The prognosis of these patients is poor.

Bronchiolitis obliterans organizing pneumonia presents as an interstitial pneumonia. It frequently occurs within 1 to 12 months post-transplantation. However, it can also occur years later. The clinical presentation is acute with dry cough, dyspnea, and fever. The chest x-ray reveals peripheral patchy consolidation, ground glass attenuation, and nodular opacities. The pulmonary function testing reveals restrictive pattern with decreased TLC and DLCO but normal FEV. Bronchoscopy is used to rule out infectious etiology. Biopsy is helpful to confirm diagnosis. Treatment usually involves corticosteroids.

Idiopathic pneumonia syndrome typically occurs within 120 days of transplantation and is related to TBI, GvHD, older age, and pretransplantation chemotherapy. Clinical presentation and radiographic findings are non-specific and difficult to distinguish from infectious etiology. Pulmonary function testing reveals restrictive pattern.

Renal Complications

The prevalence of renal dysfunction after allogeneic stem cell transplantation is unclear. The risk factors include older age at transplantation, female gender, hypertension after transplantation, low pretransplantation GFR, use of fludarabine, and exposure to radiation. Substances that may be involved in renal dysfunction include chemotherapy prior to transplantation as well as the conditioning regimen and antibiotics, antivirals, and antifungals. Furthermore, cyclosporine and calcineurin inhibitors have been recognized as a potential agent by causing tubular atrophy, interstitial fibrosis, and calcineurin inhibitor arteriolopathy.

Endocrine Complications

Hypothyroidism is common post-transplantation but responds well to supplementation and has been attributed to chemotherapy as well as exposure to TBI.[39] As previously mentioned, the risk of diabetes among allogeneic transplant survivors is increased three fold compared to siblings.[32]

Genitourinary Complications

Infertility is also a frequent complication post stem cell transplantation, which is related to a combination of chemotherapy in the conditioning regimen and radiation. A thorough and frank discussion with the patient about these issues is recommended. Furthermore, sexual dysfunction is also a common complication of treatment.[40]

Musculoskeletal Complications

There are two major musculoskeletal complications of transplantation are osteoporosis and osteonecrosis of the joints. The odds ratio of development of osteoporosis in survivors is 3.1.[32] The increased risk of osteoporosis has been attributed to chronic corticosteroid use. There is also an increased risk of osteonecrosis of the joints due to chronic corticosteroid use.

Ophthalmologic Complications

Ophthalmologic complications include cataract formation and dry eyes. Cataract formation has been attributed to TBI and corticosteroid use and is unfortunately very frequent. Dry eyes usually can improve with time and respond well to artificial tears.

Secondary Malignancies

Finally, there is an increased risk for a secondary malignancy. The risk of secondary malignancy was 3.6 times more likely in survivors than in the general population.[30] Of the 17 subsequent malignancies in a cohort, 14 were solid non-hematopoietic malignancies with one patient presenting with a therapy-related leukemia, one patient presenting with a non-Hodgkin lymphoma, and one patient presenting with a secondary malignancy of unknown etiology. A retrospective analysis of a total of 28,874 hematopoietic stem cell transplantation survivors found 189 cases of secondary solid malignancy.[41] The overall risk of secondary malignancy was found to be twice the risk of the general population. The risk also appears to increase over time, with the risk at three fold at 15 years. The risk of non-squamous cell carcinoma was also contingent upon the age of the person at the time of the transplant. Patients younger than 30 had a nine fold higher risk of developing non-squamous cell carcinoma compared with older patients. Male gender and chronic GvHD were risk factors for squamous cell carcinoma of the skin and oral pharynx. The risk of melanoma was increased in patients who had received prior radiation as well as T-cell depleted conditioning regimen suggesting that immunosuppression was a culprit. Thyroid cancer was increased among those with a history of radiation exposure, young age, female gender, and chronic GvHD. The risk of breast cancer was also increased six fold that of the general population. Therefore, there is substantial evidence that long-term survivors need to be monitored closely for the development of a secondary malignancy.

CONCLUSIONS

More than one hundred years since its initial description in the medical literature, the treatment of AML remains controversial and challenging. The prognosis is varied depending on the disease biology as well as on the patient-related factors. Our understanding of the heterogeneity of AML has helped in defining the prognosis and the role of allogeneic stem cell transplantation. Standard treatment with intensive chemotherapy and possible stem cell transplantation offers the potential for cure in some patients.[9] However, the morbidity and mortality of these treatments must be considered in the treatment decision. With reduced-intensity transplantation and as the overall population lives longer, we can expect the population of long-term survivors of leukemia to increase. Long-term survivors of leukemia require close monitoring for long-term consequences of their disease and treatments. Further study into the survivorship of leukemia is warranted as more patients are living longer. A coordinated approach to caregiving is required between the hematologist and the primary care physician.

REFERENCES

1. Appelbaum FR, Gundacker H, Head DR, et al. Age and acute myeloid leukemia. *Blood* 2006; 107(9): 3481–3485.

2. Surveillance, Epidemiology and End result (SEER) database. Available at: http://seer.cancer.gov.

3. Miller KB and Pihan G. Chapter 60: Clinical Manifestations of Acute Myeloid Leukemia. In: Hoffman R, Benz E, Shattil, S, Furie B, Silberstein L, McGlave P, Heslop H, eds. *Hematology: Basic Principles and Practice* 5th ed.. Philadelphia: Churchill Livingston Elsevier; 2009: 933–963.

4. Deschler B and Lubbert M. Acute Myeloid Leukemia: Epidemology and Etiology. *Cancer* 2006: 107: 2099–2107.

5. Ley TJ, Ding L, Walter MJ, et al: MNMT3A mutations in acute myeloid leukemia. *New Engl J Med* 2010:363,2424–2433.

6. Swerdlow SH, Campo E, Harris NL, et al. *WHO classification of tumours of haematopoietic and lymphoid tissues* 4th ed. Lyon: International Agency of Research on Cancer IARC; 2008: 439.

7. Dohner, H, Estey EH, Amadori S, et al. Diagnosis and management of acute myeloid leukemia in Adults: recommendations from an international expert panel, on behalf of the European LeukemiaNet. *Blood* 2010; 115: 453–474.

8. Breems DA, Van Putten WL, De Greef GE, et al. Monosomal karyotype in acute myeloid leukemia: a better indicator of poor prognosis than a complex karyotype. *Journal of Clinical Oncology.* 2008; 26: 4791–4797.

9. Yanada M, Garcia-Manero G, Borthakur, el al. Potential cure of acute myeloid leukemia. *Cancer* 2007; 110: 2756–2760.

10. Cheson BD, Bennett JM, Kopecky KJ, et al. Revised Recommendations of the International Working Group for diagnosis, Standardization of Response criteria,

Treatment outcomes and reporting standards for therapeutic trials in acute myeloid leukemia. *Journal of Clinical Oncology* 2003; 21: 4642–4649.

11. Fernandez HF, Sun Z, Yao X, et al. Anthracycline dose intensification in acute myeloid leukemia. *New England Journal of Medicine* 2009; 361: 1249–1259.

12. Grimwalde D and Hills RK. Independent Prognostic factors for AML outcomes. *Hematology.* 2009; 385–395.

13. Juliusson G, Antunovic P, Derolf A, et al. Age and acute myeloid leukemia: real world data on decision to treat and outcomes from the Swedish acute leukemia registry. *Blood* 2009; 113: 4179–4187.

14. Kantarjian HM, Ravandi F, O'Brien S, et al. Intensive chemotherapy does not benefit most older patients (age 70 years or older) with acute myeloid leukemia. *Blood* 2010; 116: 4422–4429.

15. Kantarjian HM, O'Brien S, Huang X, et al. Survival advantage with decitabine versus intensive chemotherapy in patients with higher risk myelodysplastic syndrome: comparision with historical experience. *Cancer* 2007; 109 (6): 1133–1137.

16. Giles FJ, Borthakur G, Ravandi F, et al. The haematopoietic cell transplantation comorbidity index score is predictive of early death and survival in patients over 60 years of age receiving induction therapy for acute myeloid leukemia. *British Journal of Haematology* 2007; 136(4): 623–627.

17. Walter RB, Kantarjian HM, Huang X, et al. Effect of Complete Remission and Responses less than Complete Remission on Survival in Acute Myeloid Leukemia: A Combined Eastern Cooperative Oncology Group, Southwest Oncology Group and MD Anderson Cancer Center Study. *Journal of Clinical Oncology* 2010; 28: 1766–1771.

18. Tilly H, Castaigne S, Bordessoule D, et al. Low-dose cytarabine versus intensive chemotherapy in the treatment of acute nonlymphocytic leukemia in the elderly. *Journal of Clinical Oncology* 1990; 8(2): 272–9.

19. Alibhai SMH, Leach M, Kermalli H, et al. The impact of acute myeloid leukemia and its treatment on quality of life and functional status in older adults. *Critical Reviews of Oncology Hematology* 2007; 64: 19–30.

20. Alibhai SMH, Leach M, Gupta V, et al. Quality of life beyond 6 months after diagnosis in older adults with acute myeloid leukemia. *Critical Reviews of Oncology Hematology* 2009; 69: 168–174.

21. Alibhai SMH, Leach M, Kowgier ME. Fatigue in older adults with acute myeloid leukemia: predictors and associations with quality of life and functional status. *Leukemia* 2007; 21: 845–848.

22. Panju AH, Danesh A, Minden MD, et al. Associations between quality of life, fatigue, and cytokine levels in patients aged 50+ with acute myeloid leukemia. *Supportive Care Cancer* 2009; 17: 539–546.

23. Schumacher A, Wewers D, Jeinecke A, et al. Fatigue as an important aspect of quality of life in patients with acute myeloid leukemia. Leukemia research 2002; 26(4): 355–62.

24. Battaglini, CL, Hackney AC, Garcia R, et al. The effect of an exercise program in Leukemia patients. *Integrative cancer therapies* 2009; 8: 130–138.

25. Chang PH, Lai YH, Shun SC, et al. Effects of a walking intervention on fatigue-related experiences of hospitalized acute myelogenous leukemia patients undergoing chemotherapy: A randomized controlled trial. *Journal of pain and symptom management* 2008; 35: 524–534.

26. Rubin EH, Andersen JW, Berg DT, et al. Risk factors for High-dose cytarabine neurotoxicity: An analysis of a cancer and leukemia group B trial in patients with acute myelogenous leukemia: *Journal of Clinical Oncology* 1992; 10 (6): 948–953.

27. Latagliata R, Petti MC, Fenu S, et al. Therapy-related myelodysplastic syndrome-acute myelogenous leukemia in patients treated for acute promyelocytic leukemia: an emerging problem. *Blood* 2002; 99(3): 822–824.

28. Ogasawara T, Yasuyama M, Kawauchi K. Therapy-related myelodysplastic syndrome with monosomy 5 after successful treatment of acute myeloid leukemia (M2). *American Journal of Hematology* 2005; 79: 136–141.

29. Lemez P, Urbanek V. Chemotherapy for AML with cytosine arabinoside, daunorubicin, etoposide and mitoxantrone may cause permanent oligoasthenozoospermia and amenorrhea in middle aged patients. *Neoplasma* 2005; 52(5): 398–401.

30. Bhatia S, Francisco L, Carter, A, et al. Late mortality after allogeneic hematopoietic stem cell transplantation and functional status of long-term survivors: report from the Bone Marrow Transplant Survivor study. *Blood* 2007; 110: 3784–3792.

31. Tichelli A, Bucher C, Rovo A, et al. Premature cardiovascular disease after allogeneic hematopoietic stem cell transplantation. *Blood* 2007; 110: 3463–3471.

32. Baker KS, Ness KS, Weisdorf D, et al. Late effects in survivors of acute leukemia treated with hematopoietic cell transplantation: a report from the Bone Marrow Transplant Survivor Study *Leukemia* 2010; 1–9.

33. Baker KS, Ness KK, Steinberger J, et al. Diabetes, hypertension and cardiovascular events in survivors of hematopoietic cell transplantation: a report from the bone marrow transplantation survivor study. *Blood* 2007; 109: 1765–1772.

34. Taskinen M, Saarinen-Pihkala UM, Hovi L et al. Impaired glucose tolerance and dyslipidemia as late effects after bone marrow transplantation in childhood. *Lancet* 2000; 356: 993–997.

35. Rackley C, Schultz KR, Goldman FD et al. Cardiac manifestations of graft-versus-host disease. *Biology of blood and marrow transplantation* 2005; 11: 773–780.

36. Tichelli A, Bhatia S, Socie G. Cardiac and cardiovascular consequences after haematopoietic stem cell transplantation. *British journal of haematology* 2008; 142: 11–26.

37. Tichelli A, Rovo A, Gratwohl A. Late pulmonary, cardiovascular and renal complications after hematopoietic stem cell transplantation and recommended screening practices. *Hematology* 2008; 125–133.

38. Patriarca F, Skert C, Sperotto A, et al. Effect on survival of the development of late-onset non-infectious pulmonary complications after stem cell transplantation. *Haematologica* 2006; 91: 1268–1272.

39. Sanders JE. Chronic Graft-versus-Host disease and late effects after hematopoietic stem cell transplantation. *International Journal of Hematology* 2002; 76: 15–28.

40. Watson M, Wheatley K, Harrison GA, et al. Severe adverse Impact on sexual functioning and fertility on bone marrow transplantation, either allogeneic or autologous, compared with consolidation chemotherapy alone. *Cancer* 1999; 86 (7): 1231–1239.

41. Rizzo JD, Curtis RE, Socie G, et al. Solid cancers after allogeneic hematopoietic stem cell transplantation. *Blood* 2009; 113: 1175–1183.

31

BONE MARROW TRANSPLANTATION SURVIVORSHIP

COREY CUTLER, MD

INTRODUCTION

Allogeneic stem cell transplantation is used increasingly to treat a variety of hematologic neoplasms, non-malignant marrow disorders, and inborn errors of metabolism. Coupled with the increased volume of stem cell transplantation over the past decade has been a steady improvement in transplant outcomes, related largely to refinement in HLA-matching, improved supportive care, and advances in infectious disease therapy. As a result, there are a growing number of long-term survivors of transplantation, and the transplant community has now recognized the importance of providing specialized care to these individuals.

In contrast to non-transplant therapy for cancer, transplant recipients (particularly myeloablative transplant recipients) undergo highly toxic therapy and are subject to several long-term complications not routinely seen after conventional doses of chemoradiotherapy. In addition, allogeneic transplant recipients are subject to the long-term consequences of chronic graft-vs.-host disease (GVHD), which may require specialized care, even when quiescent or resolved, for many years. In order to address the requirements of the long-term transplant survivor, specialized transplantation survivorship care is required. Drawing from almost all fields of medicine and allied health sciences, the model for stem cell transplantation survivorship medicine is a paradigm for cooperation among medical subspecialists.

Continued medical care for transplantation survivors is critical. In one large report of transplant survivors, 10% of two-year transplant survivors subsequently died of non-relapse related causes.[1] Despite this, it is estimated that five-year survivors of transplantation have long-term survival that approaches survival rates in age-matched populations,[2,3] again underscoring the need for long-term transplant survivorship care.

This chapter will discuss an overview to the care of the stem cell transplant survivor, focusing on issues that require attention at approximately one year from transplant onwards.

COORDINATION OF CARE

There are comprehensive consensus guidelines that recommend the appropriate screening studies to monitor for the long-term complications of stem cell transplantation,[4] however, interpretation of the recommended tests (Table 31.1)

TABLE 31.1 RECOMMENDED ANNUAL SCREENING TESTS: DANA-FARBER CANCER INSTITUTE TRANSPLANT SURVIVORS CLINIC

Blood Tests

Hematology

  Complete blood count

  Serum ferritin

Renal

  Urinalysis and urine microalbumin

  Kidney function testing (BUN/creatinine)

Endocrine

  Fasting lipid profile

  Vitamin D level

  TSH & free T4

  Fasting glucose and Hemoglobin A1c

  Testosterone & Sex hormone binding globulin level (Male)

  Follicle stimulating hormone & Luteinizing hormone (Female)

Immunology/Infectious Disease

  CD4 count

  Immunoglobulin levels

  Hepatitis B/C viral load

Radiology and Other Tests

  Electrocardiogram

  Echocardiogram or Exercise stress testing (in selected patients)

  Pulmonary function testing and oxygen diffusion capacity

  Bone Densitometry

  Schirmer test and intraocular pressure measurement

often lies outside the realm of expertise of the transplantation physician, and some require consultation with subspecialists. Some centers discharge patients several months after transplantation to the care of the referring hematologist/ oncologist or primary care physician. For these patients, arranging standardized long-term follow-up can be even more problematic, since primary care physicians may not be aware of the long-term complications of transplantation[5] or have access to subspecialists who do. For this reason, we advocate a multispecialty clinic that can cater to the individual needs of the long-term transplant patient. In this multispecialty clinic, transplant survivors are offered one-stop shopping with access to a number of subspecialists with an interest in transplant survivorship. Unfortunately, this multispecialty clinic model may not be practical in centers with low stem cell transplant patient volume. In the absence of a multispecialty clinic, centers should develop a plan for screening patients for the long-term complications of transplantation, based on the individual patient history.

When determining the appropriate subspecialists and referrals for transplant survivorship care, a number of factors need to be taken into consideration, such as the age and gender of the patient, the chemoradiotherapy given prior to transplant to treat the malignancy, the donor type (autologous versus allogeneic), the agents used in pre-transplant conditioning therapy, the transplant conditioning intensity (myeloablative versus reduced-intensity), and the occurrence of early complications after transplantation.

INDIVIDUAL ORGAN SYSTEM LONG-TERM COMPLICATIONS OF TRANSPLANTATION

While the emergence of chronic health conditions cannot be altered with screening practices alone, it is hoped that the severity and consequences of the resulting conditions can be altered. Each of the following organ systems has known long-term complications and appropriate screening or preventative actions can reduce the resultant morbidity and mortality of these conditions.

Cardiovascular

Survivors of stem cell transplantation are known to have inferior long-term cardiovascular health when compared with their non-transplant siblings.[1] Studies have estimated the prevalence of cardiovascular complications of transplantation to be between 3.6% and 6.8%.[6,7]

Several determinants of cardiovascular health are affected after transplantation. Hypertension is common after transplantation,[6] and is often related to the prolonged use of corticosteroids and calcineurin inhibitors (cyclosporine or tacrolimus), as well as chronic renal dysfunction. Other risk factors for cardiovascular morbidity include pre-transplant anthracycline chemotherapy (associated with delayed non-ischemic heart failure) and mediastinal radiation therapy (associated with accelerated coronary atherosclerosis). In addition, diabetes and dyslipidemia (discussed below), both of which occur with elevated frequency after transplantation, are both associated with an increased incidence of cardiovascular events such as myocardial infarction, cerebrovascular disease, and congestive heart failure.

Preliminary data suggest that long-term cardiovascular health is equivalent regardless of conditioning intensity, even though it has been postulated that cardiac outcomes after reduced intensity transplantation would be superior when compared with myeloablative transplantation.[8] Since classic risk factors for cardiovascular morbidity appear to be implicated in post-transplantation cardiovascular disease,[9] appropriate screening and counseling techniques can be used to prevent mortality from cardiovascular disease after transplantation. Regular measurement and control of blood pressure, nutritional counseling and obesity control, counseling for smoking cessation, and control of diabetes are all critical. Electrocardiography should be performed routinely to screen for asymptomatic coronary disease, and selected patients should be referred for echocardiography or exercise stress testing.

Respiratory

There are several potential causes of impaired lung function after transplantation, including lung injury from total body irradiation, chemotherapy, infection, and the inflammatory pneumonitides. Reduced intensity transplantation is associated with similar infectious and non-infectious pneumonitis risks, however, the chemoradiotherapy insults are generally less severe. Bronchiolitis obliterans, often considered the pulmonary manifestation of chronic GVHD, is noted uniquely after allogeneic transplantation and has a major impact on lung function and survival after transplantation. Both early post-transplant[10] and pre-transplant lung function[11] are important predictors of lung impairment and mortality after transplantation.

Pre-transplant lung function testing is performed routinely, and considerations should be made to repeating these tests early after transplantation to establish a new baseline. A repeat assay at one year is recommended for long-term survivors of transplantation. Careful attention to residual airflow obstruction and diminished oxygen diffusion capacity can be useful in detection of ongoing inflammatory lung processes. Smoking cessation counseling should be provided to all transplant survivors.

Renal

Chronic renal disease after transplantation is common and is often multifactorial in etiology. The relative contribution of radiation injury, chronic calcineurin inhibitor use, hypertension, and microangiopathy (the latter two often a result of calcineurin inhibitor use) can often not accurately be differentiated. In addition, membranous glomerulopathy and other autoimmune-like diseases of the glomerulus have been associated with chronic GVHD in allogeneic transplant recipients. Finally, patients (particularly those with multiple my-eloma) may have clinical or subclinical renal disease prior to transplantation, which increases the risks of post-transplant renal dysfunction.

The incidence of renal disease after transplantation varies widely, with estimates as low as 4.4% up to 38% in long-term allograft survivors.[12,13] While initially presumed that total body irradiation-free reduced intensity preparative regimens would be associated with a reduced incidence of chronic renal injury, this does not appear to be true.[14]

Presenting signs of chronic renal injury include reductions in the glomerular filtration rate and proteinuria. While serum creatinine and BUN are checked frequently after transplantation, urinary measurements of protein excretion are not, and therefore should be considered for long-term transplant survivors.

Endocrine

Diabetes/Metabolic Syndrome

Type II diabetes is very prevalent after stem cell transplantation. The Bone Marrow Transplant Survivors Study documented a 3.65 fold increase in the rate of diabetes among allogeneic transplant recipients, but not autologous recipients, likely due to the frequent use of corticosteroids as well as the routine use of calcineurin inhibitors after allogeneic but not autologous transplantation.[15] The incidence of diabetes was as high as 30% in a smaller survivorship cohort at two years from allogeneic transplant, and among those with diabetes any time after transplant, nearly one third still had diabetes at the two year mark from transplantation.[6] The association with diabetes and hyperlipidemia and hypertension (the metabolic syndrome) is common after transplantation since the individual components of this syndrome share several common risk factors.[16] Untreated metabolic syndrome is associated with accelerated cardiovascular disease (see Cardiovascular, above) and must be recognized early for effective intervention. Therefore, screening for diabetes using fasting glucose and glycosylated hemoglobin measurement is warranted in all transplant survivors. Similarly, fasting lipid concentration measurement is recommended.

Thyroid

Hypothyroidism is very common after transplantation, and the incidence of clinical hypothyroidism increases with time, with a relative risk of over two when compared with healthy sibling controls.[17] Chemotherapy-only conditioning regimens cause clinical hypothyroidism, however, total-body irradiation regimens have a much higher incidence, with single fraction irradiation being a greater risk than fractionated dose regimens. All transplant survivors should have thyroid hormone assays at one year from transplantation and at least annually thereafter. Earlier assays can be performed if clinical suspicion exists, but the clinician must be aware of the possibility of the sick-euthyroid syndrome early after transplantation.

Bone Health

It is known that accelerated bone loss occurs after both autologous and allogeneic stem cell transplantation.[18] Factors associated with increased loss of bone mineral density include the use of post-transplant steroids, conditioning intensity, and hypogonadism. The routine use of calcium or calcitonin after transplantation has not been shown to prevent the loss of bone mineral density,[19] however the use of bisphosphonates can prevent some, but not all, of the bone mineral loss.[20] Dual energy x-ray absorptiometry is a recommended screening test for all patients one year after transplantation. Special attention should be paid to those patients at increased risk for avascular necrosis of a major joint.[21]

Reproductive Endocrinology

Temporary or permanent hypogonadism is common after both autologous and allogeneic transplantation (although more common in women than men), and myeloablative allogeneic transplantation almost always causes permanent sterility, although rare exceptions to this rule have been noted. Retained spermatogenesis appears to be more common than preservation of ovarian function, particularly in men transplanted at a younger age, and without persistent chronic GVHD.[22] In addition to changes in sex hormone levels, loss of libido, erectile dysfunction, and dyspareunia are common, although seldom discussed. Screening for sex hormone levels with appropriate replacement therapy is recommended one year or earlier, and then again later as needed after transplantation and sexual health counseling is appropriate where needed.

Oral

There are several potential long-term complications of transplantation that can arise in the mouth. Chronic dry mouth (xerostomia) can be a complication of total body irradiation therapy, focal irradiation prior to transplant (for patients with lymphoma involving the head and neck) and chronic salivary gland GVHD. Chronic xerostomia significantly increases the risk of developing accelerated dental caries, particularly along the gum line and in between teeth. In addition, chronic xerostomia, mucosal chronic GVHD, and sclerodermatous GVHD involving the oral aperture are all associated with difficulty with mastication and swallowing, which can result in chronic malnutrition.

Appropriate screening for the chronic oral complications of transplantation by an oral medicine specialist or dentist is recommended 6–12 months after transplantation, and at least twice annually thereafter.

Ophthalmologic

Chronic dry eye (keratoconjunctivitis sicca) is a common complaint after transplantation. Ocular dryness may be the result of the loss of lacrimal gland function from either chronic GVHD or total body irradiation. In addition to topical therapy with lubricating drops, temporary or permanent punctal occlusion can be helpful. Other common complications of total body irradiation include the development of cataracts, which occurs nearly universally after radiation-based preparative regimens, although there is an increased incidence of this complication even among non-TBI based preparative regimen recipients. Cataract development is a particularly common long-term complication of pediatric transplantation as well.[23]

The specialized management of ocular often includes the use of corticosteroid eye drops. The prolonged use of ocular steroids increases the risk of glaucoma after transplantation, so routine pressure measurements of the anterior chamber are required. Other increasingly recognized complications of the anterior and posterior chambers of the eye include uveitis, choroiditis, infectious retinitis, and retinal microvascular disease.

While some screening for the ocular complications of transplantation can be performed by the transplant physician (basic visual acuity, Schirmer test for tear production), ocular care after transplantation must be performed by an ophthalmologist knowledgeable in the potential complications of transplantation. Initial evaluation at one year, or earlier if there are changes in visual acuity should be performed, and annual screening thereafter is required.

Dermatologic

Being the most common organ involved in acute and chronic GVHD, the skin requires specialized care after transplantation. When examining the skin and skin-derived structures (i.e. nail beds, hair) careful examination for the early signs of GVHD (follicular erythema, dyspigmentation, focal inducation, joint contracture) should occur. Long-term cutaneous recommendations include counseling for prevention of sun burn and damage (dermatoheliosis) and to prevent severe dryness (xerosis), a risk factor for GVHD and cutaneous infections.

Infectious Disease

Transplant recipients remain at risk for opportunistic infections long after normal hematopoiesis returns and leukocyte numbers normalize, due to lymphocyte naivete and restricted immunologic repertoires. Vaccination strategies after transplant continue to evolve, and are based largely on consensus recommendation rather than rigorous scientific data.[24,25] Screening studies that address immunologic reconstitution after transplant include the measurement of immunoglobulin levels and a CD4 count one year after transplantation. Persistent low T cell counts are an indication to continue immune prophylaxis and persistent hypogammaglobulinemia is an indication for replacement therapy. In addition, Hepatitis B and C viral load measurement at the one year mark after transplant is reasonable, particularly in those patients who were heavily transfused, who were seropositive prior to transplantation, or who had seropositive donors. Continued immune prophylaxis with antiviral and antipneumocystis therapy beyond one year from transplantation should occur in the presence of chronic GVHD, in the presence of very low CD4 counts (ie < 100/μL) or in those who remain on immunosuppression. Special considerations for functionally or anatomically asplenic patients should be made.

SCREENING FOR SECONDARY MALIGNANCIES
AFTER TRANSPLANTATION

Stem cell transplant recipients develop secondary solid malignancies at a rate twice that of age-matched population controls.[26,27] This is in addition to the elevated rate of secondary myelodysplastic disorders encountered after autologous stem cell transplantation, particularly when total body irradiation is used in the preparative regimen.[28]

The site with the highest odds ratio when compared with age-matched controls is the oral cavity, where there is a seven-fold risk increase in long-term survivors.[27] Common presenting features of intra-oral malignancy include non-healing ulcers, mucosal growths, and induration. Early cancerous lesions may appear very similar to GVHD and are identifiable as malignancies only with tissue biopsy.

As with the oral mucosa, there is an excess of pre-malignant and true malignant neoplasms of the skin noted after transplantation, and complete skin examination is required for monitoring against this complication. It is postulated that the elevation in the rate of malignancies of both the skin and the mouth is due to a defect in tumor surveillance related to chronic immunodeficiency after transplantation. While screening for all malignancies is likely to be impractical and associated with a high false-positive rate in all transplant survivors, targeted screening, including complete dermatologic evaluation, intraoral examination, mammography in women exposed to chest radiation, cervical cancer screening, and other targeted interventions where appropriate is likely to reduce the mortality from secondary cancers in transplant survivors.

PSYCHOSOCIAL HEALTH AND LIFESTYLE MODIFICATION

In addition to careful attention to the physical complications of transplantation, special care must be given to psychological health of the transplant survivor. It is known that GVHD has a major impact on the quality of life of transplant survivors,[29,30] but even in the absence of GVHD, significant psychological distress can occur.[31] While often dismissed as being less important than physical complications of transplantation, depression after transplantation has been associated with inferior outcome,[32] and therefore patients should undergo screening and appropriate counseling should depressive symptoms occur. In addition, transplant patients may have deficits in cognition that can only be revealed on detailed neuropsychological testing, so involvement of mental health providers in the long-term care of the transplant survivor is essential.

Other factors may prevent the normal transition back to normalcy after transplantation. Patients must learn to deal with new issues with exercise tolerance and exercise physiologists may be helpful in this setting. Nutritional counseling can also be useful, as transplant patients often have prolonged disturbances in taste and may require diet modification to ensure adequate caloric intake. Obesity counseling from a nutritionist is also useful, where indicated, since transplant patients have increased rates of cardiovascular disease. Finally, sexual health should be addressed with transplant survivors. Often linked to endocrine issues, sexuality after transplantation is most often neglected for a variety of reasons.

CONCLUSIONS AND FUTURE DIRECTIONS IN TRANSPLANT SURVIVORSHIP

Once deemed experimental and medically aggressive, stem cell transplantation is now an accepted form of therapy for even early stage hematologic malignancies, and as such, transplant volumes continue to increase. Along with the increase in transplant volume, survival statistics after transplant continue to improve, leading to a large number of transplant survivors faced with a large number of potential complications of transplantation. Survivorship after transplantation is a collaborative affair, since the spectrum of post-transplant issues is vast, and generally beyond the scope of any single physician. The multi-disciplinary model for transplant survivorship care can be adapted to many clinical program settings, and is a useful starting point for most programs. The growth of survivorship research in transplantation will undoubtedly lead to new recommendations in the coming years as the estimates and impact of complications of transplantation continue to be elucidated.

Among others, transplant survivors may have specific needs in the following areas:

- Cardiology and vascular medicine
- Respiratory medicine
- Nephrology
- Endocrinology (including bone and sexual/reproductive health)
- Oral medicine
- Ophthalmology
- Dermatology
- Infectious disease
- Nutrition
- Exercise physiology
- Cognitive and psychosocial health

For centers in which patients have been discharged, and the long-term care is done elsewhere, it is important to ensure that the results of screening tests are reported to both the transplant team and current medical provider. In addition, the responsibilities for follow-up of the individual test results should be clearly delineated. Finally, a comprehensive plan for future screening and monitoring tests should be devised, and the plan should be clearly communicated to the primary treating team. As part of the plan, it is crucial to report long-term adverse events back to the transplant center to help shape future long-term follow-up plans.

REFERENCES

1. Sun C-L, Francisco L, Kawashima T et al. Prevalence and predictors of chronic health conditions after heamtopoeitic cell transplantation: A report from the Bone Marrow Transplant Survivor Study. Blood 2010;116(17):3129–3139.

2. Nivison-Smith I, Simpson JM, Dodds AJ, Ma DD, Szer J, Bradstock KF. Relative survival of long-term hematopoietic cell transplant recipients approaches general population rates. *Biol Blood Marrow Transplant* 2009;15(10):1323–1330.

3. Martin PJ, Counts GW, Jr., Appelbaum FR et al. Life Expectancy in Patients Surviving More Than 5 Years After Hematopoietic Cell Transplantation. *Journal of Clinical Oncology* 2010;28(6):1011–1016.

4. Rizzo JD, Wingard JR, Tichelli A et al. Recommended screening and preventive practices for long-term survivors after hematopoietic cell transplantation: joint recommendations of the European Group for Blood and Marrow Transplantation, the Center for International Blood and Marrow Transplant Research, and the American Society of Blood and Marrow Transplantation. *Biol Blood Marrow Transplant* 2006;12(2):138–151.

5. Shankar SM, Carter A, Sun CL et al. Health care utilization by adult long-term survivors of hematopoietic cell transplant: report from the Bone Marrow Transplant Survivor Study. *Cancer Epidemiol Biomarkers Prev* 2007;16(4):834–839.

6. Majhail NS, Challa TR, Mulrooney DA, Baker KS, Burns LJ. Hypertension and Diabetes Mellitus in Adult and Pediatric Survivors of Allogeneic Hematopoietic Cell Transplantation. *Biology of Blood and Marrow Transplantation* 2009;15(9):1100–1107.

7. Tichelli A, Passweg J, Wojcik D et al. Late cardiovascular events after allogeneic hematopoietic stem cell transplantation: a retrospective multicenter study of the Late Effects Working Party of the European Group for Blood and Marrow Transplantation. *Haematologica* 2008;93(8):1203–1210.

8. Chow EJ, Baker KS, Friedman DL et al. Population-Based Analysis of Late Cardiovascular Morbidity and Hospitalizations After Hematopoietic Cell Transplantation. ASH Annual Meeting Abstracts 2009;114(22):517.

9. Armenian SH, Sun CL, Mills G et al. Predictors of Late Cardiovascular Complications ináSurvivors of Hematopoietic Cell Transplantation. *Biology of Blood and Marrow Transplantation* 2010;16(8):1138–1144.

10. Walter EC, Orozco-Levi M, Ramirez-Sarmiento A et al. Lung Function and Long-Term Complications after Allogeneic Hematopoietic Cell Transplant. *Biology of Blood and Marrow Transplantation* 2010;16(1):53–61.

11. Parimon T, Madtes DK, Au DH, Clark JG, Chien JW. Pretransplant Lung Function, Respiratory Failure, and Mortality after Stem Cell Transplantation. *Am J Respir Crit Care Med* 2005;172(3):384–390.

12. Choi M, Sun CL, Kurian S et al. Incidence and predictors of delayed chronic kidney disease in long-term survivors of hematopoietic cell transplantation. *Cancer* 2008;113(7):1580–1587.

13. Ando M, Ohashi K, Akiyama H et al. Chronic kidney disease in long-term survivors of myeloablative allogeneic haematopoietic cell transplantation: prevalence and risk-factors. *Nephrology Dialysis Transplantation* 2010;25(1):278–282.

14. Al Hazzouri A, Cao Q, Burns LJ, Weisdorf DJ, Majhail NS. Similar risks for chronic kidney disease in long-term survivors of myeloablative and reduced-intensity allogeneic hematopoietic cell transplantation. *Biol Blood Marrow Transplant* 2008;14(6):658–663.

15. Baker KS, Ness KK, Steinberger J et al. Diabetes, hypertension, and cardiovascular events in survivors of hematopoietic cell transplantation: a report from the bone marrow transplantation survivor study. *Blood* 2007;109(4):1765–1772.

16. Majhail NS, Flowers ME, Ness KK et al. High prevalence of metabolic syndrome after allogeneic hematopoietic cell transplantation. *Bone Marrow Transplant* 2008;43(1):49–54.

17. Baker KS, Gurney JG, Ness KK et al. Late effects in survivors of chronic myeloid leukemia treated with hematopoietic cell transplantation: results from the *Bone Marrow Transplant Survivor Study. Blood* 2004;104(6):1898–1906.

18. Yao S, Smiley SL, West K et al. Accelerated Bone Mineral Density Loss Occurs with Similar Incidence and Severity, But with Different Risk Factors, after Autologous versus Allogeneic Hematopoietic Cell Transplantation. *Biology of Blood and Marrow Transplantation* 2010;16(8):1130–1137.

19. Valimaki MJ, Kinnunen K, Volin L et al. A prospective study of bone loss and turnover after allogeneic bone marrow transplantation: effect of calcium supplementation with or without calcitonin. *Bone Marrow Transplant* 1999;23(4):355–361.

20. Kananen K, Volin L, Laitinen K, Alfthan H, Ruutu T, Valimaki MJ. Prevention of Bone Loss after Allogeneic Stem Cell Transplantation by Calcium, Vitamin D, and Sex Hormone Replacement with or without Pamidronate. *J Clin Endocrinol Metab* 2005;90(7):3877–3885.

21. Campbell S, Sun CL, Kurian S et al. Predictors of avascular necrosis of bone in long-term survivors of hematopoietic cell transplantation. *Cancer* 2009;115(18):4127–4135.

22. Rovo A, Tichelli A, Passweg JR et al. Spermatogenesis in long-term survivors after allogeneic hematopoietic stem cell transplantation is associated with age, time interval since transplantation, and apparently absence of chronic GVHD. *Blood* 2006;108(3):1100–1105.

23. Gurney JG, Ness KK, Rosenthal J, Forman SJ, Bhatia S, Baker KS. Visual, auditory, sensory, and motor impairments in long-term survivors of hematopoietic stem cell transplantation performed in childhood. *Cancer* 2006;106(6):1402–1408.

24. Guidelines for preventing opportunistic infections among hematopoietic stem cell transplant recipients. *MMWR Recomm Rep* 2000;49(RR-10):1–7.

25. Ljungman P, Cordonnier C, Einsele H et al. Vaccination of hematopoietic cell transplant recipients. *Bone Marrow Transplant* 0 AD;44(8):521–526.

26. Lowe T, Bhatia S, Somlo G. Second Malignancies after Allogeneic Hematopoietic Cell Transplantation. *Biology of Blood and Marrow Transplantation* 2007;13(10):1121–1134.

27. Rizzo JD, Curtis RE, Socie G et al. Solid cancers after allogeneic hematopoietic cell transplantation. *Blood* 2009;113(5):1175–1183.

28. Brown JR, Yeckes H, Friedberg JW et al. Increasing Incidence of Late Second Malignancies After Conditioning With Cyclophosphamide and Total-Body Irradiation and Autologous Bone Marrow Transplantation for Non-Hodgkin-Æs Lymphoma. *Journal of Clinical Oncology* 2005;23(10):2208–2214.

29. Andrykowski MA, Bishop MM, Hahn EA et al. Long-term health-related quality of life, growth, and spiritual well-being after hematopoietic stem-cell transplantation. *J Clin Oncol* 2005;23(3):599–608.

30. Pallua S, Giesinger J, Oberguggenberger A et al. Impact of GVHD on quality of life in long-term survivors of haematopoietic transplantation. *Bone Marrow Transplant* 2010;45(10):1534–1539.

31. Rusiewicz A, DuHamel KN, Burkhalter J et al. Psychological distress in long-term survivors of hematopoietic stem cell transplantation. *Psycho-Oncology* 2008; 17(4):329–337.

32. Loberiza FR, Rizzo JD, Bredeson CN et al. Association of Depressive Syndrome and Early Deaths Among Patients After Stem-Cell Transplantation for Malignant Diseases. *Journal of Clinical Oncology* 2002;20(8):2118–2126.

33. Hoffmeister PA, Madtes DK, Storer BE, Sanders JE. Pulmonary function in long-term survivors of pediatric hematopoietic cell transplantation. *Pediatr Blood Cancer* 2006;47(5):594–606.

34. Hoffmeister PA, Hingorani SR, Storer BE, Baker KS, Sanders JE. Hypertension in Long-Term Survivors of Pediatric Hematopoietic Cell Transplantation. *Biology of Blood and Marrow Transplantation* 2010;16(4):515–524.

35. Hoffmeister PA, Storer BE, Sanders JE. Diabetes Mellitus in Long-Term Survivors of Pediatric Hematopoietic Cell Transplantation. *Journal of Pediatric Hematology/Oncology* 2004;26(2).

INDEX

Fruits and vegetables, 118, 119; nutritional issues, 121–22
FSAD. *See* Female sexual arousal
disorder
Functional Assessment of Cancer Therapy (FACT), 291

Gabapentin, 211, 287
Gastrointestinal distress, 288–89
Gastrointestinal health, 288–89
Gastrointestinal malignancy: active
disease surveillance, 230–31; acute
toxicities, 226; chronic toxicities,
226–29; defining survival, 222;
financial issues, 230; incident cases,
by age group, 223; medical concerns, 225–29; neurologic effects,
226–27; psychologic concerns,
229–30; survival rates, 224; by age
group, 225; treatment complications,
228. *See also* Colon cancer
Gastrointestinal stromal tumor (GIST),
258–61
Gastrointestinal tract cancer, 301–2
Gemcitabine, 226
Gender: LiveSTRONG survey, 15; survivor time-line, 87
Genetic counselors, 69
Genetic disorders, 327
Genetic mutations, 322–23; *BRCA,*
214; *BRCA2,* 198
Gestational surrogate/carrier, 197
GIST. *See* Gastrointestinal stromal tumor
Glucarate, 120
Glutamine, 211
GOG Lap 2 trial. *See* Gynecologic On-
cology Group Lap 2 trial
Gonadotoxicity, 256
Graft-*versus*-host-disease (GVHD),
342, 345–46; complications from,
347–49
Gray Cancer Center survivors, 66–67
GVHD. *See* Graft-*versus*-host-disease
Gynecological malignancies: psycho-
social issues/sexual aspects of,
290–92; risk factors, 283–84;
surveillance recommendations, 292;
therapy for, 284–90; local, 284–86;
systemic, 286–90

Gynecological neoplasms, 283
Gynecologic Oncology Group (GOG)
Lap 2 trial, 285
Gynecology, 283–92

Hartford hospital: cancer survivorship
program, 65–72; mission of, 65
Hartford Hospital's Helen & Harry Gray
Cancer Center: cancer survivorship
services, 67–72; community hospitals and, 65
Head and neck cancers, 264–76; chemotherapeutic regimen toxicities,
267–68; chronic toxicities, "new
normal," 268–76; HPV, 264–65;
long-term survivors, specific complications of, 269–76; QOL tools,
268; radiation-associated toxicities,
267; rehabilitation intervention and,
108, 109; sexuality, 275; smoking,
266; surgery, 266–67; surveillance,
276; survivor, 265–66; treatment,
266–67
Head and neck squamous cell carcinoma (HNSCC): late stage, 265;
surveillance recommendations, 276;
treatment and prognosis, 264–65
Health care providers, 21; barriers related to, 99; co-survivors and, 157,
158, 159
Health promotion, 7
Health-related quality of life (HRQOL),
268
Hematologic damage, 210
Herceptin, 137
HiDAC. *See* High-dose cytarabine
High-dose cytarabine (HiDAC),
329–30
HL. *See* Hodgkin's lymphoma
HNSCC. *See* Head and neck squamous
cell carcinoma
Hodgkin's disease, 137, 297–306;
ABVD therapy, 298; chemothera-
pies, 297–99; incidence of, 297; ra-
diation field size, 297; SEER: Crude
Incidence Rates, 297, 298; survival
estimates, 299
Hodgkin's lymphoma (HL): coordinated
care, 305–6; follow-up guidelines,

About the Editor and Contributors

Editor KENNETH MILLER, MD, is Staff Oncologist at Sinai Hospital of Baltimore, and Instructor in the Department of Medicine at Harvard Medical School, and a Live**STRONG** Scholar. He is immediate past director of the Live**STRONG** Survivorship Clinic at Dana-Farber Cancer Institute, Boston, and immediate past director of the annual Harvard Continuing Medical Education course on cancer survivorship. Dr. Miller has been a medical oncologist for 20 years and is founding director of the Connecticut Challenge Cancer Survivorship Program at the Yale University Cancer Center. He has authored numerous journal articles and one previous book, *Choices in Breast Cancer Treatment: Medical Specialists and Cancer Survivors Tell You What You Need to Know.*

BRITTANY ALGIERE, BS, is a research assistant at the Dana-Farber Cancer Institute and a recent graduate of Northeastern University.

BINJA BASIMIKE, BS, is a student intern at the Dana-Farber Cancer Institute from Northeastern University.

IRIT BEN-AHARON, MD, PhD, is a Medical Oncologist and researcher at the Institute of Oncology, Davidoff Center, Rabin Medical Center Petah-Tiqva, Israel.

RICHARD N. BOYAJIAN, NP, RN, MA, APRN, is the clinical director of the Adult Cancer Survivorship Program at the Dana-Farber Cancer Institute.

NANCY CAMPBELL, MS, is an Exercise Physiologist for the Adult Cancer Survivorship Program of the Dana-Farber Cancer Center.

SUSANA CAMPOS, MD, MPH, is an Assistant Professor of Medicine at the Harvard Medical School and the Clinical Director for Gynecologic Malignancies at the Dana-Farber Cancer Institute.

FURHA COSSOR, MD, is a Hematology and Oncology Fellow at the Tufts Medical Center in Boston, MA.

COREY CUTLER, MD, MPH, FRCP(C), is Assistant Professor of Medicine at the Harvard Medical School and Medical Director, Lance Armstrong Bone Marrow Transplant Survivors Clinic of the Dana-Farber Cancer Institute.

MATTHEW S. DAVIDS, MD, is an Instructor in Medicine at the Harvard Medical School and an attending physician in the Lymphoma Program at the Dana-Farber Cancer Institute.

AYMEN ELFIKY, MD, is an Instructor in Medicine at the Harvard Medical School and a member of the Genitourinary Cancers group of the Dana-Farber Cancer Institute.

DAVID C. FISHER, MD, is an Assistant Professor of Medicine at Harvard Medical School and an attending physician in the Lymphoma Program at the Dana-Farber Cancer Institute.

SUZANNE GEORGE, MD, is an Assistant Professor Medicine at the Harvard Medical School and the clinical director of the Center for Sarcoma and Bone Oncology Dana-Farber Cancer Institute.

AMY GROSE, MSW, LICSW, is a senior clinical oncology social worker at Dana-Farber Cancer Institute, working in pediatric and adult oncology and survivorship. She also has a private practice specializing in mindfulness, bereavement, and survivorship.

ROBERT HADDAD, MD, is an Associate Professor of Medicine and the Acting Director of the Head and Neck Oncology Division of the Dana–Farber Cancer Institute.

LINDSAY HAINES, BS, received her degree from Yale University. She has served as a research intern for the Dana-Farber Cancer Institute's Cancer survivorship Program and is presently attending the Mount Sinai School of Medicine in New York.

ABIGAIL HUEBER, DI/E, is a Dietetic Intern at the Dana-Farber Cancer Institute/Brigham & Women's Hospital.

LINDA A. JACOBS, PhD, RN, AOCN, is the Director of the LIVE**STRONG** Survivorship Center of Excellence, Living Well After Cancer Program of the Abramson Cancer Center and a Clinical Associate Professor at the University of Pennsylvania.

DEEPA JEYAKUMAR, MD, is a Oncology and Hematology fellow at Tufts Medical Center in Boston, MA.

STACY KENNEDY, MPH, RD, CSO, LDN, is a Senior Clinical Nutritionist at the Dana-Farber Cancer Institute/Brigham & Women's Hospital.

JOSEPH LEHRBERG, BA, is a program assistant at the Dana-Farber Cancer Institute.

SEWANTI LIMAYE, MD, is an Instructor in Medicine at the Harvard Medical School and an attending Physician in the Head and Neck Oncology Group at the Dana–Farber Cancer Institute.

ANDREA MARRARI, MD, is a clinician in the Center for Sarcoma and Bone Oncology Dana-Farber Cancer Institute.

MARY McCABE, RN, is the Director of the Memorial Sloan Kettering Cancer Center Adult Cancer Survivorship Program.

NADINE JACKSON McCLEARY, MD, MPH, is an Instructor in Medicine, Harvard Medical School and a Medical Oncologist in the Gastrointestinal Cancer Center Dana-Farber Cancer Institute.

CHRISTIAN McEVOY, MPH, is a Program Director for the Connecticut Challenge in Stamford CT.

KENNETH B. MILLER, MD, is a Professor of Medicine and the Associate Chief of the Hematology/Oncology Division, Tufts Medical Center.

ANDREA NG, MD, is an Associate Professor of Medicine at the Harvard Medical School and an Attending Physician in Radiation Oncology at the Dana-Farber Cancer Institute.

STEPHANIE NUTT, MA, MPA. is a Program Specialist | Evaluation & Research LIVE**STRONG** in Austin, TX.

ALMA PETROVIC, MD, MPH, is a Director of Programs at Screening for Mental Health, Inc.

JENNIFER POTTER, MD is an Associate Professor of Medicine at the Harvard Medical School.

RUTH RECHIS, PhD, is the Director of Evaluation & Research for LIVE **STRONG** in Austin, TX.

KATHRYN RUDDY, MD, is an Instructor in Medicine at Harvard Medical School and a Medical oncologist at Dana-Farber Cancer Institute.

ANDREW L. SALNER, MD, FACR, is the Director, Harry and Helen Gray Cancer Center PI, NCI Community Cancer Center and PI, Lance Armstrong Foundation Survivorship project at Hartford Hospital in Hartford, CT.

HESTER HILL SCHNIPPER, LICSW, OSW-C, is the Chief of Oncology Social Work at the Beth-Israel Deconness Medical Center in Boston, MA.

JULIE K. SILVER, MD, is an Assistant Professor at the Harvard Medical School and Chief Editor of Books for Harvard Health Publications.

LISA SCHULZ SLOWMAN, OTR, MS, OT/L, CHT, is the President of Oncology Rehab, Inc., in Boston, MA.

SHERRI STORMS, RN, MSN, is the Project and Survivorship Coordinator for the Lance Armstrong Foundation Survivorship project at Hartford Hospital.

CARRIE TOMPKINS STRICKER, PhD, RN, AOCN, is the Director of Clinical Programs & Oncology Nurse Practitioner at the LIVE**STRONG** Survivorship Center of Excellence Abramson Cancer Center and a Clinical Assistant Professor Nursing University of Pennsylvania.

CARLY STROICH-EISLEY, RN, APRN, is a Survivorship Nurse Practitioner for the Lance Armstrong Foundation Survivorship project at Hartford Hospital.

USHA THAKRAR, MPH, is the Program Administrator, Perini Family Survivors' Center and Director, Clinical Programs, Pediatric Oncology Dana-Farber Cancer Institute.

ASHLEY VARNER, MSW, MBA, LCSW-C, is the Senior Director, Caregiving Programs for Cancer Support Community.

FREDERICA M. WILLIAMS, MBA, is the President & CEO, Whittier Street Health Center in Boston, MA.

KAREN WINKFIELD, MD, PhD, is an Instructor at the Harvard Medical School and an Assistant in Radiation Oncology for Lymphoma, Leukemia & Transplant Services at the Massachusetts General Hospital.